Praise for *ChefMD's Big Book of Culinary Medicine*

"Every one of us has an internal doctor, a natural inner leader who can keep us healthy. Dr. La Puma teaches you how to eat the right food so your inner doctor can do its work. Learn how to eat well and feel well at the same time."

—JACK CANFIELD, coauthor of *Chicken Soup for the Body and Soul*

"John La Puma has a way of bringing the science and pleasures that should come from healthy eating together on the same plate. As a fascinating blend of both chef and physician, his passion and talent come through with practical and enticing tips on how to shop, cook, and eat. In this engaging book, he shows us that healthy food can be both good for you and bring delicious pleasure to our lives."

—JESSE ZIFF COOL, author, restaurateur, and advocate of sustainable agriculture

"Using your knife and fork can save your life. In *ChefMD's Big Book of Culinary Medicine,* John La Puma, M.D., tells how, making it easy, fun, and stunningly delicious. He makes the healthiest eating irresistible."

—DANA JACOBI, author of *The Essential Best Foods Cookbook*

"Through the culinary wizardry of Dr. John La Puma, not even your taste buds will know that you're eating 'good for you' food. You can live well, and long, with his guidance."

✦ —MEHMET OZ, M.D., author of *YOU: Staying Young* and *YOU: The Owner's Manual*

"Dr. John La Puma and Rebecca Powell Marx show you how to spend a little more time in the kitchen so you'll have many more years with your family and friends . . . and better-tasting food on your table."

—JEFF REIN, CEO of Walgreens

"John taught me how to cook and how to make healthy food taste terrific. Get this book and he'll share that brilliant wisdom and practical advice with you. Your body and your taste buds will thank you for it."

—MICHAEL ROIZEN, M.D., chief wellness officer of the Cleveland Clinic and coauthor of four #1 *New York Times* bestsellers, including *YOU: Staying Young*

"What a concept! Dr. La Puma's approach is radically different, and the results are not only healthier, but more delicious."

—DR. ART ULENE, TV health commentator and former *Today* show "Family Doctor"

"Dr. La Puma brings to your table a rare combination of medical experience and culinary skills. Anyone's health and meals will both benefit by reading this book."

—WALTER C. WILLET, M.D., PH.D., chair, Department of Nutrition, Harvard School of Public Health

ChefMD's
Big Book of Culinary Medicine

Chef MD's
Big Book of Culinary Medicine

A FOOD LOVER'S ROAD
MAP TO LOSING WEIGHT,
PREVENTING DISEASE,
AND GETTING REALLY
HEALTHY

BY JOHN LA PUMA, M.D.,
and Rebecca Powell Marx

THREE RIVERS PRESS
NEW YORK

ChefMD is a trademark and the ChefMD colophon is a registered trademark of ChefMD, LLC.

Library of Congress Cataloging-in-Publication Data
La Puma, John.
  Chef MD : the food lover's guide to culinary medicine / John La Puma and Rebecca Powell Marx.—1st ed.
    p. cm.
  1. Nutrition. 2. Diet therapy. 3. Cookery (Natural foods) I. Marx, Rebecca Powell. II. Title.
RA784 L3 2008   613.2—dc22 2007041789

ISBN 978-0-307-39463-7

Printed in the United States of America

Design by Helene Berinsky

10 9 8 7 6 5 4

First Paperback Edition

CONTENTS

We are most grateful to John's patients and Rebecca's friends: Each group gave us the courage to explain why food works, and to reveal the pleasures of culinary medicine, too often buried beneath the fears and uncertainty about what to eat.

We thank Karen Levin of Highland Park, Illinois, for her terrific recipe-development and -testing skills. Karen's brilliant reinvention of good-for-you food is just what culinary medicine needs. And Elsa Dixon's ability to help crystallize the complex so it becomes accessible is priceless.

To create the most scientifically accurate book possible on culinary medicine, we relied on medical experts and researchers who dug deep to help us, especially Marilyn Acquistapace, Stefanie Bouma, Julie Hopper, Dr. Laura Jana, David Green, Elizabeth Ko, Katherine Seward, and J. T. Yu. Dr. Bruce Tiffney of the extraordinary College of Creative Studies and Dr. Paula Bruice and Gary Greinke of UCSB kept John connected to one of the best educational institutions in the United States. Dr. Dan Nadeau and Dr. John Foreyt's enthusiasm for what people can do for themselves—with gusto—excites us, and Drs. Mike Roizen and Mehmet Oz gave us daily inspiration, in motivating YOU to understand that you can control your genes.

We are also grateful to Barbara Henry for her gourmet insight and welcoming care; to Dr. Kathleen Zisser of East West Medicine for providing space for the Santa Barbara Institute; and to Mark

Palmer of Sales Insights and Dr. Allen Schaffer, who have created innovative, personal models of how to truly help people with business.

Special continued thanks to Chefs Rick Bayless, Tracey Vowell, Kevin Karales, Geno Bahena, and the staff of Frontera Grill and Topolobampo for championing great food and creating a commitment to local farmers. Bill and Delia Coleman of Coleman Family Farms and Bill and Barbara Spencer of Windrose Farms radiate happiness with every moment they farm and teach, and Drs. George Bifano, Helmuth Billy, Andy Binder, John Petrini, Tim Rodgers, and Jay Winner encourage medical success with every referral.

Bob Levine and Kim Schefler got us to the right place, and to the audience this work needs. Dr. David Schiedermayer's insightful, inspiring review of the final manuscript made sure the medical facts were accurate, though he bears none of the responsibility for any that may have slipped past. We thank the entire team at Crown for their support from the start, and for dedicating themselves to making it work. Special thanks to our editor, Heather Jackson, whose easy way and great confidence are just what an author needs to do the best work and keep doing it. Her assistant, Heather Proulx, kept everything on track, and Selina Cicogna saw that it got into your hands. Judy Hansen, Kathy Seidel, and Ann Rohlen all encouraged this complementary partnership. Gary and Meme Hopmayer helped us understand that understanding others' needs is a way to success in life, for which we will be forever grateful. Mike Lynch, Drs. Scott Nelson, Tanya Remer Altmann, and Bruce Dan of the NAMC thankfully fostered a community where thinking outside the box is the norm.

We are indebted to our wonderful colleagues at Marx Creative and *Health Corner*—especially David Marx, for his tone tweaks, enthusiasm, and his openhearted support of the idea that food can be fun and tasty, and still be good for you. We thank Bob Marx for his steady hand, confidence, and care; Kurt Walbrandt for his writing; Jim Vaughn and Lauren Burke for their direction; Jimmy Bohan and Ann Kammerer for their design; Florida Perry-Smith for her style; Kristin Arnett, Vinnie Besasie, Danielle Bernard, Amy Bruss, Terry Crumble, Tony Cutraro, Chiquita Eubanks, Bob Gregory, Dianne Hue-Freese, Jennifer Janz, Margaret Johnson, Duke and Betty Marx, Jean Mulvaney, Bradd Romant, Patrick Haley, Mike Luce, Chris Maisa, Jodi Olson, Emily Rasbornik, Jim Rude, Kelswe

Stoehr, Michael Thompson, Rob Wernette, Telana Wilson, David Zale, and ChefMD Nurse Kristen Crumble. Brian Behrens and Barry Houlehen developed ChefMD.com brilliantly. We thank Shawna Muren and Jon Gass of Whole Foods; Tom Balisteri, Jr., Tom Balisteri III, and Jimmy Balisteri of Sendik's. It really does take a village to create a top-quality TV show and segment, and these people are the best. And a special thanks to our colleagues on *Health Corner,* Leeza Gibbons, Dr. Jamie Haysman, and especially Lisa Thornton, M.D., without whom we wouldn't have been able to share this book with you. Brad Backer, Darci Middaugh, Sue Kahn, and Roger Fox made sense of it all. Jeff Rein, George Riedl, Craig Sinclair, Bob Rosenbarger, Bonnie Gordon, Katie Dalquist, and especially Connie Splitt and Brodie Bertrand are our angel Ambassadors to Walgreen's, a great company.

John thanks the beautiful Annie Kratz, not just for your business acumen and manuscript reviews, but for your kindness and love. And Linda La Puma for great editing and insight.

To Rebecca's lifelong friends Kathy Coakley, Karen Trimble, Meg Schoenecker, Jeanne Siebert, Nancy Nesslar Schultz, Margie Wieglow Wilson, Laurie Jankowski, and Aaron Zick: you are beautiful souls.

A special note of love from Rebecca to her dad and mom, Roland and Marlene, and her sisters, Susan and Diane. Roland's valiant fifty-year struggle with juvenile diabetes often left her family with the question, "What do you eat for that?" When Rebecca met John La Puma, as she likes to say, "on the corner of food and medicine," she knew we could build a tribute to her dad. Rebecca dedicates this book to people like him everywhere who have the courage to smile and be joy-filled, even when their bodies are failing. With "culinary medicine," food will never be your enemy again. It will be as it should be . . . delicious and flavor-filled "food as medicine." And to Rebecca's husband, David, and children, Michaela, Gabrielle, and Zach: you are my lifelines. My love for you is boundless.

The New Art and Science of Culinary Medicine

Within every patient there resides a doctor and we as
physicians are at our best when we put our patients in touch
with the doctor inside themselves.

—ALBERT SCHWEITZER, M.D.

I wrote this book so you can learn to listen to your body like a doctor and create great flavor like a chef. No one knows your body like you do. But you might not know that you can eat *delicious* food to help prevent and control common medical conditions.

I love food and cooking and food markets. I also love being a doctor. I have known since age fifteen what I wanted to do with my life, and I became an internist and medical ethicist. But fifteen years ago I was thirty-five pounds overweight, with newly sprouting gray hair and a big gut. I knew I was aging because of how I was eating, and I needed to eat healthier meals. I began to study nutrition, but while healthy meals may be virtuous, they're not much fun for me unless they taste incredibly good, leave me satisfied, *and* help prevent disease. My lifelong love affair with food landed me in cooking school.

Since cooking school I've blended what I learned in medical school with my training as a chef and my research in nutrition and created what I truly believe is a revolutionary new field: culinary medicine.

Culinary medicine—which I define as food that deliciously prevents and controls common conditions—helped me lose those extra thirty-five pounds, and I now feel younger at fifty than I did at thirty-five. In *ChefMD's Big Book of Culinary Medicine,* you'll find terrific foods and recipes that work like medicine, and as a complement to prescription drugs and your doctor's wise counsel. And like taking prescription medicine or seeing your own doctor, consistency counts. Eating the ChefMD way helps prevent conditions before they start, and helps control them when you already have them.

Your Doctor Inside

I'm going to help you learn to see food as your body sees it. You have the right to know what's in your food and how it will affect your body, because I believe that when you have high-quality, unbiased, scientifically sound information, you can make better choices. Seize the Inner ChefMD moment with that part of you that instinctively knows what will be healthy and delicious.

I've been able to write about food and medicine before, in *The RealAge Diet* and *Cooking the RealAge Way* with Michael Roizen, M.D., and have provided recipes for *YOU: The Owner's Manual* by Mehmet Oz, M.D., and Michael Roizen, M.D.

But here in *ChefMD,* I write delicious culinary prescriptions to help you find the doctor inside. These prescriptions can help you achieve optimal health; can help you prevent and control conditions from asthma to heart disease to breast cancer; and can even help you beat some of them outright. You'll get the most from the best foods, avoid the wrong foods, and learn how to eat so you will feel full and fully satisfied. Every meal, every day. And when you can't use the finest ingredients, I'll show you how to make the most of what you do have.

Why Weight?

Perhaps you are familiar with the French paradox. You know: saturated fats, no workouts at the gym, and little heart disease. Well, have you heard of the American paradox? Less fat in our diet, one workout fad after another, and we're still getting fatter by the minute. On average, we gain a pound a year, every year, after age thirty-five. One in three people born in 2000 in the United States will develop diabetes at some point in their lives. Increases of 75 percent in China and 134 percent in India are forecast by 2030. And it's because we are all eating the wrong foods.

The Standard American Diet (SAD, isn't it?) is killing us. Luckily we now have the opportunity to use food that works like tasty medicine.

What's in It for You?

For years I practiced culinary medicine without putting a name to it. I didn't start calling myself a ChefMD until I met my business partner, Rebecca, a television producer and journalist. Her husband coined the term *ChefMD*, and she convinced me to write this book, do a regular segment, "What's Cookin' with ChefMD?" on her television show, and form a company. She also taught me that people always want to know "What's in it for me?" (WIIFM, pronounced "wiffum"). A longer, easier, healthier, higher-quality life is what's in it for you.

The Keys

There are three keys to unlocking culinary medicine. They are: bioavailability (body-ready food), avoiding anti-nutrients (hidden toxins), and achieving satiety (feeling full and fully satisfied). I devote a chapter to each so you can fully understand and use them. The first key involves getting the most out of the best foods: making them "body ready" or "bioavailable." It's not a new concept to medical science, but it's a new concept as I apply it to food and it's truly groundbreaking. Throughout the book, I'll highlight facts you never knew about food and bioavailability and how to get the most out of what you eat. I call these facts Little Bites.

Unfortunately, our world and our food are full of hidden toxins—but once you know where they are lurking, you can get them out of your diet. This is the second key of culinary medicine: avoiding anti-nutrients. My tips on staying away from anti-nutrients are found in Noxious Nots.

❋ **LITTLE BITES**

Bake pizza hotter or longer? Either one gives you more antioxidants! Baking a pizza crust at 550°F for 7 minutes instead of 400°F for 14 minutes increases antioxidants—and their body readiness—by up to 45 percent. Baking at 400°F for 14 minutes instead of 7 minutes does the same thing.

❋ **LITTLE BITES**

Just have to hit the drive-through for your favorite fries or burger? Grab a fistful of almonds twenty minutes before your drive-through rendezvous. Within minutes, the antioxidants in the almonds begin to block the artery-stiffening and inflammatory effect of the saturated and trans fats in the fast food.

✂ NOXIOUS NOTS

Genetically modified foods have genes from an animal, plant, virus, or bacteria inserted. Those new genes do what all genes do: they tell other genes what to do, or they make new proteins. By using genetic modification, scientists have added flounder genes to tomatoes so that they stay fresh longer, made soybeans resistant to weed killer, and even put jellyfish genes into potatoes, which glow in the dark when they need to be watered. Too bad they can't grow a plant that does the dishes!

Should we be worried about these foods? I say yes. A recent study showed that rats fed biotech giant Monsanto's MON863 maize for ninety days showed "signs of toxicity" in the liver and kidneys. It's not known how these foods will affect humans. You've almost certainly already been eating them without knowing it—the U.S. government does not require food manufacturers to label food that contains genetically modified ingredients. Foods that contain corn or its by-products (corn oil, cornstarch, corn flour, high-fructose corn syrup) most likely contain genetically modified ingredients.

What can you do? Buy organic.

◉ SATIETY SOLUTIONS

Cold cooked potatoes have resistant starch not found in hot potatoes. What does this mean to you at the dinner table? The cold potatoes' resistant starch causes a slower glycemic response to a meal, so your blood sugar doesn't spike. Your gut satiety proteins glucagon-like peptide 1 (GLP-1) and peptide YY (PYY), made by your body to regulate your feeling of fullness, move in nicely. So if you want to feel full faster and stay full longer, cold cooked potatoes might help.

See my recipe for Garlicky Potato Salad with Spinach and with Lemon on page 135.

One of the reasons traditional weight-loss diets don't work is that you feel deprived and hungry and then go off them. I have one word for you: satiety. Satiety (pronounced suh-tie-uh-tee) and the science behind it will help you never, ever feel deprived again. It's the third key to culinary medicine and simply stated, satiety is feeling satisfied and gratified but not overly full after a meal.

We can stop the craziness of eating supersize portions and still feeling hungry. So I've peppered the book with ways to make food more satisfying to you, without adding calories. I call these nuggets Satiety Solutions.

You have the ability to listen to your body and train the doctor inside. You actually don't need to go to medical school for this, because your body already knows a lot. But you do need better information, and you need to pay attention to how foods make you feel, not to mention which foods will help keep your chin up and your weight down.

Why? Because the link between being overweight and having heart disease, cancer, diabetes, stroke, and dying way before you're ready is well known. Since I'm a ChefMD who practices culinary medicine, that link is always top of mind for me. So, while this isn't a diet book, every recipe I develop is not only delicious, it's completely satisfying and low in calories. Throughout the book I'll roll out what I call The Skinny On . . . tips you might not know about weight loss.

After you read *ChefMD*, I hope you'll never look at food the same way again—or cook the same way. Food that works like medicine is powerful and should be a great pleasure to eat, choose, and enjoy. If I could, I would come to your kitchen and cook with you. While I spent years in cooking school and working in a great restaurant to learn about flavor, the good news is that you don't have to. With *ChefMD*, you'll learn what I know. What you eat and how you eat it can help you look and feel better than you ever have, no matter what your current condition.

You may be thinking: I'm too busy, too tired, not ready, have no time, the kitchen is a mess. Why not just throw a hunk of something animal on the grill, turn up the heat, and put it in the middle of the plate? Because there is good news here, too—new tools and new and excellent prepared foods make it easier than ever to unlock the healing power and flavor not just of meats but of vegetables, whole grains, and legumes as well.

For my recipes, I keep it simple. Ten or fewer ingredients total, less than thirty minutes to cook, and no hole in the middle of the plate where there used to be your dinner. I'll equip you with a pantry, fridge, and freezer also stocked with great meals that need ten minutes or less to prepare, with grab-on-the-go ideas built in.

Throughout *ChefMD*, I'll mix in culinary tips, which I call Doctor It Up!

One Small Change Changes Everything

My patients who have made small changes and stuck with them look and feel better than they thought possible and actively prevent medical problems. What you eat and how you eat it can help you look and feel better than you ever have, no matter what your current condition.

Consider my patient Emily. Emily was having problems with her knees. I told her that losing some weight would help. She didn't want to "go on a diet." I agreed because if you go on a diet you have to go off it, too. So, instead of drinking the sixteen-ounce cola she

---

❦ THE SKINNY ON . . . BEANS!

If you eat foods high in resistant starch instead of most crackers and pastries, you burn more fat all through the day, because you use the fat before you can store it. Legumes (lentils, peas, soybeans, and beans) have more resistant starch than any other foods: that's why you'll find them in my Spicy and Rich Sausage and Kidney Bean Chili (page 107); my Roasted Red Pepper, Wine, and Red Lentil Soup (page 105); and my Shrimp and Egg Burritos with White Beans and Corn (page 106).

✚ DOCTOR IT UP!

So, you say you don't like whole-wheat couscous or you think whole-grain rice isn't flavorful enough? Try pan toasting! It doesn't add calories, but it does add toasty flavor. Add the couscous or rice directly to a dry sauté pan, with no liquid, and heat over a medium heat. Stir briskly for a few minutes until the grain lightly browns. Let cool for a moment to avoid spatters, add your liquid and cook. This simple tip adds nutty, warm flavor to your dish. Try my Butternut Barley Risotto with Goat Cheese and Toasted Almonds on page 111.

had each noon and night, she began having a small glass of red wine at dinner with her husband. Soon she had lost four pounds by doing just that one thing.

She felt so much better that she went on to make more small changes and lost over thirty pounds and has kept them off for over two years. Her knees feel great and she now plays tennis with her husband three times a week. It wasn't just losing the extra two hundred calories per day that made the difference. The glass of wine also set a different tone for their dinners. The couple started having better conversations, and Emily said she naturally ate less because she was more satisfied.

Here's the math. A sixteen-ounce soda has two hundred calories. Thirty-five hundred calories is one pound of fat. That means that by eliminating just one soda from your diet each day, you can reduce your calories by more than thirty-six thousand, or over ten pounds in six months.

As part of discovering the doctor inside, you will need to build a kitchen prescription medicine chest, otherwise known as your pantry! And I will help you there, too. There are fifty powerful and satisfying foods you *must* have on hand in chapter 4. This is one medicine chest you can raid guilt-free. Plus, there are fifty recipes and fourteen days of menus in chapter 5!

Every day, we face choices about food: what to choose from the menu; what to buy at the grocery store; and what to make for breakfast, lunch, and dinner. I call each one of these choices a Fork in the Road, a decision point about which way to send your body. Do you turn left or right? Do you make a good choice or a bad choice? I want to help you make an informed choice, the best choice you can. Why not be more careful, get higher quality, great flavor, and better health all at once? Replace bad habits with good ones and make your life easier.

The eight-week program (in chapter 6) gives you a step-by-step plan for optimal health. The radical good news is that at almost any age you can become a vibrant and superhealthy person just by what you put on your dinner plate—even if you are in your eighties or nineties. In chapter 7, you're going to find the best answers I know to "What do you eat for that?" for forty common conditions and meet some of my patients.

Laughter is some of the best medicine. I like Dennis Miller's humor and he has perfected the art of the rant so I decided to steal it, although Dennis Miller is clearly a whole lot funnier.

ChefMD Rant: Why Don't They Teach Doctors About Food?

They don't teach doctors enough about food in med school and I think that's crazy. This year 900,000 Americans will die from heart disease, 500,000 from cancer, 200,000 from complications of diabetes, and 150,000 from a stroke. Over 1.6 million of us will die from diseases affected in some way by diet.

Your doctor surely knows that you shouldn't eat too much saturated fat or too many sugars. She or he is certainly aware that fiber is a good thing, and so are antioxidants. But most physicians are un-schooled in the finer points of nutrition. And it's not their fault.

I had fewer than four hours of nutrition training in the three thousand lecture hours of medical school. Out of the 116 medical schools in America, 68 have no requirement for nutrition classes. At those schools you can actually graduate and walk out with your medical degree without a single class hour in "eating right." And those other 40 percent with nutrition class requirements? They require an average of just two credits, basically one course, about nutrition. One course! Are you kidding me?

In the years ahead, every medical school in America needs to teach nutrition and cooking as a required part of its curriculum. A physician walking out of medical school with a diploma should know enough to be on his or her way to being a ChefMD, too. How your body "sees" the food you put in your mouth directly affects your health and how you feel.

I'm a ChefMD and I hope the first of many. I'm not saying that physicians need to quit their practices, go to culinary school, and do nutrition research like I have. They shouldn't have to. If medical schools taught physicians about food and cooking—not just nutrients and nutrition—it would radically change health care. I envision a day when thousands of physicians have the knowledge and training to call themselves ChefMDs. Think of how health care would change.

FORK IN THE ROAD: LEARN THE CALORIES IN EVERYDAY FOODS

My business partner travels a lot. Her favorite airline serves warm, doughy chocolate chip cookies made fresh on most flights. She'd always eaten two and often four mindlessly, just like most people on the plane. How many calories were in one of those (one ounce) irresistible cookies? A hundred and twenty calories and six grams of fat. She was at a fork in the road. If she ate four cookies, she ate half the total amount of saturated fat she should have for the whole day. Plus, the 480 calories in four tiny cookies represented well over an hour of walking on her treadmill at 3.5 miles per hour at a fifteen-degree incline. Which would you choose?

■ ■ ■

Forever, people have been looking for the fountain of youth. In the 1500s, the Spanish explorer Ponce de León wandered around southern Florida looking for it. There really is a fountain of youth and old Ponce didn't need to sail across the Atlantic Ocean from Spain to find it. It was right there in front of him all along. It was in his kitchen and it's in yours, too.

I tag my television segments by saying, "The fountain of youth starts in the kitchen." And I truly believe it. The kitchen is the heart of your home, and at the center of your health. *I believe that you can transform your life and your health with what you eat and I am committed to showing you how to do that.*

Your food should be body ready, fully satisfying, and delicious. That is the essence of "culinary medicine" and is at the heart of the ChefMD plan. The word *medicine* is derived from the Latin *ars medicina,* which means "the art of healing." In *ChefMD* you'll learn to find the doctor inside; unlock the healing power of irresistible foods; and add more pleasure, fun, ease, and energy to your life. Please join me. A whole new world of great food, great times, and great health—better than you thought possible—awaits you.

Part One

Understanding Culinary Medicine

CHAPTER 1

Enhancing Bioavailability: ABSORB MORE OF THE GOOD STUFF

Sex is good, but not as good as fresh, sweet corn.
—GARRISON KEILLOR

Bioavailability—Test Your ChefMD IQ

1. Is cooking vegetables better nutritionally than eating them raw?
   Yes _____   No _____
2. Does thawing frozen vegetables before cooking them help to maintain their nutritional value?
   Yes _____   No _____
3. Do you generally eat your fruits with the skin off?
   Yes _____   No _____
4. Do you generally eat your vegetables with the skin on?
   Yes _____   No _____
5. Is it true that eating a few almonds before eating a sausage will help block the negative effects of its saturated fat?
   Yes _____   No _____
6. Do you know how to sauté, steam, simmer, marinate, dry rub, roast, and grill?
   Yes _____   No _____
7. Do you use herbs and spices liberally?
   Yes _____   No _____

8. Do you usually use a low-fat or nonfat salad dressing on your salad?

Yes ____   No ____

9. Is milk chocolate more nutritious than dark chocolate?

Yes ____   No ____

10. Can cocoa lower blood pressure?

Yes ____   No ____

Scoring: Give yourself 1 point for each correct answer.

1. **Yes:** Cooking usually unlocks vitamins from the fiber in vegetables, and less cooking is usually better. When you boil your veggies many of the nutrients end up in the water. You keep the nutrients when you steam.

2. **No:** Studies show that frozen vegetables maintain a much higher level of nutrition when cooked frozen.

3. **No:** Bet you knew this. Much of the nutritional value of fruit is in the skin.

4. **Yes:** Bet you knew this, too. Like fruit, much of the nutritional value in vegetables is in the skin.

5. **Yes:** Eating a few nuts before eating meat will help block the negative effects of the meat's saturated fat.

6. **Yes:** These are healthful ways of preparing foods.

7. **Yes:** Herbs and spices contain an incredible array of antioxidants and, of course, great flavor.

8. **No:** There's a surprise. Use full-fat dressings or add a bit of healthy fat (avocado, walnuts, almonds, olives) to your salad.

9. **No:** Dark chocolate good, milk chocolate bad (more on that later).

10. **Yes:** Just thirty calories worth of dark chocolate daily can help.

Total score (0–10): _____

8–10 points: Your Inner ChefMD is smart and cookin'.

4–7 points: Your Inner ChefMD is almost ready for prime time. Read this chapter to hone your skills.

0–3 points: Your Inner ChefMD needs to go to culinary medical school. Read this chapter immediately!

Food is like sex. When done well, it engages all five senses; it taps into our most primal needs and urges and it's among the greatest pleasures you can experience. And like sex, eating good food is a celebration, and an affirmation of life.

Would you watch TV while having sex? If it was great sex, probably not. So why would you grab a burger while running through an airport or eat a hot dog while sitting in front of the tube?

It's so much more satisfying to enjoy and savor the experience of eating good, fresh, nourishing food than to eat mindlessly. And like sex, eating a meal is usually better if you're doing it with someone you love.

You know you should eat more fruits and vegetables—you've been hearing it since you were a small child and didn't want to eat your peas. Now that you're a grown up, your brussels sprouts probably still get left behind on the plate, and the last piece of fruit you had was the maraschino cherry out of a mai tai. You know that if you ate more fruits and vegetables, you'd be healthier. But what you may not know is that how you look and feel is also affected by your food's bioavailability. Say what?

What Is Bioavailability?

Bioavailability is a word borrowed from pharmacology, the study of drugs and their effects on the body. In pharmacology, bioavailability means the amount of a particular drug the body actually absorbs into the bloodstream, not just the amount you take. It's how much medicine is available for your body to use.

With respect to food, bioavailability *means body ready: the nutrients absorbed and available for your body to use.* Naturally, you want to maximize the body readiness of healthy nutrients for your system. Let me give you some examples.

Say it's a beautiful summer day and you stop by your local farmers' market to pick up a watermelon. You get it home and you kind of wish the watermelon were cold, but you don't want to wait for it to cool down in the refrigerator. Take heart. Watermelon that's been stored at room temperature has up to 40 percent more lycopene and up to 139 percent more beta-carotene than watermelon out of the cooler or your fridge. Store and eat your watermelon at room temperature to maximize those powerful antioxidants. And here's a little bonus. The lycopene and beta-carotene in harvested watermelon actually increase over time—

for up to two weeks. So let that freshly picked melon mellow to maximize its nutrients.

Sure, you already know that boiling vegetables reduces their nutritional value. But if you're going to boil your vegetables, and I'd prefer you steam them, do it in as little water and for as short a time as possible. *Reducing the amount of water and the cooking time reduces nutrient loss and maximizes bioavailability.*

I'm sure you've noticed how the color of the water turns slightly yellow when you're boiling a yellow vegetable and tints green when you boil a green vegetable, right? That's the flavonoids leaching out of your meal. Flavonoids are brilliant antioxidant compounds in vegetables that give them their fabulous colors and activate your DNA repair system, helping to protect you from cancer. Save that water and use it to make soup or cook pasta.

Here's an example of how to maximize the body readiness of vitamin C in your fruit. *Buy whole fruit and cut it up yourself.* Although it's easiest to grab the packages of presliced fruits your grocer has conveniently prepared, studies show that preslicing fruit can reduce its vitamin C content over time. Cantaloupe, kiwi, and pineapple seem particularly prone to vitamin C loss when precut. Precut fruit costs you more and you get less nutrition. I'd call that a double whammy. So, know your fruit: for cantaloupe, kiwi, and pineapple, go whole and slice your own.

The concept of body readiness is vital to the ChefMD plan, because it is the missing link to being simultaneously overweight and undernourished, as so many people now are.

Why? *Because our food is increasingly less nutritious than it used to be—and not just processed fast foods.* Researchers recently looked at data from the USDA from 1950 and 1999 on the nutrient content of forty-three different crops of fruits and vegetables. They found that six out of thirteen nutrients had declined in these crops over the fifty-year period: protein was down by 6 percent, calcium by 16 percent, phosphorus by 9 percent, iron by 15 percent, riboflavin by 38 percent, and vitamin C by about 20 percent. Furthermore, they found a strong correlation between high yield in wheat crops and a loss of nutrients in the wheat, such as zinc and phosphate. This was also true of high-yield commercial broccoli and its level of calcium.

And it's not just vegetables. A British study showed that chicken in 2004 contained a third less protein than chicken in 1940. The

You may think the best lettuce is at the bottom of the pile at the grocery but you'd be wrong. Choose leaf lettuce from the top rather than the bottom: these heads of lettuce have more flavonoids. Why? Because the grocery store lights help them retain or even increase their nutrients.

twenty-first-century chicken also had more than twice as much fat and a third more calories.

Wow. We've become much better at producing larger and larger quantities of food, but bite for bite its nutritional value is smaller and smaller.

We don't know the precise reason for this decline in nutrition over the past decades. Greater crop yields are seen by some as the culprit. Whatever the reason, I want to help you to absorb more nutrients from the food you eat—because the fact of the matter is that there are fewer nutrients in it.

How much you eat; what other foods you eat at the same time; and how you cook, store, and choose food all affect how much you absorb from what you eat and how well your body can use it.

Some people point out that your genes dictate how you absorb nutrients, and how unfair that is. Some people eat a healthy diet and die at fifty; others eat that same diet and thrive past one hundred. That's the diet-gene paradox: our genes determine how we absorb what's in food that's good for us, and not so good for us. But the amazing thing is that food can tell your genes what to do, and with better bioavailability, you can get even more from what you eat—no matter what your genes.

Sadly, *there are also barricades to bioavailability.* Say, for example, you're trying to get more leafy greens in your diet, a wonderful thing to do. You've hit on a crunchy green, completely virtuous salad, with beautiful red peppers, green peppers, a grape cherry tomato or two, with a low-cal squeeze of lemon or store-bought fat-free dressing. You're sitting pretty, having maybe 125 calories in a bowl as big as your head and headed to weight-loss heaven. You may feel virtuous when you sit at your desk at lunchtime with that lunch, and maybe also feel a little jealous when you see your co-worker's Philly cheese steak.

What you might not know is that the fat-free dressing is actually keeping you from absorbing the carotenoids in that green salad that can help stave off cancer. Locked up inside that salad is nearly every antioxidant you've ever heard of. You're getting less than you could—unless you eat that salad with avocado, or with walnuts or roasted walnut oil, or extra-virgin olive oil, or nearly any other good-for-you fat.

Why? Because the oil makes the lutein in the green peppers, the capsanthin in the red peppers, the lycopene in the tomato, even the limonene in the lemon more body ready for you. Each of them is optimally absorbed with a bit of fat. Even reduced-fat dressing won't let you get as many of these valuable nutrients as you could. You've been running from fat—who knew you might actually need it?

Later in the book, I'll teach you to make a simple and delicious dressing for my Parmigiano Caesar Salad with Shrimp (page 121): the olive and walnut oils give you healthy fat, fight fatty buildup in the arteries, offer great flavor, and save you from the sugars that may be in that bottled fat-free dressing. And there is an added benefit to this particular salad dressing: its garlic contains allicin, a substance that can fight hardening of the arteries. The garlic clove has to be exposed to air to make the allicin active, and you'll do that when you crush it for the dressing. Why not take the simple steps to unlock all the goodness that salad has to offer?

I guarantee that an hour after your salad, you'll feel fine, while Mr. Philly Cheese Steak may be passed out on his desk. All of those saturated fats from his sandwich are now lying like melted cheese in his arteries, constricting them and not allowing them to dilate, which in turn doesn't let his muscles get enough oxygen, making him fatigued. So now he's out cold like a fish on ice at the Pike Place Market.

The foods we eat affect our bodies for good or for bad. With the ChefMD approach, you give up none of the richness, satisfaction, and flavor to get more from what you eat. You absorb more of the cancer-fighting, stroke-slaying, heart-disease-stopping antioxidants that only work when they come from food, not pills. That's what this book is all about: the celebration of healthful recipes that extract all the goodness from every delicious morsel and every juicy bite. But before we go further, let me offer a very short overview of what you need to know about nutrition.

The Basics of Nutrition

Most of us were too busy passing notes or throwing spitballs to pay attention when they taught us nutrition in grade school, so you may not remember that there are only six types of nutrients: protein, carbohydrates, fat, vitamins, minerals, and water.

However, there are also literally thousands of compounds in

food that are not technically nutrients. We talk about them as nutrients, but they are really other kinds of beneficial compounds.

They're as important as the original six, because they regulate many of the basic metabolic and physiologic processes that govern how your body works, how your brain works, how your muscles work, and more. And in food, these compounds are metabolized at many different levels in the body, and present a powerful package of nutrition—more than any one nutrient by itself.

Your nutrients have to be in a form that can be recognized by the body to be absorbed. For example, if you swallow a piece of metal containing iron because you're only eight and your brother dared you to do it, the body will not recognize it and will not absorb the iron. But if you eat a piece of liver, the body will recognize the iron it contains and absorb it.

We need certain nutrients to avoid developing serious diseases such as cancer, diabetes, and atherosclerosis (hardening of the arteries), and that need is constant. But the ability of our bodies' systems to get essential nutrients to where they are needed fluctuates. Like nutrition itself, bioavailability is complicated. But we can make it work for us with what we know now. And every day, scientists and physicians are discovering new and exciting ways to get the most out of what we eat.

Now that you understand the basic concepts of nutrition and bioavailability, I'll explain the three factors you can use to maximize your food's bioavailability:

1. Freshness and quality
2. Food combinations
3. How food is processed and cooked

Once you understand these factors, you will be able to unlock the secrets to getting more from what you eat.

FACTOR 1: FRESHNESS AND QUALITY

The first step in absorbing more of the good stuff from your food is to buy the best-quality food you can afford. When it comes to freshness and quality the first rule of thumb is to buy foods that look most similar to their original form. You don't see square bread-crumb-covered halibut swimming around in the ocean, right? I guess then we'd call them stick fish. And what about chicken fingers? Since when do chickens have fingers? In the ChefMD plan, fruits, vegetables, dairy, whole grains, legumes, certain fish, tea, wine, dark chocolate, and nuts have the real star power, with lean meats playing a supporting role.

Fruits and Vegetables

I'm crazy about fruits and vegetables—as a chef, a doctor, and as someone who loves to eat good food. When you look at the vibrant and beautiful palette found in most fruits and vegetables don't you think Mother Nature is trying to tell us something? There's a reason it's not called mad broccoli disease. I know that when you start to learn the secret benefits of produce and how easy they are to choose and prepare, you'll come to love them more.

When shopping for fruits and vegetables, use at least three senses: sight, touch, and smell.

Look for rich color. Strong color means strong medicine. A red bell pepper, for example, is red because of its many carotenoids. There are at least six antioxidant carotenoids in red peppers; green and yellow peppers have only three. Rich color will also look prettier on your plate, and what brings pleasure in eating is not just taste—it's the whole sensory experience. Food that delights the eye will be more likely to delight the palate.

Freshness is the most important thing to look for because most nutrients decline as food ages. But if you live somewhere that doesn't have a lot of fresh produce during the winter, frozen fruits and vegetables are great substitutes. The good news is they don't lose many nutrients from being frozen—and some don't lose any.

Feel the weight. Unlike us, being heavy is a good thing for produce. As a general rule, being heavy for its size indicates ripeness and sometimes natural sugar content—sugars that sweeten your meals, often without spiking your blood sugar, insulin, or inflammation levels. Hold the vegetable or fruit to get a sense of its weight—it should be heavy in your hand for its size—and also to determine its firmness, and any soft spots, which often mean it has overstayed its welcome.

Smell the flavor. Many fruits, like ripe, voluptuous peaches and ripe cantaloupes, have wonderful scents. But if they don't have

❋ **LITTLE BITES**

You know broccoli is good for you, but you still don't like it. Well, you may not have tried BroccoSprouts. They are a special strain of broccoli sprouts which are delicious on top of salads. Researchers at Johns Hopkins School of Medicine found that one serving of BroccoSprouts provides as much cancer-fighting sulforaphane as one and a quarter pounds of adult broccoli. So if you want to fight free radicals, try adding BroccoSprouts. One ounce contains 4 percent of the recommended daily value of dietary fiber, 15 percent of the recommended amount of vitamin C, and 2 percent of the recommended intake of calcium. If you can't find them, ask your grocer to order them. See my recipe for Bison Steak and Broccoli Salad on page 110.

much smell, they probably won't have much taste. Your nose is sometimes ahead of your eyes. That gorgeous, perfect conventionally grown strawberry may taste like watery Styrofoam. The mystically fragrant, oddly shaped, smaller organic strawberry will likely explode with flavor.

You might wonder if the nutrients in organic food are better than those in nonorganic food. Food chemists from the University of California–Davis have discovered that organically grown tomatoes have significantly more vitamin C than conventional tomatoes. The same chemists found no appreciable nutritional differences between conventional and organic bell peppers. A different study showed that tomatoes grown with organic fertilizer had a higher antioxidant level than those grown with conventional fertilizer. In 2001, a review comparing the nutritional value of organic and conventional produce concluded that organic produce had on average 27 percent more vitamin C, 21 percent more iron, 29 percent more magnesium, and more than 13 percent more phosphorous than conventional produce. An extract from organic strawberries has been shown to be more effective in treating cancer cells of both the colon and breast than an extract from conventionally grown strawberries.

All fruits and vegetables are good, but some are better than others. The Environmental Working Group (EWG) examined U.S. Department of Agriculture (USDA) studies of forty-six conventionally grown fruits and vegetables from 1992 through 2001. The EWG labeled the top twelve with the most pesticide contaminants "the Dirty Dozen." They are peaches, strawberries, apples, spinach, nectarines, celery, pears, cherries, potatoes, sweet bell peppers, raspberries, and imported grapes. Buy these organically: the EWG says you drop your pesticide exposure by 90 percent by doing so. The twelve with the least contaminants are asparagus, avocados, bananas, broccoli, cauliflower, corn, kiwi, mangoes, onions, papaya, pineapples, and peas.

And even though vegetables and fruits get their minerals from the soil, other factors add to their nutrient content, such as the strain of plant. For example, some strains of broccoli are just packed with more cancer-fighting glucosinolates than others—remember the BroccoSprouts?

You get tired after a trip across the country, and so does produce. To

Try sardines to keep your mind sharp into the future. Fish oil helps reduce mental decline in old age. The amount of fish oil in sardines varies according to season; it's lowest in the spring. The best time to eat fresh sardines is in September and October, when they are both tastier and more abundant.

get the most nutrients, buy organic and locally when you can. But what if you live in New York and are given the choice between a locally grown, conventionally grown salad and an organic one that was shipped from California, as nearly half of all U.S. vegetables are? Does the freshness of a local conventional green—one grown, say, within a leisurely day's drive from home—outweigh the slight increase in minerals and other nutrients in the organic one? Or does the handling and shipping after harvest affect food's nutritional value even more than how it was grown? Since these are nearly impossible questions to answer universally, it's a choice you must make for yourself. Whether to buy organically or locally is up to you. Look for produce that is local and organic or grow a little of your own.

FACTOR 2: FOOD COMBINATIONS

At Chef Rick Bayless's world-class restaurant Topolobampo in Chicago, I was fortunate to cook once weekly for nearly four years. I worked as a very small part of a great team—that was the way we did our best work. Nutrients are the same—they do their best work as a team.

In nature, phytonutrients (that is, nutrients from plants) are like many basketball players—they're often looking to make an assist. Scientific research shows that the way nature gives us phytonutrients is the best way to get them. The mixtures found in whole foods and in food combinations are more effective than single phytonutrients packaged in pills in getting real health effects. Why? Perhaps because many different chemicals in food reach your cells through different cellular windows: some come in with water, some with fat, and some through the side door.

The same is true for food combinations. Like a riffing jazz band, many fruits and vegetables play off and with each other. *They become more powerful culinary medicine in combination with other fruits and vegetables than when they are eaten alone.* Nutrients, when absorbed through foods eaten together, form "crime-fighting teams" that cruise your body like good Terminators, looking for bad guys like cancer cells to take out.

Looking for foods to combine can be fun (chips and dip count on feast days). Try one of my favorite flavor tricks: match two different foods of the same type and color—for example, two vegetables that are yellow, two fruits that are red, and two herbs that are green. You might combine tomatillos and serranos, raspberries and strawberries, or mint and fresh dill—all delicious duos. And nutritious ones.

What are the health effects? Researchers have found that a combination of broccoli and tomatoes offered more powerful protection against cancer than just eating either vegetable alone. The same effect was not achieved by eating broccoli and taking lycopene supplements extracted from tomatoes. *It's only these whole foods eaten in combination that give you the health benefit.*

This explains why studies that look at isolated nutrients like beta-carotene frequently fail to show impressive results. Since nutrients—especially isolated antioxidants—aren't nearly as powerful by themselves, testing one single nutrient from any vegetable probably won't show anything remarkable. *And thus far, very few single, purified, isolated nutrients have been shown to make a big difference. Only food.*

When you eat broccoli and tomato, for example, you're not just eating glucosinolates and lycopene, respectively. You're eating hundreds of protective phytonutrients that help prevent chronic diseases like prostate cancer. Glucosinolates help your body detoxify poisons, including carcinogens. Lycopene is a carotenoid, a natural antioxidant coloring normally concentrated in the prostate and testes. Eating lycopene in food (not in supplements) is associated with a lower prostate cancer risk. In animals, tomato carotenoids can reduce testosterone levels, which can slow prostate cancer. The equivalent of a cup of tomato sauce and a cup and a half of broccoli daily is all it takes to get the benefit, according to the research. Try my Broccoli, Cheese, and Kalamata Olive Pizza on page 101.

Some of the best food on earth combines powerful flavors and powerful medicine: Chinese, Thai, Italian, Mexican, even home-cooked American food—nearly every cuisine except most American fast food. It's fascinating to me that across the globe, in different cultures with different foods, people have used the doctor inside to combine foods in the healthiest way possible without even knowing it! For example, when making sushi, the Japanese mix the rice with vinegar before forming the little rice ovals on which the raw fish sits.

Researchers in Japan have discovered that adding vinegar to sushi rice decreases the glycemic index of the rice by 20 percent to

✳ LITTLE BITES

Eat leeks, cauliflower, and green beans fresh, or cook them while still frozen, as they will lose more than 55 percent of their folate if you let them thaw.

35 percent. (You knew there was a reason you like sushi.) A lower glycemic index means the rice stays in your stomach longer; lowers the insulin response in your body; and creates a more even blood sugar level, less hunger, and less weight gain.

People in India have long eaten curries that include both turmeric (every curry powder has turmeric) and onions. It has recently been shown that curcumin (the yellow pigment in turmeric) and quercetin (the flavonoid found in onions, tea, and apples), when taken in combination, make an extremely powerful treatment for colon cancer. In one study, researchers gave patients with hereditary colon polyps 480 milligrams of curcumin with 20 milligrams of quercetin daily for six months. The patients saw the average number of their polyps fall by an incredible 60 percent. And the average polyp size shrank by 50 percent. This is an example where the supplement does seem to match the food. But especially in India, food is acknowledged as the best medicine.

Perhaps no one is more clever with food combinations than the people of Mexico. They have known for centuries to soak dried corn in lime water, which allows the hull to separate from the grain, and causes nutrients to be released inside the corn, including iron, copper, zinc, and niacin. Calcium increases by a whopping 750 percent. Somehow these people knew this combination to be healthier than not soaking and cooking the corn. Then they went on making

✚ DOCTOR IT UP!

Curry is a ChefMD power food. Turmeric, found in curry powder and in mustard, also helps to prevent formation of the damaging amyloid plaques found in the brains of Alzheimer's disease patients. India consumes 80 percent of the world's turmeric and has the lowest Alzheimer's rates in the world. But that's not all. Ten subjects who took five hundred milligrams of curcumin a day for only seven days demonstrated an 11.6 percent decrease in total serum cholesterol and 29 percent increase in high-density lipoprotein (HDL) cholesterol—the good kind! That's down with the total and up with the healthy.

Turmeric is also in mustard, but mustard's not usually for breakfast. Or is it? Try deviled eggs for breakfast. Hard-boil 12 eggs. Peel, under cold water, so the shells come off easily. Split in half, lengthwise. Lose the yolks. Blend together ¼ cup silken tofu, ¼ cup thick Greek yogurt, a few minced chives, a scant teaspoon of Dijon mustard, salt and pepper to taste, and ⅛ teaspoon turmeric: the filling should be vibrant yellow. Fill the egg white halves. Serve with my Garlicky Potato Salad with Spinach and Lemon (page 135) and some coffee or tea, and you're good to go. It tastes so much better than clunky mayonnaise and heavy yolks—and it doesn't have the saturated and trans fats, so you'll have a lot more energy and zip!

tortillas and tamales for centuries. And with good reason—authentic Mexican food is delicious and nutritious.

FACTOR 3: HOW FOOD IS PROCESSED AND COOKED

You knew I was going to say that foods that have been commercially processed to within an inch of their lives are not usually a good ChefMD choice. How could most nutrients possibly survive a tomato's long journey from hanging on the vine to ending up in your freezer as the filling in a football-shaped pizza roll?

You can enjoy and enhance prepared food using a method called speed scratch cooking. What is speed scratch cooking? It's adding fresh ingredients to high-quality prepared foods to change everyday food into great food. What you do yourself, at home, dramatically improves the flavor and body readiness of your foods. Plus, once you get the hang of it, it's fun.

For example, in Saffron Scallop, Shrimp, and Chickpea Paella (page 128), I call for organic, fire-roasted diced or crushed tomatoes and store-bought cooked brown rice. Why? Because the preparers have done all the work for you, with high-quality ingredients that are deeply flavorful, just ready to be surrounded by your own olive oil, minced garlic, saffron, and seafood. Total cooking time? Fifteen minutes. Dab a slice of crusty whole-wheat bread in a little olive oil, and you'll slow down how quickly you absorb the carbs from the meal. If you use conventional chicken in this recipe instead of shrimp, trim the fat: it's where the hormones are stored. And if you're drinking tea instead of wine with this dinner, but don't want the caffeine, just pour off the water from the first thirty seconds of soaking your tea bag: the caffeine goes with it.

Processing has a bad rap, but some traditional food processing is actually good for you. Traditional processing is artisanal and preserves food through a natural process so that it can be eaten later (such as fermenting milk to make yogurt, or fermenting cabbage to make sauerkraut). Traditional processing often makes the food better tasting and its nutrients more body ready. Small-scale processing—locally produced, labeled, and named—is often artisanal. Industrial processing methods, conversely, frequently use chemical preservatives; neutralize flavor so that sugar, salt, and artificial flavors must be added; and destroy or diminish nutrients. That's to be avoided.

There are easy ways to getting more from your food when you

cook. Steaming vegetables with a little bit of water, stock, juice, or wine, whether on the stovetop or in the microwave (which I love to do) with a glass or ceramic container, preserves most of their nutrients; boiling does not. Steaming in the microwave actually helps most vegetables keep their nutrients, not lose them.

✛ DOCTOR IT UP!

Roasting is a great option for cooking vegetables and can do wonderful things to their flavor and texture. It's also very simple. To roast vegetables like potatoes, cauliflower, and beets, chop them into bite-sized chunks, toss them in a bowl with a little olive oil using the best cooking tools you have—your hands. Roast them until tender in a 425° F oven on a baking sheet lined with parchment paper. Or, you might cut a butternut squash in half, put it cut side down on a sheet pan in a 425° F oven for 40 minutes, toss out the seeds, scoop out the flesh, and eat it mashed with cinnamon, nutmeg, and a splash of orange juice—simple and delicious as a side dish.

Grilling and sautéing are two other wonderful ways to cook vegetables without allowing nutrients to slip away. And sautéing can bring out the lovely color in some vegetables, such as snow peas— try my Ginger Peanut Grilled Chicken with Sweet Potatoes and Sugar Snap Peas on page 117. Cooking vegetables in broth for a soup is another great way to preserve all the goodness because you eat the broth, too, as is pureeing them and making them into dips, sauces, and dressings.

The nutrients in many vegetables are better absorbed once they are cooked. The fiber in a carrot is more available when it has been softened by almost any cooking method, which also makes its beautiful beta-carotene more absorbable. Cooked spinach has more vitamin K than does fresh; cooked corn has more vitamin C than raw corn. Raw vegetables, especially cruciferous ones, are also great, but just a touch of cooking many vegetables helps them become body ready.

Unlike a visit from your in-laws, your ChefMD Eight-Week Program for Optimal Health (see chapter 6) doesn't have to turn your life upside down. It can be made up of small changes such as a cup of cocoa instead of a slice of cake, a piece of fine, dark chocolate

---

❋ LITTLE BITES

Leave the skins on vegetables whenever you can—many of the nutrients are just beneath, and the skin gives you fiber and your food texture.

instead of a cookie, or a roasted, curried sweet potato instead of a hot potato with butter and sour cream. These are not acts of self-denial, but better, more successful choices. *Vitality and better health are possible at any age, and often through small, surprising, and relatively simple lifestyle changes.*

For example, the flavonoids in food seem to help prevent breast cancer, so you should drink tea instead of alcohol if you are trying to prevent breast cancer. You want omega-3s to lubricate your joints and mitigate the symptoms of osteoarthritis, so you should enjoy wild Alaskan salmon, walnuts, and flax. You might want to drink fortified nonfat milk or soy milk to have plenty of vitamin D in the southbound lane to prevent colon cancer. Vitamin D is added by the dairy, not the cow, so either beverage will give you what you need. I'll go into what to eat to prevent specific conditions and symptoms in detail in chapter 7. But the point is you don't want your car running on empty. You want your gas tank to be full of the healthful nutrients that can help keep you disease-free.

Food is such a powerful medicine in the fight against medical problems ranging from attention deficit hyperactivity disorder to Alzheimer's, it's astonishing to me how few of us know about bioavailability and the fact that we can fight serious diseases with just a few simple and easy changes in our diets.

Because there are fewer nutrients in our food now than there were fifty years ago, we've got to make every meal a chance to put our health first. The best way to safeguard your health is to eat a wide variety of quality foods in the best combinations.

Celebrate that there is part of you—your doctor inside—that already wants to make healthy choices. It wants you to get every bit of goodness you can out of your foods. It also wants you to avoid the bad stuff—which is what we'll discuss in the next chapter.

✻ **LITTLE BITES**

Everyone knows that tomatoes are good for you, possibly because of the carotenoids inside. Lycopene is reported to protect against heart disease and prostate and cervical cancer. But did you know that cooked tomatoes release more lycopene than uncooked tomatoes? And when you add a bit of healthy fat, like olive oil, your body absorbs the lycopene more readily—four times more, in fact. That's how you maximize the body readiness of carotenoids from a tomato: cook and eat it with a little healthy fat.

CHAPTER 2

Avoiding Anti-Nutrients: AVOID BAD GUYS IN YOUR FOOD

Don't dig your grave with your knife and fork.

—ENGLISH PROVERB

Nutrients and Anti-Nutrients—Test Your ChefMD IQ

1. Do you take megadoses—more than 100 percent of the recommended daily value of nutrients in your multivitamins?
   Yes _____   No _____
2. Besides the "feel good" factor, is buying from local farmers important to your health?
   Yes _____   No _____
3. Are organic food items actually better for you?
   Yes _____   No _____
4. Do you eat commercial fast food more than once per month?
   Yes _____   No _____
5. Are foods that are white generally good for you?
   Yes _____   No _____
6. Are artificial sweeteners bad for you?
   Yes _____   No _____
7. Do you eat breaded, deep-fried, or charred foods less than once per month?
   Yes _____   No _____
8. Can you, at a glance, tell the difference between saturated and unsaturated fats?
   Yes _____   No _____

9. Is filtered water better for you than tap or bottled water?

   Yes _____   No _____

10. Is it generally good to marinate poultry or meat before cooking it?

    Yes _____   No _____

11. Is it safe to cover and then microwave fatty food in plastic wrap?

    Yes _____   No _____

12. Is heating an empty nonstick pan at medium temperatures generally safe?

    Yes _____   No _____

Scoring: Give yourself 1 point for each correct answer

1. **No:** Surprise! Avoid megadose vitamins—you shouldn't overdose on anything.

2. **Yes:** Buying local has huge and very real health benefits. More on that later in the book.

3. **Yes:** Bet you guessed that's right. Besides being pesticide-free, organic foods are generally higher in nutrition.

4. **No:** When it comes to fast food, less is more.

5. **No:** White foods like white potatoes, enriched flour, white bread, white rice, sugar, and so on are too often nutritional losers.

6. **Yes:** Why would you want to eat something with the word artificial in it? Do you eat artificial meat, artificial bananas, artificial water?

7. **Yes:** You already know that stuff's not good for you.

8. **Yes:** Unsaturated fats are good for you and saturated fats are, well, less so. Upcoming: how to spot them at a glance.

9. **Yes:** Generally speaking, most bottled water is tap water, and filtered tap water is even safer.

10. **Yes:** Marinating can protect you from toxic chemicals formed while cooking.

11. **No:** Emerging research suggests that plastic's chemicals can enter your food when you microwave fatty food in soft plastic and plastic wrap, including phthalates or "synthetic hormones."

12. **Yes:** Low and medium temperatures are okay. High temps are not.

Total score (0–12): _____

10–12 points: Your Inner ChefMD is smart and cookin'.

5–9 points: Your Inner ChefMD is almost ready for prime time. Read this chapter to hone your skills.

0–4 points: Your Inner ChefMD needs to go to culinary medical school. Read this chapter immediately!

Nobody wants his or her spouse to cheat—but if your spouse *is* cheating, wouldn't you want to know about it? Nobody wants something awful in their food—but if there *is* something awful in your food, wouldn't you want to know about it?

I want you to know exactly what's going on in your body—even if it's not pretty—so that you can take action. Once you know, then you can do something about it—namely, get those anti-nutrients out of your life!

There are so many things we can't control: hurricanes, drunk drivers, and whether or not the guy you're stuck next to on the plane has had a bath in the past week. It's great that we can control what goes into our bodies. In the last chapter, we looked at the good stuff in food. Now we're going to look at some of the not-so-good stuff.

Saturated Fats

My divorced friends say the most dangerous food in the world is a wedding cake. I say it's anything made with lots of saturated fat, which, come to think of it, could include a wedding cake. Saturated fats are nonessential fats, which means that the body can make them on its own, so you need very little. One exception: women with anovulatory infertility who may need more saturated fat. *The National Academy of Sciences says we should minimize our intake of food with saturated fats, as they raise bad cholesterol (low-density lipoprotein, or LDL) and increase the risk of cardiovascular disease.*

Foods with a lot of saturated fat are meats, butter, lard, coconut oil, cottonseed oil and palm oil, full-fat dairy products (especially cream and cheese), and some prepared foods. Think *sat* rhymes with *fat*, because these foods can pack on the pounds. At least the makers of prepared foods are required to put the saturated-fat content on their labels. Your local steak house is not. Neither is the corner bakery, the neighborhood deli, or street vendors, as charming as these delicious places can be. So when it comes to your saturated-fat intake, it can be hard to know how much you're getting.

Let me talk science for a minute. There are four common saturated fats: (1) stearic acid found in chocolate and in animal fats like dairy, meat, lard, and tallow; (2) palmitic acid found in palm oil, chocolate, and meat; (3) lauric acid found in coconut; and (4) the worst of all when it comes to raising your LDL level—myristic acid, found in dairy products and coconut.

Some people argue that these fats raise not only LDL cholesterol but also HDL ("good") cholesterol, thus keeping that important ratio between the "bad" and the "good" cholesterol even. However high LDL is high LDL, and bad for your heart, brain, skin, and sexuality. While it's true that stearic acid does not raise LDL levels, it does raise fibrinogen and C-reactive protein levels in the blood. Fibrinogen and C-reactive protein are both indicators of inflammation, which may actually cause heart disease—the number-one killer in this country—and also increases the risk of breast cancer. Not what you want! Dr. Ken Cooper of the Cooper Institute says that high levels of C-reactive protein may be worse than high levels of LDL for your heart and that high levels of C-reactive protein put you at increased risk of a sudden, fatal heart attack.

"So, Dr. John, where's the good news?" you ask. *Studies show that replacing saturated fats in the diet with unsaturated fats (like those in nuts and avocado) will increase your ratio of HDL to LDL cholesterol.* That means eating the ChefMD way—olive oil instead of butter, a portobello "steak" or grass-fed beef or bison instead of a fatty, grain-fed ribeye, salsa instead of sour cream—can reverse the tread marks left on your arteries by all the steaks in years gone by.

Omega-6 (Linoleic Acid)

Omega-6 is saturated fat's evil brother. Together they are the Lyle and Eric Menendez of fats, causing death and destruction through inflammation, clogged arteries, and heart disease.

Like saturated fat, we need some omega-6, but most Americans already get far too much of it. Where is all this omega-6 coming from? Before World War II, cattle were grass-fed in pastures, but today most cattle are fed industrial corn or grain. The starch in the

The thrill of the grill is to get great flavor and to minimize nasty carcinogens before you cook. There are five ways: First, nuke that steak for sixty seconds before you cook it, pour off the amino acids that leak out, and it will have 90 percent fewer cancer-causing heterocyclic amines (HCAs) than if you'd tossed it straight on the fire. HCAs are formed inside well-done and grilled meats. Second, cook at low temperatures—you'll keep the juiciness and minimize the HCAs. Third, marinate your burgers in a low-sugar, lower-fat marinade or coat them with a dry spice rub: you barricade the meat against HCAs, which can also affect DNA. Fourth, cut off any char, because it's carcinogenic. Toxic polycyclic aromatic hydrocarbons (PAHs) form in well-done meat and charred meat, and in the fat that flames up. And last, eat all your grilled meat with cruciferous vegetables on the side. The phytochemicals of broccoli, kale, brussels sprouts, cauliflower, and watercress help your liver detoxify the carcinogens in well-done meat.

corn and grain converts to fat, which in corn-fed cattle is mostly saturated and omega-6 fats. Starch produces the white marbled, high-sat-fat meat that Americans love, and that can give you twice your daily allotment of saturated fats in a single serving. Corn-fed beef—even beef "finished on grain"—is higher in saturated fat and omega-6s and lower in protein and omega-3s than grass-fed beef.

You only need about two or three times the omega-6 than you do omega-3. Remember this ratio by the fact that six is twice of three. You may need even less: hunter-gatherers had a ratio of one to one. But many Americans get closer to thirty times as much omega-6. Scientists believe that very high levels of omega-6s can lead to fatal health problems like those caused by too many saturated fats. Like so many other changes in our diet over the past hundred or so years, we are getting much less omega-3 than we should. *Omega-3 can reduce inflammation; omega-6s increase it.* Like corn-fed cattle, farmed salmon is much higher in saturated fats than wild salmon, and like cattle, farmed salmon are fed industrial corn that promotes omega-6s and reduces other nutrients. A study published in January 2004 in *Science* found that in most cases consuming more than one serving of farmed salmon per month could elevate your risk of cancer because it contains so much omega-6.

My ChefMD prescription? Go for the best nutrition *and* the best flavor. When you choose beef or salmon, eat only grass-fed beef, bison, and wild salmon. (All Alaskan salmon, by the way, is wild salmon.)

Irradiated Meat

Most of us have some vague idea that conventionally farmed animals aren't kept in very good conditions—appalling is a better word—but don't like to think about it too much. After all, most people like animals. But let's put aside the animals' concerns for a moment, and think of our own.

Animals have bacteria in their waste, and these bacteria get spread around the feedlot from animal to animal. They also get transferred onto the cuts of meat by machines during the slaughtering process. So the meat you bring home from the grocery has bacteria on it. And when we're talking about bacteria like *E. coli* 0157, that's a chilling thought. Remember all the recalls?

For the most part, bacteria are killed when the meat hits a hot pan. But commercially ground meat gets the bacteria ground into it—and usually from many different animals, and sometimes from different countries, all at once.

How is the meat industry dealing with this fact? It's allowed to irradiate meat. Irradiating meat does get rid of a lot of but not all of the bacteria in ground meat, reducing the risk of food poisoning and increasing shelf life. But it also gives the meat a slight taste of burnt hair. Another burger, anyone? And it's a new enough practice that we don't yet know enough about it. A recent study on the chemicals that irradiation creates in meat has led the European parliament to call for further studies.

By buying irradiated meat—carried by about three thousand supermarkets in the United States, and the federal school lunch program—we are paying to clean up a mess that never should have been made in the first place. If slaughterhouses were forced to keep more hygienic conditions, and process cattle more safely, we wouldn't have to bring gamma rays or electron beams into the kitchen just to try to keep ourselves from getting sick from bacteria, insects, and pathogens that shouldn't be there in the first place. Sometimes when I'm dealing with commercially ground meat I feel I should be wearing a protective full body suit and radiation-resistant gloves, like a scientist at a nuclear plant.

To top it all off, the government is considering labeling irradiated meat "pasteurized," to make it more appealing to folks who don't want to buy irradiated meat. That's deceptive. Right now, markets usually identify irradiated meat as irradiated, as well they should.

Spices keeping meat safer may explain the traditional use of spices in countries with warm climates such as India, the Caribbean, and the Middle East. Perhaps, through trial and error, cooks in those regions realized that spicing up meat could make it last longer and, of course, taste scrumptious. Check out the recipe for Cumin-Crusted Salmon over Silky Sweet Potatoes on page 115.

Hormones

Hormones are fun. They are what made us misbehave as teenagers, and what can make us misbehave now, as adults, especially if we

✳ **LITTLE BITES**

Clove, garlic, cinnamon, oregano, and sage may do more than just give food delicious flavor. Researchers at Kansas State University found that these spices may help stop the growth of *E. coli* bacteria in uncooked meat.

When uncooked hamburger meat was mixed with *E. coli* and between two to five teaspoons (to reach a ratio of 7.5 percent spice to 92.5 percent ground meat) of either powdered clove, cinnamon, garlic, oregano, or sage, clove was found to have the most potent effect. It reduced bacteria by more than 99 percent. Cinnamon reduced them by 80 percent; garlic by 75 percent; oregano by 50 percent; and sage by 37 percent. Researchers pointed out that people can still get sick from meat that is 99 percent free of *E. coli*.

You're standing in front of the dairy case, wondering whether to buy organic or regular milk. Is the organic really worth the extra cost?

Let's do the math. At my local Trader Joe's, a gallon of nonorganic no-rBST milk is $2.99. A gallon of organic milk is $5.99—twice the price, which might be what is making you hesitate. But let's look closer. There are sixteen eight-ounce glasses of milk in a gallon. A glass of nonorganic milk costs $0.19, and a glass of organic milk is $0.38. That's a difference of $0.19 per glass. The government recommends three servings of dairy a day. If you get two of those servings as milk, that's a cost of $0.38—less than the price of a postage stamp. It's worth the price of a stamp to send your body a message of good health.

If you are at risk for prostate or breast cancer (and who isn't?), and if your immune system is impaired or if you just want to protect it (and who wouldn't?), you want to spare your body from chemical assault whenever you can. The choice of which milk to buy is like the glass door on the dairy case itself—open and shut. Buy the organic.

meet someone we really like and we're both single (and for some people, even when they're not, which is usually a bad idea). But when it comes to our food, hormones are no fun at all.

The cartons of milk you buy may proudly state that the milk has been produced without the use of the growth hormone called re-combinant bovine somatotropin (rBST). But you may also know that rBST has been approved for use in cows by the Federal Drug Agency (FDA). So how do you know if it's harmful or not? The answer is that rBST is probably not harmful in and of itself. It also won't make you grow. Cows given routine injections of it, however, also may receive antibiotics to fight infection from those injections, and then you've got antibiotics on your breakfast cereal. Also, cows treated with rBST have a higher level of an insulin-like growth factor (IGF-1) in their milk, which may increase the rate of prostate and breast cancers in people.

What can you do? *Buy milk and other dairy whose packages say they come from cows that have not been treated by rBST.* Better yet, buy organic or soy! The cows will love you for it.

Synthetic Chemical Pesticides

A pesticide is anything that destroys, repels, or keeps away a pest. So in a sense, the cubicle wall between you and your annoying co-worker is a pesticide.

But of course, when we speak of pesticides, we think of farming. For the last ten thousand years, since a man in Jericho first grew a wheat plant and a bird came along and stole a grain, farmers have been battling to keep nature from stealing, damaging, or destroying their crops. In addition to birds, farmers must fight fungi, weeds, insects, slugs, snails, rodents, and viruses. This battle between man and beast raged until the 1940s, when DDT was discovered. Then farmers simply began dumping chemicals on all those pests.

Unfortunately, in the time since, those highly toxic chemicals have wreaked havoc with our health, both by being in the food we eat and in the environment in which we live. *Researchers continue to uncover the links between pesticides and several types of cancer, neurological and reproductive disorders, birth defects, and asthma.* While nobody has proven once and for all that the pesticides farmers use today cause fatal illness, synthetic chemical pesticides are toxic chemicals made to kill, and they're in conventional food. You don't have to be a research genius to see the connection.

Pesticides aren't just used on crops—they are used in livestock and fish farming, too. A study released in the journal *Environmental Science & Technology* reported much higher levels of some cancer-causing chemicals as well as flame retardant in farmed salmon as compared with wild. How about a nice yummy glass of flame retardant?

No surprise, I'm sure, that I recommend organic foods, since organic farmers don't use synthetic chemical pesticides. If organic produce is unavailable, use running water or a fruit and vegetable wash to clean the produce—they're equally effective. *Buying local helps, too,* as you don't know what additives they are using in say, China, which supplies vitamin supplements and additives to many industrial food processors (enriched bread, anyone?) or which herbicides and fungicides might accompany your well-traveled green peppers.

Antibiotics

Antibiotics kill bacteria. Before antibiotics, doctors often treated infections with poisons such as strychnine, which killed the bacteria by killing the patient. Do you think this was around the time that someone invented medical malpractice insurance? Antibiotics were considered "magic bullets" because they did not have this unwanted side effect. And they've saved countless lives since. But now they're posing a health threat of their own.

Conventionally raised livestock and farm-raised salmon in the United States are frequently fed antibiotics in their feed not because they are ill or to prevent disease but because low doses of antibiotics make them grow faster. In animals, low doses of antibiotics in animal feed are called "antimicrobial growth promoters," or AGPs. They help animals get bigger faster, so they can be slaughtered sooner, saving farmers money.

Although it may seem gross to eat meat from an animal that has been given antibiotics, the antibiotics won't hurt you. But what might are antibiotic-resistant infections that arise because of the AGP. These are caused by "super-bugs"—antibiotic-resistant bacteria that also cause infections in people. "The reason to buy meat

Love baseball? Well, if you want to knock one out of the park for your health, you might want to switch your snack.

Nitrites are used in many packaged, cured meats (ham, bacon, pastrami, salami), and they also exist in beer and nonfat dry milk. They fight bacteria and also give cured meat a fresh, pink hue. Without nitrites, meat would turn brown. Sodium nitrate is often added to processed meats, too, and nitrates readily convert to nitrites. This is a problem. Because when nitrites react with amino acids and heat, they form nitrosamines, which are carcinogens.

The take-home lesson? If you buy them at all, buy cured and packaged meats such as bacon and salami that are nitrate- and nitrite-free. Consider avoiding processed red meat altogether and limiting red meat: it increases colon and rectal cancer risk. More about that later.

without antibiotics is not because the antibiotics in the meat are transferred to the person, but because of how the antibiotics increase the number of antibiotic-resistant bacteria," said Dr. Stuart Levy, director of the Center of Adaptation Genetics and Drug Resistance at Tufts University Medical School, in a January 17, 2001, *New York Times* article.

Antibiotics and antibiotic-resistant bacteria are found in the air and soil around farms, surface and ground water, wild animal populations, and on meat and poultry in the supermarket. *Because a lot of people don't know how to handle meat safely, these antibiotic-resistant bacteria can wind up cross-contaminating other foods in their kitchen.*

If you think super-bugs are a thing of the future that we can deal with later, think again. Americans are now at risk of a highly contagious bacterial infection called methicillin-resistant staphylococcus aureus (MRSA). Roughly 130,000 of us are infected with MRSA each year, and 5,000 die from it, including one of every twenty infected hospitalized patients.

Professional athletes are especially at risk, and football players, who often get cuts during play, are being hit the hardest. Since 2003 the Redskins, Rams, and Browns have reported multiple cases of staph infections such as MRSA. Five different Browns have been stricken, including Brian Russell, who got two separate staph infections in one season. Cleveland wide receiver Braylon Edwards got staph and faced possible amputation of his arm. Scary, huh? And sadly, anyone who shares hygiene facilities with others is at risk, such as people who work out at a gym, are in the military, are in prison, or are in a nursing home.

Once again, Europe's ahead of us when it comes to food safety issues. The European Union banned the nontherapeutic use of antibiotics in agriculture in 2006, and Sweden banned AGPs in 1986. In 2003 the World Health Organization recommended that all countries phase out the use of AGPs. The Pan American Health Organization recommends the same thing.

What to do? *Buy meat that is labeled "certified organic."* And don't be misled by a meat label that says "natural." (After all, botulism is natural.) The USDA even allows meat from animals given growth hormones and antibiotics to be labeled as "natural," a fact that many people don't know.

"Most people are shocked to find that the 'natural' label is essentially meaningless and has nothing to do with the way animals are raised. It only pertains to the handling of meat after slaughter," said Gene Baur, president of Farm Sanctuary, the nation's leading farm animal shelter and advocacy organization.

Sugar and High-Fructose Corn Syrup

It's part of our happiest childhood memories—the lollipop given by Grandma, the cotton candy at the Ferris wheel, the ice-cream cone melting faster than we can eat it on a hot summer afternoon. It's hard to imagine that something that seems so innocent could be doing such damage to our health.

It's not the teaspoon of sugar you put into your morning cup of coffee that's doing all the damage. It's the sugar that other people put into your food that is making the waistband of your jeans too tight. Forget that those Cocoa Krispies are organic or that that Krispy Kreme donut is whole grain. These are actual products on the market—I'm not making them up. The sugar blast they give could knock the neighbor's kid off his skateboard.

But not every food with sugar screams out "I'm sugary!" Commercial processing of almost any whole food will blunt its flavor. How do processors get some taste back into the food? By putting sugar in it. And you can't trust your taste buds to tell you when, since many processed foods with sugar don't taste sweet—like mayonnaise or pickles, for example. When you start reading labels, you'll be amazed how many products contain sugar. In a list of ingredients, most words that end with "ose"—such as glucose—and any "syrup" refer to a sugar. The exception are some starches, like amylose. But sucrose, lactose, fructose, glucose, dextrose, galactose, maltose, sorbose, xylose, ChocolateCakeose, JellyBellyose—all sugars!

Too much added sugar in any form is not good for your body as it adds calories, has no helpful nutrients, and forces your body into an insulin and inflammatory response that can eventually backfire as asthma, gout, rheumatoid arthritis, and diabetes, just to name a few. And we're drowning in sugar, especially kids and young people, who are targeted by food companies with high-sugar foods. For example, a large Mr. Misty Slush from Dairy Queen has 280 percent of the recommended daily allowance for sugar. That's enough to wire

✛ DOCTOR IT UP!

You only need to use a little sugar in a dessert if you know how to give it a flavor boost. I love to make a sweet sauce with just a little brown sugar, balsamic vinegar, and juniper berries! It makes a great dressing to put on sliced fruit, especially strawberries, while indulging your sweet tooth and saving your real teeth and the rest of you from too much sugar. It's even great drizzled on my Quick Steel-Cut Oats with Apples, Ginger, and Walnuts (page 97).

your kid for days! The Center for Science in the Public Interest recommends ten teaspoons per day as a limit—the average American teenage boy gets thirty-four.

There is one particularly evil member of the sugar family—the Jeffrey Dahmer of sugars—high-fructose corn syrup (HFCS). HFCS is perfect for frozen foods that have been heavily processed because it keeps food from getting freezer burn. It's good for baked goods that need to have a long shelf life, and it's in those not normally sweetened, like bread. It's cheap, it's great for weight gain, and we eat way too much of it, which is the real problem. *Some scientists think that the body processes HFCS differently than it does regular corn syrup and that it decreases our metabolism by tampering with our metabolic hormones.* It also forces the liver to kick more fat out into the bloodstream, raising your triglyceride level.

No ChefMD recipes contain any product with HFCS—and you'd be amazed at how many we tossed out because they did.

Peter Havel, a nutrition researcher at the University of California–Davis, has shown that HFCS affects leptin, a hormone made by the body's fat cells. Simply put, leptin is the master switch that tells your brain to stop eating; HFCS seems to disable that switch. Havel's research also shows that fructose doesn't stop ghrelin, a hormone that increases your hunger and appetite.

This double whammy means that you will keep eating past the point when you would normally stop, because your "I'm full" safety system has been disabled. You don't get the message to stop eating. The end result? *Your body is tricked into wanting to eat more food and, at the same time, to store more fat.*

What can you do? Eat as little cane sugar as you can, and avoid HFCS. Check the label on every packaged food you buy, and if HFCS is listed, put it back on the shelf. If it's in your pantry, fridge, or freezer (Danger, danger Will Robinson!), toss it. Replace them with better versions of the food. In restaurants, avoid dishes with glazes or sweet sauces, especially in national chain restaurants where such sauces are shipped in on pallets and railcars. Or cook at home, where you actually know what's in your food because you're the one who put it there!

Finally, try to avoid artificial sweeteners. It's not just that they have been linked to migraines and have no nutritional value. It's that they change what your taste buds think is sweet. Pretty soon, it's hard to tell the difference between what is sweet and has no

⊗ NOXIOUS NOTS

Nothing seems more wholesome than a loaf of whole-grain bread. Who knew you had to watch out for HFCS? And now here's another danger lurking in that loaf: potassium bromate.

Potassium bromate is used to strengthen bread dough and let it rise higher. Bromate causes cancerous tumors in rats. It is considered a category 2B (possibly carcinogenic to humans—to be or not to be, indeed!) carcinogen by the International Agency for Research on Cancer.

So what can you do? Read the label. Fortunately, many bakeries are taking potassium bromate out of bread. Shop at a local bakery where you can speak to the baker about what goes into the bread: he or she wants good things for customers, too. If you don't have a local bakery, contact the company that bakes the bread you eat and ask if they use potassium bromate.

calories and what is sweet and is calorie-dense and nutrient not. And guess who overeats and doesn't know it?

Trans Fat

What movie monster frightens you the most? Michael Myers from *Halloween*? Freddy Krueger from *Nightmare on Elm Street*? The shark from *Jaws*? How would you feel if you came across one of them in real life? That fear and dread is the same feeling I want you to have when you come across our next anti-nutrient—the Grand Poobah of ugly, unwanted, getting-you-to-the-grave-faster additives to American food—trans fat.

Trans fat, also called trans-fatty acids, is formed when hydrogen is added to liquid vegetable oils to make them more solid. Food processors love to use trans fats because they give food a longer shelf life, and also give foods—for example, bread—a softness that many people like.

Most trans fat is found in processed food—shortenings, stick (or hard) margarine, cookies, crackers, snack foods, fried foods, doughnuts, pastries, and baked goods. Often, food is fried and deep-fried in partially hydrogenated oils. Some trans fat is also found naturally in small amounts in meat and dairy products.

According to the FDA, the average American gets almost six grams of trans fat a day. Trans fat raises your "bad" LDL cholesterol levels and lowers your "good" HDL cholesterol levels, causing your arteries to become clogged and increasing your risk of developing heart disease and stroke. *Unlike saturated fats and omega-6s, we don't need any of it at all. Ever.*

WHICH CHOLESTEROL IS GOOD AND WHICH IS BAD?

Michael Roizen, M.D., author of the RealAge series of books, invented a great way to remember which cholesterol is bad: H in HDL stands for "healthy" and L in LDL stands for "lousy."

Luckily, trans fats are easier to identify than ever before. Trans fat used to be called the "hidden" fat, because food manufacturers were not required to list it on their labels.

Happily, that has changed. The new labels list trans fat content separately on the Nutrition Facts panel of all packaged foods when there is half a gram or more present, thereby saving us from having to rely on our powers of clairvoyance.

What to do when faced with artificial trans fat? Act like you're facing the zombies from Dawn of the Dead, *and run for your life!* Or, um, just put the package back, and no one will get hurt.

MARGARINE—BETTER THAN BUTTER?

When margarine came onto the market fifty years ago, it was touted as a healthy alternative to butter. Then we discovered that trans-fatty acids that come from hydrogenating oil to make margarine solid at room temperature were worse for your heart than the saturated fats found in butter. To butter lovers who had forced themselves to eat margarine, this seemed like a cruel joke.

Now a new generation of cholesterol-lowering butter-substitute spreads made from plant sterols and stanols are advertised as being trans-fat-free. But can we believe these claims? Not necessarily. The government allows food manufacturers to advertise any product that has less than half a gram of trans fat as being free of trans fat, which means that you may be eating trans fats even when you think you are not.

What to do? You might look to a caramel-flavored Benecol Smart Chew instead of margarine, because for just eighty calories and no fat at all, you get the daily recommended amount of plant sterols. Or try the light versions of spreads such as Smart Balance, Benecol, or Take Control. They do not have any trans-fatty acids. Better yet, have a naturally fat-free spread like apple butter on your toast, or a healthy, flavorful fat like artisanal extra-virgin olive oil on your vegetables.

Enough About Food. What About My Water?

Why would someone pay the water department for water, then shell out five bucks for a bottle of Evian? (Answer: try spelling Evian backward.) We are made mostly of water, and having plenty of fresh, available drinking water is far more vital to our survival than food.

Unlike so many people in other countries, we have both hot and cold water at our fingertips with the turn of a faucet. But how safe is the water coming out of your tap? Let's look at the five most common and potentially problematic contaminants in the water you drink:

1. *Chlorine:* When chlorine reacts with organic waste products in water, it forms trihalomethane, which may increase the risk of bladder and rectal cancers.

2. *Agricultural chemicals:* Synthetic pesticides, herbicides, and fungicides can seep into water through old or cracked pipes.

3. *Lead:* Lead leaches into the water from lead solder in old pipes. Lead solder was banned in the United States in 1986, and lead-based paint in 1977, but if your house was built or painted before then, you may have lead in your pipes—both the pipes in your house and the pipes in your body. Lead solder may have been used in the pipes of the municipal system. The possible effects of long-term exposure to lead are serious, especially for kids under age six, and include kidney disease, cancer, and stroke.

4. *Radioactive water:* If you live near or downstream from an old radioactive dumping site, it's possible that radioactive material in the ground could seep into your water supply.

5. *Nitrates:* Fertilizers with nitrogen, including animal or human waste, can put nitrates into your water, especially if you have a well. Nitrates can cause cancer.

器 NOXIOUS NOTS

What can perfume, some massage lotions, and a sex toy lead to? I know what you're thinking, but that's not it. The answer is they can lead to serious health problems. All of them contain chemicals known as phthalates (pronounced "tha-lates"). And—most important for the doctor inside to know—phthalates are used in some plastic food packaging. New research shows that low-dose exposures to phthalates may be reducing testosterone levels in men, which is a cause of rising obesity rates, since low testosterone levels appear to increase belly fat in men.

What can you do? You could start by not buying food that's packaged in plastic, right? Fresh produce such as melons don't need any packaging at all; cuts of meat can be wrapped in paper by the butcher. And don't microwave fatty foods in soft or take-out plastic containers, which can cause phthalates to leach into the food. While phthalates have not been conclusively shown to cause cancer, the EPA says phthalates "can be reasonably anticipated to be carcinogenic." Ouch.

Up to 20 percent of a child's lead exposure is through the water supply. If you are concerned about the safety of your water, filter your water, using a simple inline filter, a pitcher filter, or best of all, a reverse-osmosis system, which is a lot easier to use than it sounds. Use only cold water for cooking and reconstituting, and run tap water for a minute before using. The hotter and longer it sits in pipes, the more lead can dissolve. Boiling your water does not help.

If you want to know more, buy an EPA-approved testing kit and call the EPA safe-drinking water hotline: 1-800-426-4791. Ask your water company to give you a copy of the tests that are routinely done on their water (the water company is required to give you this) so that you can see if the contaminants in your water are coming from the public supply or from inside your system.

What About Bottled Water?

I'm sure you've heard about the debate over bottled versus tap water. Many bottled waters are simply municipal water with a few minerals added for flavor. Buying them on top of paying your water bill makes as much sense to me as paying a company to allow you to breathe air. Some people, however, love the taste of bottled water, or they like its convenience or the bubbles. *If buying bottled water gets you to drink more water, and you don't mind the expense, and you can recycle all those bottles, go for it.*

But you should know that city water is highly regulated and monitored for quality. Bottled water is not. Also, bottled water is monitored by the FDA, but the 60–70 percent of bottled water that is sold in state is exempt from federal regulation. And tests on one thousand bottles of 103 different brands of bottled water found man-made chemicals, bacteria, and arsenic in 22 percent of the bottles.

Personally, I drink mostly filtered tap water. Fill an aluminum or hard plastic water bottle, and wash it both inside and out after each use. Take one with you when you go out. That's not only H$_2$O—that's what I call H$_2$O2Go!

Ready for some science? A calorie is the amount of energy it takes to raise one liter of water one degree centigrade. Half a liter is just about sixteen ounces. If you drink sixteen ounces of ice water, your body will need to burn 17.5 calories to bring the water to body temperature. Do this twice a day for year, and you lose three pounds. Hey, it's just ice water!

Whew . . . we got through it. Did you get it all? It's really very simple. Remember, all you have to do is minimize your intake of stearic acid, palmitic acid, lauric acid, myristic acid, and linoleic acid, and avoid recombinant bovine somatotropin, synthetic chemical pesticides, antibiotics, high-fructose corn syrup, trans fat, nitrates, chlorine, and lead.

What's that? You're having trouble keeping track of it all? That's okay—you don't have to remember all the science. Here's all you need to do:

- Buy minimally processed foods whenever possible.
- Buy food that is recognizable as the plant or animal it came from.
- Eat a diet rich in organic fruits and vegetables.
- Choose whole-grain baked goods and find out what's gone into them.
- Eat wild salmon instead of farmed salmon.
- Eat lean grass-fed organic beef or bison instead of corn-fed beef.
- Eat antibiotic-free, certified organic poultry.
- Precook or marinate meat before high-temperature cooking.
- Choose hormone-free, low-fat, or nonfat organic dairy products.
- Filter your drinking water.
- Cook at home whenever possible.

That's it! I hope you feel like I did when I learned about all the toxins in my food and water—very excited that I now had a chance to get them out of my diet.

Enough of the serious stuff—it's time for some fun. In the next chapter, we'll talk about what you *can* get more of from your food—satisfaction!

CHAPTER 3

The Science of Satiety: FEEL FULL FASTER

> My doctor told me to stop having intimate dinners for four.
> Unless there are three other people.
>
> —ORSON WELLES

Satiety—Test Your ChefMD IQ

1. Do you eat foods high in fiber, such as fruits, vegetables, and whole grains almost every day?

   Yes ____   No ____

2. Do you eat foods high in resistant starch almost every day?

   Yes ____   No ____

3. Do you eat foods containing lots of water, such as soups and salads, especially at the start of lunch or dinner, almost every day?

   Yes ____   No ____

4. Do you eat healthy oils and fats almost every day?

   Yes ____   No ____

5. Do you eat foods rich in lean protein, without visible fat, almost every day?

   Yes ____   No ____

6. Do you eat breakfast almost every day?

   Yes ____   No ____

7. Do you nearly always eat three meals a day, and do those meals always take you at least twenty minutes to eat?

   Yes ____   No ____

8. Does your breakfast nearly always have a protein-containing food like nuts, tofu, eggs, chicken, turkey, or cheese?

   Yes _____   No _____

9. Do you often eat meals either standing up or on the go?

   Yes _____   No _____

10. Do you like to smell the aromas of your food before eating it?

    Yes _____   No _____

Scoring: Give yourself 1 point for each correct answer.

1. **Yes:** Know the benefits of soluble and nonsoluble fiber. One helps lower cholesterol while the other helps your digestive system.

2. **Yes:** I'll show you what resistant starch is and why it's a very good thing.

3. **Yes:** By "volumizing" you can eat a lot and feel fuller longer without taking on extra calories.

4. **Yes:** There's such a thing as healthy fat, and you should have some every day.

5. **Yes:** Where's the beef? Here's good news! Protein keeps you satisfied.

6. **Yes:** Eat breakfast almost every day. It gets you going on the right track *and* it'll help you lose weight.

7. **Yes:** The only way to eat the ChefMD way is slowly. It's less stressful and you'll eat less, guaranteed.

8. **Yes:** Protein is very important at breakfast.

9. **No:** Sitting and relaxing through a meal is powerful medicine.

10. **Yes:** The aroma of your food is a huge part of the flavor.

   Total score (0–10): _____
   8–10 points: Your Inner ChefMD is smart and cookin'.
   4–7 points: Your Inner ChefMD is almost ready for prime time. Read this chapter to hone your skills.
   0–3 points: Your Inner ChefMD needs to go to culinary medical school. Read this chapter immediately!

Do your clothes seem to be shrinking? Even the clothes you haven't washed lately? If so, this chapter is for you. It's about the third key of culinary medicine—satiety—and it's really pretty simple. *Satiety is feeling full and fully satisfied after a meal and staying satisfied until your next meal*—without snacking, munching, and mindless eating. It is a small medical word that offers big benefits if you understand how to achieve it. Fortunately, we are learning more and more about how satiety works and ways we can have fun reaching it.

Satiety is a key component of successful weight loss, but satiety is vital for more than just weight loss. It's vital for preventing common conditions. When you eat high-quality food and feel full and fully satisfied without feeling stuffed, you've eaten to the point of satiety. You've eaten less food than if you had gorged mindlessly. You've eaten fewer of the anti-nutrients that can threaten your health. If you control satiety, you control your salt intake if you have high blood pressure, your sugar and starch intake if you have diabetes or prediabetes, and your food-borne carcinogen and immunity threats if you are at risk of breast or prostate cancer.

Satiety is determined by two things: how fast or slow you eat, and what you eat.

First, know your hormones. Your satiety center is at the back of the brain in the hypothalamus. It is controlled by two opposing brain chemicals—cocaine- and amphetamine-regulated transcript (CART) and neuropeptide Y (NPY). CART tells the hypothalamus to increase metabolism, lessen appetite, and increase insulin so that energy can be burned. NPY does the opposite. Leptin, a hormone made by your belly fat, tells your body you've had enough food. Cholecystokinin (CCK), released by your intestines when food with fat is inside, tells the brain you're full. And ghrelin, a hormone your stomach produces when it's empty, makes you hungry. Really hungry.

Hunger and Satiety

There are two kinds of satiety. One is short term, which means you're full after finishing this meal, right now. The other is long term, which means you'll be full until four to six hours from now, when you should be hungry again. If you're lustfully dreaming about Mom's meat loaf sooner than four hours after you've finished a meal, you're eating the wrong foods or the wrong amounts of the right foods.

It's usually the wrong amounts of the right foods. Most people on diets feel hungry, and they hate it. One week into a diet and even your cat's kibble starts to look tasty. You try to battle the feelings of hunger with sheer willpower, but it just doesn't work. One day you're walking down the street, and your hunger sneaks up behind you and pushes you through the front door of a doughnut shop and then begs for a baker's dozen, including the holes. This is just a fact of diet life.

But the ChefMD approach to hunger and satiety is different: it offers a different baker's dozen of thirteen Satiety Solutions, which work together so you can achieve pleasant fullness faster, with fewer calories. You won't go hungry. You achieve satiety.

Satiety isn't just about feeling full—it's about true satisfaction, or feeling pleasantly full with genuinely delicious food.

What are the tricks for reaching satiety faster, and keeping it longer? My goal is for you to learn to listen to your body. No one knows your body like you do. Stop eating not because everyone else at the table has stopped eating or you have already cleaned your plate, but because you are pleasantly satisfied. Don't listen to anyone who says your habits are too ingrained. Replace bad habits with these ways to keep yourself on track.

Satiety Solution 1: Engage All of Your Senses

When we think of a sensory response to food, we think of taste, and we'll get to that. But the other senses are used when we eat, too, even when we're not aware of it. The sooner you engage your other senses—smell, feel, sight, and sound—the sooner you can reach satiety.

SMELL

Smell well to eat well. Three-quarters of how well you taste certain foods actually comes from how you smell them. The Asthma and Allergy Foundation estimates that up to forty million American adults and children have allergic rhinitis, an allergic reaction to mold, dander, dust, or pollen. Rhinitis irritates the inside of the nose and causes mucus to form, reducing your ability to sense flavors. Common medications, chemical exposures, lead and silver fumes, and even polyps in the nose can alter your sense of taste. If this is you, see your doctor.

With its greasy kielbasa, fried cheese, and potato pierogis, Polish cuisine isn't exactly known as health food. But maybe it should be. Why? Because the traditional Polish diet is heavy in fermented cabbage—aka sauerkraut. When cabbage ferments, it forms isothiocyanates (natural mustard oils), which is what gives cabbage a little sharpness and also helps prevent breast cancer and maybe prostate cancer, too. Women who consume at least four servings per week of fermented cabbage are 72 percent less likely to develop breast cancer than those who only consume 1.5 servings per week.

Not wild about ordinary sauerkraut? Try mine—Sauerkraut with Onion, Apple, and Toasted Caraway (page 136). Or for something really spicy, try Korean kimchi—fermented cabbage and radish with a chile kick. Shredded fresh cabbage is a great option, too, with its cancer-fighting glucosinolates. For a delicious, all-in-one cancer-fighting meal, try my Grilled Citrus Trout over Crunchy Mediterranean Slaw on page 118.

There is a famous cooking school and prankster experiment in which a nose-pinched, blindfolded student or volunteer is fed a slice of onion and then a slice of crisp pear. Nearly all the time, he or she cannot tell the difference in taste. Because there is no smell. *And if you cannot smell well, you do not taste your food fully.*

Smell adds to satisfaction when you slow down to enjoy the aroma of your food. Inhale the aroma of each food before you eat it. Don't just gulp a drink or dig into a plate full of food. Take the time to notice what scents you can find in your dinner, drink, or snack. This will help you taste deliberately, notice color, see what is on your plate, and feel more satisfied. You'll appreciate more. And you'll also slow your rate of eating.

FEEL

Texture is an important part of food appreciation and can speed you up, slow you down, and even count you out. Biting into a mushy tomato or a stale piece of bread is awful, and you may even spit the food back out. Food manufacturers know this and spend millions trying to create foods that have the right, as they call it, "mouthfeel." Mouthfeel for butter should be smooth and round. Mouthfeel for fresh carrots is crunchy. Mouthfeel for an orange segment is juicy and bright. None of these are flavors: they are textures.

Luckily, in the ChefMD Eight-Week Program for Optimal Health (see chapter 6), great texture is built in. Mother Nature won't let you down. Imagine biting into a juicy dripping peach, a succulent and smooth melon slice, or a crisp green apple. Fruits, nuts, and vegetables, when good quality and well prepared, have texture that can work for you. *As you might guess, crunchy and chewy textures slow you down and help you eat more deliberately and more joyfully.* But that doesn't mean silky smooth is out: a Strawberry Pomegranate Blender Blaster (page 144) is creamy, rich, and thick. Combining textures (try my Maple Syrup Triple Berry Parfait—page 141) is a little-known secret to enjoying food more fully: the parfait is crunchy, smooth, and refreshing all in one.

SIGHT

Food that looks good sends a very strong message to the brain about how good the food is going to taste. People eating in the dark have a quite dim eating experience and less appreciation of their food.

Take the time to present food beautifully. Plated food seems more precious and a smaller serving can seem appropriate, almost like a present. Simple garnishes, like chopped parsley, sliced almonds, a sprinkle of cheese or sesame seeds, give dishes a visual flair. When we expect food to taste good because of how it looks, it usually does, because the eyes—and not just the stomach—affect satiety. We can feel just as satiated—remember, pleasantly full, *not* stuffed—with a small amount of beautiful and delicious-looking food as we can from a bigger amount of less appetizing-looking food.

SOUND

The *ssss* of a steak hitting the hot grill and popcorn's sound when it pops both promise flavors that can make your mouth water. Even the snap of topping and tailing fresh green beans has an auditory satisfaction all its own. *Enjoy the sound of your food—it can enhance its flavor.*

Sound of the Sea, a dish on the menu of the three-Michelin-starred Fat Duck restaurant in England, comes with an iPod that plays sounds of the ocean and breaking waves that patrons listen to while eating this dish that features seafood and edible seaweed.

Chef Heston Blumenthal, the owner of Fat Duck, told *Square Meal* magazine that he had conducted a series of tests with experimental psychologist Charles Spence at Oxford University that showed that sound could enhance taste. He said that listening to sounds of the ocean made the dish stronger and saltier than when, for example, one listened to barnyard noises.

A restaurant patron agreed, according to a BBC News article. "It definitely adds to the experience—the whole thing sets your senses going," she said. If you want to try this the next time you have seafood, you can listen to the ocean for as long as you like on the Red Lobster Web site (www.redlobster.com). Just click on "Fun Zone" and "Sounds of the Sea." And if you are trying to slow down your eating and improve satiety, NPR has thought-provoking programs that can make you pause and take notice. Listen to David Sedaris or Garrison Keillor tell a story while you eat, and watch how you slow down.

♥ THE SKINNY ON . . .
THE POWER OF SMELLS

Trick your mind and stomach with your nose—satiety can be achieved by smelling a food for approximately as long as it would take to chew it during a meal.

◎ SATIETY SOLUTION

Pick one main dish to improve how quickly you feel full. If you eat just one food you get what is called sensory-specific satiety. You've been eating, eating, eating one food and you have had enough of it already. That's why some diet books ask you to eat the same thing, over and over again. In contrast, variety makes you overeat. So maybe you shouldn't serve the chicken cordon bleu, the lobster thermidor, and the flaming crown roast au vin blanc all on the same night. Maybe my one recipe for Cumin-Crusted Salmon over Silky Sweet Potatoes (page 115) would be better.

Satiety Solution 2: Eat Long Fats

Eat long, liquid fats. By *long*, I do not mean that melted mozzarella that is stretched three feet between your slice of pizza and the pizza box—I mean *long* in that the fat molecule is at least ten carbon molecules long like those in olive, fish, canola, and nut oils.

Why long, liquid fats? When fat in food reaches the small intestine, the CCK hormone is released, which can help you feel full in three different ways—through your nerves, stomach, and brain. But only fat molecules at least ten carbons long effectively release CCK. Many foods contain long liquid fats: walnuts, fish, and flax are great choices. Since the food label won't tell you if the fat is ten carbons long, you need to know which foods—for example, fruits, fish, seeds and nuts—have them.

What type of fat you eat really does matter for satiety. Both short-chain solid, saturated fats (fats that are solid at room temperature)—like those in lunch meats and pastries—and trans fats worsen insulin resistance. Both saturated and trans fats cause the hormone NPY to be released from the brain. NPY then accelerates reward eating and causes you to overeat. That's right: *eating the wrong fats can actually make you hungrier.* In contrast, long-chain liquid, unsaturated fats (fats that are liquid at room temperature) improve insulin sensitivity and help you reach satiety.

My prescription? *Consciously, deliberately use the right fats when you love them, when you can see them, and when you can taste them.* Put avocado on top of taco filling, so you can see it. Sprinkle toasted walnuts or almonds onto low-fat yogurt. Drizzle the finest extra-virgin olive oil on top of a gazpacho soup. With the right fats you'll feel full and stop eating because you're satisfied.

Satiety Solution 3: Eat Lean Protein

Calorie for calorie, nothing is more filling than lean protein. There are three reasons. First, high-protein foods slow the movement of food from the stomach to the intestine. This means you'll feel full longer and get hungry again later rather than earlier. Second, protein's gentle, steady effect on blood sugar avoids the edgy rise and hunger-bell-ringing fall that occurs after you eat sugar or a starch like bread

---

◉ SATIETY SOLUTION

Wild salmon, sablefish, mackerel, herring, sardines, rainbow trout, anchovies, walnuts, almonds, flax, avocado, olives, olive oil, hazelnuts, and macadamias will all help you reach satiety. Their fats are the right stuff. And they are all absolutely delicious.

✳ LITTLE BITES

Little Miss Muffet was on to something with her curds and whey. Whey protein is very lean and whey protein powder is usually flavored as chocolate or vanilla. Lean protein increases your insulin sensitivity, improving blood sugar and reducing stored fat. Whey goes way back. An old Italian proverb goes, "If everyone were raised on whey, doctors would be bankrupt."

or crackers. And third, the body uses more energy to digest protein than it does to digest anything else.

The Nurses' Health Study investigated the link between protein and heart disease or stroke. In this fourteen-year study, women who ate the most protein (about 110 grams per day) were 25 percent less likely to have a heart attack or to have died of heart disease than the women who ate the least protein (about 68 grams per day). Whether the protein came from animals or vegetables or whether it was part of a low-fat or high-fat diet didn't seem to matter. *It's good to know that not only will eating foods with protein not harm your heart, they might actually help it.*

Certain proteins, like those in whey (the liquid that remains after milk has been curdled and strained to make cheese) are most satiating. Whey goes right through to the small intestine, where it triggers CCK and GLP-1 (glucagon-like peptide 1) release, both of which tell your brain to tell you stop eating. The way to a man's heart may be through his stomach, but it's also the way to his brain. These hormones are probably what help you to stop eating after you drink a whey shake or sprinkle whey powder on your cereal.

If you don't want to have whey by itself, try cheeses that are high in whey, such as ricotta, gjetost (a Norwegian cheese), Manouri and Mizithra (both Greek), and Requeson (Latin American). Or have a protein-rich cheese stick or a yogurt in the morning. Lean beef, poultry, and fish—whether fresh water or cold water marine—are other good sources of protein that can help keep you full. So are beans, nuts, whole grains, and soy.

Satiety Solution 4: Eat the Right Carbs

Eat carbs with resistant starch—starch that is slow burning and keeps your blood sugar level. Resistant starch is different from regular starch: with resistant starch, your blood sugar and insulin levels do not spike. Your appetite-inducing hormone ghrelin doesn't spike. Your appetite-suppressing hormone leptin rises. You stay satisfied longer.

All starch is not created equal. Most starch in the Western diet is made up of the amylopectin molecule. In fact, half of all commonly consumed carbs are this standard starch: white and wheat bread, white rice, most breakfast cereals, some instant oatmeal, crackers, and chips. These starches quickly convert to glucose in your

SATIETY SOLUTION

A liquid that is viscous or thick, like a smoothie, helps expand the stomach. Drinking the same volume of, say, water doesn't do the trick: water doesn't have the staying power of a thick liquid in the stomach. To turn off hunger, try my Tangy and Cool Buttermilk and Avocado Breakfast Smoothie (page 99).

bloodstream—pure sugar, and you get a sugar rush. Your pancreas blasts out insulin, your blood sugar crashes, and after an hour or two, you're hungry again. You snack, usually on something starchy or sugary, and the calories add up. And after all this yo-yoing, your body stops being able to handle insulin properly, and your risk for diabetes, metabolic syndrome, and inflammatory diseases goes up. Way up.

But resistant starch is different. *Resistant starch is called resistant because like dietary fiber it "resists" digestion in the small intestine.* It stays there longer and you feel fuller. It's made up of the amylose molecule. Amylose is digested in the colon, farther downstream—not in the stomach or the small intestine. It actually helps protect the colon, once it is digested. Resistant starch has barely one calorie per gram, not four, like regular starch.

And it is found in tasty foods. Legumes like lentils are the single largest source of naturally occurring resistant starch. Minimally processed whole grains like brown rice, barley, whole wheat, quinoa, steel-cut oats and buckwheat, and beans like kidney, navy, and adzuki, all have resistant starch. So do bananas (especially ones that are still a little green). And some cooked and then cooled foods have resistant starch: cooked-and-chilled pasta, cold rice as in sushi, and cooked, cold potatoes.

Resistant starch burns more slowly and helps you lose weight. As little as forty grams of whole grain has a meaningful amount of resistant starch—just a bowl of oatmeal (have a full cup of steel cut), or three-quarters of a cup of brown rice. As researchers learn more about it, resistant starch is quickly gaining attention as an ideal way to add fiber to a wide range of foods.

Most people on the standard American (Western) diet eat too few foods with resistant starches—perhaps five to ten grams a day. No one really knows the exact range as resistant starch is too new a discovery in food. You won't usually see resistant starch in a list of food ingredients; it may be labeled as fiber, starch, cornstarch, or maltodextrin. If you like to bake, you can order resistant starch at www.foodinnovation.com.

Foods rich in resistant starch appear to help you burn fat up to twenty-four hours later. Why? No one knows. But what is known is that once resistant starch gets to the colon, your body ferments it and produces an anticancer agent called butyrate—yet another great health benefit.

Satiety Solution 5: Get More Foods with Fiber

To reach satiety faster, eat more fiber-rich foods. Only plant foods have fiber, and most foods that are high in fiber are low in calories. Fiber helps you lose weight because it displaces other less-satisfying calories. More fiber-rich foods means lower insulin levels and slow, steady digestion. And when fiber reaches the halfway point inside of your gut, between the small and large intestines, it slows down the digestive process and sends the body a signal that it's full.

Look for prepared foods with five or more grams of fiber per serving. *Buy breads and cereals that have the word* whole *first.* Some of the best high-fiber foods are berries, beans, whole grains, and of course, fruits and vegetables with the skin on.

The body needs fiber to work, and there are two kinds: soluble and insoluble. Soluble fiber works on the bloodstream and on your appetite. It helps smooth out how quickly blood sugar rises, binds extra cholesterol so it can't oxidize and rust, and protects the inside of your arteries. It also lowers your cholesterol. Insoluble fiber, on the other hand, works on the gut—it keeps food moving through, getting rid of waste, excess, and toxins. Both types of fiber need enough water to do their jobs.

Soluble fiber can be found in oat bran, dried beans and peas, nuts, barley, flaxseed, oranges, apples, and carrots. Insoluble fiber can be found in green beans, leafy greens, the skins of root vegetables, whole-wheat bread, corn bran, seeds, and nuts.

✤ DOCTOR IT UP!

Ancient Greek physicians used olive oil to heal ulcers. As recently as thirty years ago in Greece, olive oil was still kept behind the counter at the pharmacist's—talk about culinary medicine!

The ancient Greeks knew something we didn't. Until recently, we thought stress caused ulcers, but the true cause of most ulcers is *H. pylori* bacteria, which infect the lining of the stomach. And a new Spanish study shows that the antioxidant compounds found in olive oil are effective against several strains of *H. pylori,* and thus may help protect you from getting an ulcer.

Keep a small bottle of extra-virgin olive oil in your fridge to keep it from going rancid and use it in place of butter or other solid fats. Try my Spicy Gazpacho with Crab on page 137 and keep your tummy in top shape.

Satiety Solution 6: Volumize

It might surprise you to learn that you eat about the same food *weight* every day. And that's actually a good thing because water has weight and adds volume to food, but it does not have any calories. This is the basis of a concept called volumetrics, popularized by Professor Barbara Rolls.

If you drink a glass of water, your body recognizes it as water and disposes of it quickly: it just filters right out of your stomach. *But if you eat a food that is full of water, your body sees it as a food and digests it more slowly.*

So if you eat food full of water, you will eat fewer calories and lose weight. And what foods are full of water? My favorites—fruits and vegetables. Also, soup. In fact, a thick, hearty, broth-based, not cream-based, soup is a super food when it comes to weight loss. Large enough portions of thick soup or smoothie stretch the very end of the stomach to turn on the hormone CCK and turn off hunger.

Again, just drinking water does not have the same effect. If you eat chicken and rice and drink a glass of water, your body identifies the water as water. But if you use that water to make a soup with chicken and rice, your body identifies the water as food and you will feel full faster—even if you chug it, which I don't recommend. People who eat soup before a meal consistently feel full sooner, eat fewer calories, and lose weight.

What does volumizing mean to you? Plump up your meals with fruits and vegetables, and eat broth-based soups. You'll achieve satiety faster. And for the sake of your waistline, stay away from quantities of water-"parched" food like cookies, crackers, pretzels, and chips.

About 80 percent of the average person's total moisture intake comes from drinking water and other liquids. The other 20 percent comes from food. The more you can reverse this proportion, the better. *Fruits and vegetables consist of at least 80 percent water.* While drinking plenty of water is good (don't forget your H_2O2Go), the water in food will fill you up in a way that plain water just can't.

Satiety Solution 7: Out of Sight Is Out of Mind

You eat more of the foods staring back at you on the counter than those in a cabinet. Working women given jars of Hershey's kisses on their desks in clear jars ate the candies 46 percent more quickly than those given chocolates in opaque jars. Women given sandwich quarters wrapped in clear plastic wrap ate more than those women given sandwiches wrapped in opaque paper.

What does this mean for you? *Store fruits and vegetables in clear containers,* near the front of the fridge, where you see them when you open the door—or, better yet, have them out in a bowl on the counter. Grape tomatoes in a candy dish, anyone? *Hide unhealthy food where you can't see it—or, better yet, toss it out.*

Satiety Solution 8: Eat Mindfully

Before you start eating, have a good look at what's on your plate so that you can start to get a sense of how much food you're really eating. Set down your fork between every couple of bites and have a sip of water or wine. Halfway through the meal or perhaps after your first soup or salad course, stretch and take a break for a few moments. You can do this on your own, or enlist someone else with whom you're eating.

Notice how long you have been eating. Has it been twenty minutes yet? How are you feeling? Are you less hungry than when you started? Are you starting to feel satisfied? If you are still hungry, keep eating, stopping at your next halfway point to take another break and see how you feel. Note what time you finish eating. Then, about a half hour after the meal ends, take another moment to see how you feel. Are you overly full? If so, make a mental note to serve yourself slightly less next time.

The point is not to eat as little as humanly possible or to cut back and feel deprived. *The point is getting to know your body and what it feels like to be fully satiated but not stuffed.* Most of us know that feeling all too well. You won't have to do this kind of self-examination forever—just for a week or two until you get a better sense of what you really need.

Satiety Solution 9: Drink from a Tall, Narrow Glass

People notice height over width (good for basketball players, bad for sumo wrestlers). In studies, people consistently thought a tall, narrow glass held more liquid than a short, wide glass and poured

🌿 **THE SKINNY ON . . . BEVERAGES**

The French say, "A meal without wine is like a day without sunshine." Sip both wine and water during dinner. Water helps you clear your palate so you taste more clearly and dilutes the effect of the alcohol, which usually boosts your appetite.

🌿 **THE SKINNY ON . . . LIQUID DIETS**

Thinking of having a liquid meal? (No, I don't mean a martini!) Better to eat solid food instead. Several studies indicate that meals containing solid food instead of thin shakes typically have a greater effect on satiety than dilute liquid meals. Even if the dilute liquid meal is the same size and same number of calories.

more into the short, wide glass thinking it was the same amount. Even veteran bartenders make this mistake.

Satiety Solution 10: Be Careful Where You Sit

If you're sitting next to someone who's eating barbequed ribs like there's no tomorrow, you'll be more likely to do the same. A better choice? Sit next to your cousin Brenda, who is slender and eats like a bird. You'll be less likely to overeat.

Satiety Solution 11: Leave Some Food on Your Plate

Many people eat until their plates are clean. Some try to eat the plate. In one experiment with soup, people didn't know they were eating from bottomless soup bowls, which slowly refilled. People in the study with regular bowls ate about fifteen ounces of soup, whereas the people with bottomless bowls ate over a quart! That's thirty-two ounces! And they did not even say they felt full, even though they ate more than double the amount in the regular bowls. Don't let your plate or bowl determine when you stop—try to listen to your stomach.

Satiety Solution 12: Tell Your Body You're Finished

Have a postmeal routine—such as brushing your teeth—to signal the brain that you're finished. This is more than just ritual: it's part of how you train your body to know when finished is finished.

Brushing your teeth helps you declare to yourself that you have finished the meal. It also helps you think twice about whether you really want to clean the leftovers off your toddler's plate or pick up an extra mini–chocolate bar on your way back to the office. And brushing gives you get the added advantage of reducing your risk for gingivitis, which, if untreated, leads to periodontal disease, tooth and bone loss, and very painful dental procedures.

Think brushing is impractical? *Carry a toothbrush in your hand-bag or briefcase: a fold-up brush and a mini–toothpaste tube is all it takes.* Use it three times daily. It takes only a half a minute, at least for this purpose, and you're finished. And you're less likely to need a false set of clackers someday.

Satiety Solution 13: Feast!

Plan to feast four times a year (e.g., birthday, anniversary, Thanksgiving, and Christmas) and then look forward to it. We have lost the idea of feasting on special occasions. One of life's greatest pleasures is enjoying our food and the company of friends and family. *Feast as it should be done, as opposed to mindless gorging—savoring the very best food in abundance, with loved ones, but just on feast day.* Doing so will send a message to your mind that life is not a state of deprivation—and perhaps a message to your body that famine is not just around the corner, and there's no need to cling to every calorie. And the next day, go back to your ChefMD plan. Give leftovers away or toss them out: feast meals are special because you have them on just one day.

When it comes to satiety, the major thing to keep in mind is to eat a proper serving of food slowly, happily, and consciously. Eating slowly will give your body time to get to satiety. Enjoy your friends' company, but shove off to the living room away from the food or, if you're going to stay at the table, remove the food that will sabotage your health efforts. Either move the food or remove yourself.

Food has always been important in my family. Even now, at age ninety-seven, my grandmother is an excellent cook. She believes, as many Italian Americans do, that a good homemade meal releases the tension of a stressful day and that your spirit sighs with pleasure afterward. Eating slowly, savoring each bite, and then spending some time in rest and reflection, is a wonderful way to eat and live.

Congratulations! You've now learned the three ChefMD keys—how to absorb more of the good stuff, how to avoid anti-nutrients, and how to feel full faster and longer. You should feel great about what you've accomplished. Now let's get out into the real world, where you can start putting these keys into practice. In the next chapter I'll show you what to keep on hand to build a more slender, more energetic, powerful, healthier, sexier, younger you!

Part Two

Becoming a ChefMD

CHAPTER 4

The Kitchen Physician Prescription:
BUILD YOUR MEDICINE CHEST

*The doctor of the future will no longer treat the human frame
with drugs, but rather will cure and prevent disease with
nutrition.*

—Thomas Edison

I have begun to think of a home kitchen in much the same way I
think of a health spa—a place where people can come to be re-
stored, feel better, experience pleasure, and become healthier. And
this is how I'd like you to start thinking about your kitchen. Your
kitchen is at the heart of your health.

In your home, you probably keep your medicine chest in the
bathroom. I'm offering a second medicine chest, one that helps prevent diseases and symptoms and that you keep right in your kitchen
cupboards, fridge, freezer, and pantry.

In this chapter, I describe fifty foods that should be part of your
kitchen medicine chest and report the best medical evidence for
what they can do for you. To create this list, our research team re-
viewed approximately three thousand culinary medicine studies—
studies done primarily in people—and rated over three hundred
foods for their medical effects. Each food had to have clear, well-
done, solid medical research demonstrating that if eaten regularly it
could prevent—and, in some cases, actually treat—specific conditions and symptoms.

These are fifty of the top foods—the ones with the most benefits. We've organized the information into nine food groups:

- Great grains
- Beneficial beans
- Vital vegetables
- Flavorful fruits
- Delicious dairy
- Nutritious nuts
- Sensational spices
- Marvelous meats, fish, and poultry
- Delectable drinks

I've highlighted just one or two health benefits for each. Enjoy them! You'll discover how easy it is to use culinary medicine to stay well and become stronger, healthier, and more vital—deliciously.

KITCHEN PRESCRIPTION GLOSSARY

AMINO ACID: A building block of protein

ANTHOCYANIN: A red-blue flavonoid that varies in color by pH; there are at least 550

ANTIOXIDANT: A molecule that prevents free radicals from damaging healthy cells

BETA-CAROTENE: An orange pigment with antioxidant effects and precursor to vitamin A

BETACYANIN: A red pigment with antioxidant effects

BETA-SITOSTEROL: A phytosterol or plant sterol

BETAXANTHIN: A yellow pigment with antioxidant effects

CAROTENOID: Pigments (yellows, oranges, and reds) with antioxidant effects; there are more than 600

CATECHIN: A flavonoid in tea and chocolate

CHLOROPHYLL: A green pigment that may have antioxidant effects

CRUCIFEROUS: Edible vegetables in the Brassica family: kale, cabbage, broccoli, brussels sprouts, and dozens more

FLAVONOID: Usually colorful plant chemicals with antioxidant, anti-inflammatory, and anticancer effects; there are over five thousand of them. Flavonoids belong to the polyphenol family

FREE RADICALS: Atoms with at least one unpaired electron that may cause cancer, heart disease, DNA damage, and aging

GLUCOSINOLATE: A compound that boosts the immune system and fights cancer; precursor of isothiocyanate

INDOLE-3-CARBINOL: A plant chemical with anticancer effects

ISOFLAVONE: One of two classes of phytoestrogens, i.e., weak estrogen-like compounds in plants

ISOTHIOCYANATE: An anticancer agent that gives a hot taste to plants such as onions and radishes

LACTOSE: The sugar in milk that can cause intolerance

LIGNAN: One of two classes of phytoestrogens, i.e., weak estrogen-like compounds in plants

LUTEIN: A yellow carotenoid that is orange-red when concentrated

MYROSINASE: An enzyme that activates sulforaphane, which has anticancer effects

PHENOLS: A class of plant chemicals that includes polyphenols, flavonoids, and capsaicin

PHYTOCHEMICAL: A chemical found in a plant

PHYTONUTRIENT: A nutrient found in a plant

PHYTOSTEROL: A plant alcohol; some phytosterols lower cholesterol

POLYPHENOLS: Chemicals such as flavonoids and tannins, responsible for the coloring and protection of some plants and that fight heart disease and cancer

PREBIOTICS: Food ingredients that nourish probiotics

PROBIOTICS: Healthy bacteria that help restore intestinal balance

QUERCETIN: A flavonoid with anticancer and anti-inflammatory effects

RESVERATROL: A plant chemical with antioxidant and anti-inflammatory effects

SAPONINS: Chemicals in waxy plant skin that stimulate the immune system

SILYMARIN: A flavonoid with antioxidant and liver-protective effects

STANOL ESTERS: Chemicals derived from plant sterols that reduce cholesterol absorbed from food

SULFORAPHANE: A type of isothiocyanate that fights free radicals

TRYPTOPHAN: An amino acid and a building block for protein

ZEAXANTHIN: A yellow-orange carotenoid

Great Grains

BARLEY

Barley is one of the oldest cultivated grains, with an earthy, nutty flavor. Gladiators in ancient Rome were nicknamed "barley eaters"—so if you're looking to have the strength of a gladiator, start eating barley.

WATER-COOLER FACT: Barley was used by ancient civilizations to make alcoholic beverages; records show that Babylonians were making barley wine as far back as 2800 BC.

WHAT'S IN IT: Barley is a very good source of soluble fiber. It contains the antioxidants vitamin E and selenium. Barley is low in fat and has no cholesterol. One cup of barley has 270 calories.

WHAT IT'S GOOD FOR: Reducing your blood pressure. Twenty-five people were fed either a whole-wheat / brown rice diet, a barley diet, or a whole-wheat / brown rice and barley diet for five weeks: blood pressures were reduced by all three whole-grain diets. Also, barley can help keep your blood sugar down. Ten overweight women were fed test meals of barley. Their blood glucose response was reduced by 59 to 65 percent. And barley is famous for lowering LDL (lousy) cholesterol and total cholesterol. A seventeen-year study of over twenty-seven thousand healthy women found that those eating three or more servings daily of whole grains, including barley, were 35 percent less likely than those eating the least whole grains to die of an inflammatory disease, such as asthma, gout, and rheumatoid arthritis.

OATS

Eighty percent of U.S. households have oats in their cupboards, and that's a good thing. But not all oats are created equally—instant oats are nearly pure starch!

WATER-COOLER FACT: Oats contain a greater proportion of cholesterol-lowering soluble fiber to insoluble fiber than any other common whole grain.

WHAT'S IN IT: Oats contain polyunsaturated fatty acids, vitamin E, and selenium. They are an excellent source of manganese; a very good source of selenium; and a good source of resistant starch, vitamin B1, soluble fiber (primarily beta-glucan), magnesium, and protein. Thicker, steel-cut oats have a lower glycemic index than rolled or instant oats, and therefore raise your blood sugar more slowly. One cup of cooked whole grain oats has 145 calories and four grams of dietary fiber.

WHAT IT'S GOOD FOR: Lowering your LDL cholesterol and guarding you against heart disease. For each gram of the soluble fiber beta-glucan in oatmeal, you get a 1.42 milligrams per deciliter total cholesterol reduction and a 1.23 milligrams per deciliter LDL reduction—a lot. Eating oats regularly is associated with a 26 percent reduced risk for coronary heart disease, according to twelve studies. In one study of almost ten thousand adults, those consuming the most fiber (twenty-one grams a day) had a 12 percent reduced risk for coronary heart disease and an 11 percent reduced risk for cardiovascular disease compared with those eating the least fiber (less than six grams a day). Oatmeal but not wheat cereal prevented arterial stiffening after a fatty (fifty grams of fat) meal in both men and postmenopausal women.

Beneficial Beans

BEANS

Beans are much more than the "musical fruit," as kids may know them. Beans are incredibly high in protein and fiber.

WATER-COOLER FACT: People who eat beans weigh, on average, 6.6 pounds less than those who do not eat beans.

WHAT'S IN IT: Beans contain folate, iron, zinc, and vitamin B1. Pinto beans have the most folate, navy beans have the most protein, and limas the most fiber. Beans are low in fat and are cholesterol-free. One cup of cooked black beans has 227 calories, but only one gram of fat, fifteen grams of protein, and fifteen grams of dietary fiber.

WHAT IT'S GOOD FOR: Lowering LDL (lousy) and raising HDL (healthy) cholesterol. A meta-analysis of eleven studies showed that bean eaters have lower total cholesterol levels by 7 percent, LDL by 6 percent, triglycerides by 17 percent, and higher HDL by 3 percent. Beans' high levels of soluble fiber and vegetable protein are thought to be the main reasons. Also, eating legumes such as dried beans, split peas, or lentils seems to lessen the growth of colorectal adenomas, which are precursors to colon cancer.

LENTILS

Once again, ChefMD has discovered that some of the oldest foods are the best. They're mentioned in the Old Testament in the story of Jacob and Esau, where Esau trades his future inheritance for a bowl of lentil soup. Probably not a wise trade but certainly a healthy one!

WATER-COOLER FACT: Lentils have the second-highest level of protein of any vegetable, second only to soybeans.

WHAT'S IN IT: Lentils are a very good source of dietary fiber and folate, and a good source of manganese, protein, vitamin B1, and

✳ LITTLE BITES

Beans have a lot of antioxidants, and the darker the bean, the more antioxidants.

✢ DOCTOR IT UP!

Soaking dried beans before cooking pours off most of the indigestible sugar that causes flatulence.

✳ LITTLE BITES

The level of vitamin C is raised 17.5 times in lentils when they are sprouted.

potassium. One cup of cooked lentils has 230 calories, no cholesterol, and no fat.

WHAT IT'S GOOD FOR: Reducing your risk of prostate cancer. A controlled study of 1,619 prostate cancer patients versus 1,618 healthy men suggested that those with the highest legume intake had a 38 percent reduced risk of prostate cancer compared with those with the lowest intake.

Vital Vegetables

BROCCOLI

When President George Bush banned broccoli from *Air Force One* in 1990, it was a dubious decision because broccoli is a health powerhouse.

WATER-COOLER FACT: Broccoli's cancer-fighting sulforaphane is formed by the enzyme myrosinase, which is activated when broccoli is chopped or chewed.

WHAT'S IN IT: Broccoli is an excellent source of vitamins A, C, and K, as well as folate and fiber; it is also a very good source of potassium, vitamin B6, and vitamin E. Frozen broccoli has 59 percent less glucosinolate than raw broccoli: glucosinolates stimulate the body's immune and antioxidant systems. One cup of steamed broccoli has forty-four calories and nine grams of dietary fiber.

WHAT IT'S GOOD FOR: Protecting you from prostate and gastric cancer. Broccoli contains indole-3-carbinol, a promising anticancer agent. In the lab, indole-3-carbinol kept human prostate carcinoma cells from multiplying, and immobilized *H. pylori*, the bacteria that causes stomach ulcers and many stomach cancers.

BRUSSELS SPROUTS

Thomas Jefferson introduced brussels sprouts to America in 1812. That was quite an overture . . .

WATER-COOLER FACT: Brussels sprouts contain a higher concentration of glucosinolates (104 milligrams per half-cup serving) than any other cruciferous (a family of plants that includes broccoli) vegetable.

✻ **LITTLE BITES**

Broccoli contains glucosinolates, which are transformed to disable toxins in the body. The younger the broccoli, the more glucosinolates.

✚ **DOCTOR IT UP!**

To increase the absorption of sulforaphane, steam broccoli briefly or even better, eat it uncooked.

WHAT'S IN IT: Brussels sprouts are an excellent source of vitamins C and K; a very good source of folate, vitamin A, fiber, potassium, vitamin B6, and vitamin B1; and a good source of omega-3 fatty acids, iron, protein, vitamin B2, vitamin E, and calcium. One cup of steamed, roasted, or boiled brussels sprouts has sixty calories, and fresh brussels sprouts have nearly four times as much glucosinolate as cooked frozen ones.

WHAT IT'S GOOD FOR: Protecting you from breast cancer if you're a woman and from colorectal cancer if you're a man. In a study of 337 Chinese women, those with the highest isothiocyanate urine levels (from cruciferous vegetables such as brussels sprouts) had a 45 percent lower risk of breast cancer. In a study of twenty men, 250 grams (just over eight ounces) of brussels sprouts and broccoli help rid the body of heterocyclic amines, carcinogens that are formed when meat is well-done.

CABBAGE

Cabbage smell is caused by sulfur being released when cabbage is cooked—too often overcooked! Eat raw or cook quickly for the least "stink."

WATER-COOLER FACT: Green cabbage contains more glucosinolates, whereas red contains more polyphenols and anthocyanins. Both are great for your health—make a salad with a little of each!

WHAT'S IN IT: Cabbage is an excellent source of vitamins C and K and a very good source of fiber, folate, vitamin B6, and omega-3 fatty acids. It is also a good source of vitamin B1, vitamin B2, calcium, vitamin A, and protein. Fermented cabbage (e.g., sauerkraut and kimchi) retain most of the glucosinolates and add healthy bacteria called probiotics to your diet, making the cabbage more digestible. One cup of shredded, boiled cabbage has just thirty-three calories.

WHAT IT'S GOOD FOR: Reducing your risk of cancer and possibly of Alzheimer's disease. In the laboratory, red cabbage protects against oxidative stress in the brain, reducing the buildup of plaque and reducing the risk of Alzheimer's. Also, a Chinese study found that women who ate the most cruciferous vegetables such as cabbage were at half the risk for breast cancer as those who ate little or none.

* **LITTLE BITES**

Use as little water as you can if you boil or steam brussels sprouts; otherwise, the glucosinolates will leak out.

* **LITTLE BITES**

The lactic acid found in sauerkraut helps you absorb iron.

* **DOCTOR IT UP!**

Red cabbage turns blue while cooking in the absence of acid: cook it briefly with wine, citrus, or vinegar to assure a bright color. To avoid discoloring pigments, don't use an iron or aluminum pot.

KALE

A cabbage is a cabbage is a cabbage . . . Well, not really. ChefMD superstar kale is one of the best.

WATER-COOLER FACT: Kale grown in the summer has more carotenoids than kale grown during the winter, but winter kale is sweeter. Store kale at room temperature; keeping it in cold temperatures (around 47° F) for five days significantly decreases its carotenoid levels.

WHAT'S IN IT: Kale is an excellent source of vitamins A, C, and K, and manganese. It is a very good source of dietary fiber, calcium, vitamin B6, and potassium. Its mature leaves are an especially rich source of glucosinolates, which activate detoxification enzymes in the liver, protecting you from carcinogens. Kale is also high in carotenoids, such as lutein and zeaxanthin. One cup has thirty-six calories.

WHAT IT'S GOOD FOR: Reducing cancer risk and possibly preventing cataracts. A study of Chinese women who smoke showed that eating cruciferous vegetables lowered their lung cancer risk by 69 percent, and in another study, colorectal cancer as well. Kale's carotenoids are stored in your eye's retina, prevent UV light damage, and reduce your risk of cataracts.

✦ DOCTOR IT UP!

Using a sharp knife to cut an onion produces fewer tears, because fewer onion cells are ruptured and exposed to air, and thus less sulfenic acid/gas reaches your eyes.

※ LITTLE BITES

Red onions have more flavonoids than yellow or white, though pink shallots have the greatest overall antioxidant activity in the onion family.

ONIONS

The ancient Egyptians buried their pharaohs with onions because they saw the onion as a sign of eternal life. Had they eaten more onions when they were alive, their life on earth may have been a bit longer.

WATER-COOLER FACT: The Latin word *unio,* meaning "one (bulb)," gives us the word *onion.*

WHAT'S IN IT: Onions are a very good source of vitamin C, dietary fiber, vitamin B6, folate, and potassium. One cup of raw onion has sixty-one calories.

WHAT IT'S GOOD FOR: Reducing cancer risk. People in southern Europe who eat the most onions showed an 84 percent reduced risk for cancer of the mouth, an 88 percent reduced risk for cancer of the throat, a 56 percent reduced risk for colorectal cancer, a 25 percent reduced risk for breast cancer, a 73 percent reduced risk for cancer of the ovaries, and a 71 percent reduced risk for prostate cancer, as compared with those who eat the least.

ROMAINE

Reach for romaine. Romaine is dark, and the darker a lettuce's green color, the more nutritious it is.

WATER-COOLER FACT: Most varieties of lettuce exude a tiny amount of a white, milky liquid when their leaves are broken. This "milk" gives lettuce its slightly bitter flavor and its scientific name, *Lactuca sativa,* which is derived from the Latin word for milk.

WHAT'S IN IT: Romaine is an excellent source of vitamins A and C and folate, and it is a very good source of fiber, vitamins B1 and B2, potassium, and iron. It contains the carotenoids alpha- and beta-carotene, lutein, and zeaxanthin. Two cups of romaine have fifteen calories. Romaine has over five times the vitamin C of iceberg and no protein.

WHAT IT'S GOOD FOR: Reducing your risk of stroke and improving satiety. A study of more than 17,500 people found that eating salad is associated with above-average concentrations of folate in the blood, and folate has been shown to reduce the risk of stroke. Three and a half cups of salad at the beginning of a meal stretch the satiety receptors in your stomach, triggering the satiety hormone cholecystokinin, or CCK, and reducing appetite.

SOYBEANS AND SOY FOOD

Until the 1970s, soybeans were used only as animal feed in the United States. Lucky animals! Thankfully, soybeans aren't just for cows and pigs anymore, something Asians have known for millennia. The healing power of soy can now be found in the West not only in miso and tofu but also in edamame, soy milk, soy hot dogs, soy sausage, soy cheese, and frozen desserts. Oh boy for soy!

WATER-COOLER FACT: Tofu was common in China by the second century BC, and the methods for making it then were pretty much the same as they are today.

WHAT'S IN IT: Soybeans are a good source of iron, phosphorus, dietary fiber, omega-3 fatty acids, magnesium, vitamin B2, and

✳ **LITTLE BITES**

The leaves on the outside of a head of romaine lettuce have the most flavonoids.

※ LITTLE BITES

The level of the isoflavone genistein is higher in fermented soybean products, especially natto, than in nonfermented soybean products, such as soy milk or tofu. It has been suggested that genistein, a weak phytoestrogen, may prevent hormone-related cancers.

potassium. One cup of cooked soybeans has 298 calories and twenty-nine grams of protein. Ordinary tofu, made like cheese, is an excellent source of tryptophan, a very good source of iron and protein and a good source of selenium, omega-3 fatty acids, and calcium. Firm silken tofu, made like yogurt, has sixty-two calories, 6.9 grams of protein, and 4 grams of fat (nearly all unsaturated) in just over three ounces. And you can whip silken tofu.

WHAT IT'S GOOD FOR: Controlling diabetes and preserving bone density. Soy foods have low glycemic and insulin response indexes, which help in controlling blood glucose and insulin levels. Postmenopausal type 2 diabetic women who ate food containing thirty grams of soy protein and 132 milligrams of isoflavones daily had reduced fasting insulin levels, insulin resistance, and levels of LDL cholesterol. Soy's isoflavones also seem to preserve bone mass in perimenopausal and postmenopausal women.

SWEET POTATOES

One potato, two potato, sweet potato more . . . Get it at the farmer's market, get it at the store. It doesn't matter where you pick it up. Just go and eat some more.

WATER-COOLER FACT: In 1992 the Center for Science in the Public Interest ranked sweet potatoes as the most nutritious vegetable.

※ LITTLE BITES

Raw sweet potato that was chopped and left to sit four hours did not lose any beta-carotene.

WHAT'S IN IT: Sweet potatoes are an excellent source of vitamin A, a very good source of vitamin C and manganese, and a good source of dietary fiber, vitamin B6, potassium, and iron. Sweet potatoes are very high in antioxidants and come in many colors. One small baked sweet potato contains three grams of dietary fiber, four grams of sugar, 8,509 micrograms of beta-carotene, 14,185 international units of vitamin A, and eighty-six calories.

WHAT IT'S GOOD FOR: Helping keep your liver healthy. Healthy adult men with borderline hepatitis who consumed a purple sweet potato beverage significantly decreased serum levels of hepatic biomarkers, which are laboratory signals of a liver problem. Also, sweet potatoes can help you avoid diabetes. Despite their sweet name, sweet potatoes help stabilize blood sugar levels and lower insulin resistance.

SWISS CHARD

What the heck is swiss chard? You know of Swiss chocolate, Swiss watches, and the Swiss Alps, but swiss chard?

Well, it isn't really Swiss at all. The French got two similar dark leafy greens confused and so the word *Swiss* was added to distinguish between them.

WATER-COOLER FACT: Swiss chard does not keep very long, but the stalks can be kept longer if they are separated from the leaves.

WHAT'S IN IT: Swiss chard is an excellent source of vitamins A, C, and K as well as magnesium, potassium, iron, vitamin E, and dietary fiber. It is a very good source of calcium, vitamin B2, vitamin B6, and protein; and a good source of vitamin B1 and folate. Swiss chard is a source of the antioxidant flavonoid quercetin. The leaves have more flavonoids than the stems, and the red leaves have the most of all. One cup of cooked swiss chard has thirty-five calories, 214 percent of the recommended daily intake of vitamin A, and 716 percent of the recommended daily intake of vitamin K.

WHAT IT'S GOOD FOR: Keeping your bones strong. Swiss chard is an excellent source of vitamin K, which helps bones absorb calcium. In Turkey, swiss chard extract is used as a hypoglycemic agent for diabetes.

✳ **LITTLE BITES**

Packaged swiss chard loses more flavonoids and vitamin C during the cooking process than does Swiss chard that has not been packaged.

TOMATOES

You say tomato, and I say tomahto, but let's not call the whole thing off. This staple ChefMD food is a building block to many recipes, and when used correctly, its healthy benefits will amaze you.

WATER-COOLER FACT: The tomato is a member of the nightshade family and is a close relation to many poisonous plants.

WHAT'S IN IT: Tomatoes are an excellent source of vitamins A, C, and K; a very good source of potassium, fiber, and vitamin B1; and a good source of vitamin B6, folate, vitamin B2, iron, vitamin E, and protein. Tomato paste and ketchup are two of the richest sources of lycopene. The lycopene in tangerine tomatoes is about 2.5 times as readily absorbed by the body than the lycopene from ordinary red tomatoes. One cup of chopped or sliced tomatoes has twenty-seven calories.

✳ **LITTLE BITES**

The whole tomato has the greatest health benefits: subjects absorbed 75 percent more lycopene and 41 percent more beta-carotene from tomato paste produced with peels than tomato paste produced without peels. Also, organic ketchup contains three times more lycopene than nonorganic ketchup. Ketchup's glutamate levels are higher than those in red tomatoes, making it an "umami" flavor booster. Umami is the fifth flavor.

WHAT IT'S GOOD FOR: Reducing your risk for heart disease and certain cancers, such as pancreatic cancer, and possibly prostate, ovarian, and gastric cancers. In a seven-year follow-up of forty thousand women, those who ate seven to ten servings of lycopene-rich foods like tomatoes per week reduced their risk of cardiovascular disease by 29 percent; those who ate more than two servings per week of oil-based tomato products reduced their risk of cardiovascular disease by 34 percent. Men who drank twenty ounces of tomato juice and ate an ounce of ketchup daily for three weeks lowered LDL by 13 percent. A three-year study reported that men who consumed a diet rich in tomatoes and tomato-based products with a high lycopene content had a 31 percent reduced risk of pancreatic cancer.

WATERCRESS

Huntsville, Alabama, is known as the "Watercress Capital of the World." Don't want to go all the way to Alabama? Just go to your grocery—watercress is one of the main vegetables in V8 juice.

WATER-COOLER FACT: The leaves of the watercress plant turn bitter when the plant starts to produce flowers.

WHAT'S IN IT: Watercress contains iron, calcium, phosphorus, potassium, vitamin A, vitamin K, and vitamin C. It also contains mustard oil, lutein, and beta-carotene. One cup of chopped watercress has four calories.

WHAT IT'S GOOD FOR: Protecting you from cancer if you are a smoker. In one study, sixty subjects, including thirty smokers, ate less than three ounces of fresh watercress every day for eight weeks. Eating watercress resulted in a 23.9 percent decrease in DNA damage to white blood cells. Changes were more significant in smokers than nonsmokers, and levels of the antioxidants lutein and beta-carotene in the blood increased by 100 percent and 33 percent, respectively. It is thought that the isothiocyanates in watercress inhibit a potent carcinogen in tobacco, suggesting that eating watercress may protect you from lung cancer if you smoke. People who have quit smoking halve their lung cancer risk with four or more raw vegetable salads weekly.

※ **LITTLE BITES**

Chopping or shredding watercress and eating it uncooked maximizes the bioavailability (body readiness) of its isothiocyanates, which break down carcinogens.

Flavorful Fruits

AÇAI BERRIES

Okay, how the heck do you pronounce this flavorful fruit? It's "ah-sigh-EE." It may be a bit hard to get your tongue around, but it is an incredibly powerful food.

WATER-COOLER FACT: The Amazonian açai berry looks like a grape or a blueberry but is smaller and darker. In South America, açai is simply pureed and served warm as a sauce or even by itself in a bowl, like a soup.

WHAT'S IN IT: One hundred grams of freeze-dried açai powder has 534 calories, 52.2 grams of carbohydrates (including 44.2 grams of fiber), 8.1 grams of protein, 1 gram of sugar, and 33 grams of fat. Açai is high in beta-sitosterol, phytosterol that competes with cholesterol for absorption, and lowers LDL. An excellent source of vitamin A and potassium, açai also contains vitamins B1, B2, B3, C, and E, as well as magnesium, copper, zinc, phosphorus, and sulfur.

WHAT IT'S GOOD FOR: Helping to protect you from leukemia and lowering bad cholesterol. Açai berry extract has been shown to kill between 45 percent and 86 percent of human leukemia cells in the lab. It acts as an anti-inflammatory, cyclooxygenase-1 and -2 (COX-1 and COX-2) inhibitor, which is linked to arthritis relief.

ARTICHOKES

Artichokes are the fruit with the heart of gold. I love artichokes.

WATER-COOLER FACT: Virtually all artichokes sold in the United States are grown in California, and 80 percent come from the county of Monterey, where Castroville calls itself the "Artichoke Capital of the World."

WHAT'S IN IT: Artichokes have vitamins A, C, and K, beta-carotene, folate, potassium, and iron. Artichokes also are rich in antioxidants and flavonoids including silymarin, which, as a dietary supplement, is widely used for liver problems. One medium artichoke has sixty calories, 6.9 grams of dietary fiber, and 4.2 grams of protein.

WHAT IT'S GOOD FOR: Assisting gastrointestinal health. In one study, artichoke leaf extract resulted in a 26.4 percent reduction in irritable bowel syndrome. Artichokes can also help lower your cholesterol. Two-thirds of an ounce of artichoke juice lowered LDL cholesterol and arterial stickiness and improved blood flow in patients with high cholesterol levels.

AVOCADOS

Avocados have been eaten for over eight thousand years in Central and South America. Although I doubt that the Central Americans of that time knew how good avocados are for you, we do now.

WATER-COOLER FACT: Avocado is a fruit, not a vegetable as many believe. Some call it "green butter."

WHAT'S IN IT: Avocados are a good source of vitamin K, dietary fiber, vitamin B6, vitamin C, folate, and potassium. They have 60 percent more potassium than bananas. They are also a food source of avocado soybean unsaponifiables, or ASUs, which are oils prescribed for osteoarthritis pain. Avocados are rich in lutein, which protects your eyes from cataracts and macular degeneration. One medium Haas avocado has 227 calories and twenty-one grams of fat, which is mostly monounsaturated.

WHAT IT'S GOOD FOR: Avocados help reduce cholesterol and triglyceride levels in healthy people, and in people with diabetes. After seven days of eating an avocado-rich diet, patients had lowered total cholesterol and LDL ("lousy") cholesterol levels, and an 11 percent increase in HDL ("healthy") cholesterol. Scientists credit the high level of monounsaturated fats and phytosterols in the avocado for this effect.

BLACKBERRIES

Blackberries, over the years, have gone by many names: brambleberries, brumblekites, and lawers. In ancient England, it was believed that blackberries should not be eaten after the middle of October because the devil would come by and spit on each bush. I'm pretty sure that's not true.

WATER-COOLER FACT: Blackberries contain the highest antioxidant content per serving size of any fresh fruit except açai.

WHAT'S IN IT: Blackberries are a good source of vitamins A, C, E, and K, as well as folate, potassium, zinc, beta-carotene, and lutein. A

☀ LITTLE BITES

Florida avocado varieties have less fat than California avocado varieties.

☀ LITTLE BITES

Frozen blackberries have almost as many antioxidants as fresh.

3.3 ounce serving has only forty-three calories. Blackberries contain antioxidants called anthocyanins, which give blackberries their deep color and protect you from free radical damage.

WHAT IT'S GOOD FOR: Helping protect you from cancer. In clinical studies, blackberry extract inhibited the growth of human colon, prostate, breast, and oral tumor cells.

BLUEBERRIES

The tiny and delicious blueberry packs an incredible antioxidant punch, but American colonists thought they made good paint. They crushed blueberries and mixed them with milk to create a Shaker gray. What a waste of a ChefMD favorite food. Couldn't they just have gone to Sears?

WATER-COOLER FACT: Blueberries are one of the only foods eaten by humans that are naturally colored blue. The bloom on the berry indicates freshness.

WHAT'S IN IT: Blueberries are a very good source of vitamin C, manganese, soluble fiber, and insoluble fiber like pectin. They are a good source of vitamin E and are high in anthocyanins.

WHAT IT'S GOOD FOR: Protecting you from a variety of cancers. Blueberries contain a high concentration of anthocyanins, colorful antioxidants that prevent free radical damage. A study of almost two thousand colorectal cancer cases found that of all the flavonoids, food with anthocyanins are associated with the greatest reduction (43 percent) in colorectal cancer risk. In addition, blueberry extract has been shown to inhibit the growth of prostate, breast, and oral tumor cells.

LIMES

British sailors are called "limeys" because in the nineteenth century they used lime juice to prevent scurvy. But limes aren't just for sailors—they're a ChefMD staple for all of us.

WATER-COOLER FACT: Limes have more citric acid than lemons. Most limes turn yellow, like lemons, on lime trees if allowed to mature, and they become slightly sweeter.

✳ **LITTLE BITES**

Wild blueberries, which are smaller in size and more tart in flavor than cultivated blueberries, contain 50 percent more total antioxidants, too.

✳ **LITTLE BITES**

Vitamin C increases the bioavailability, or body readiness, of non-heme dietary iron. So put a squeeze of lime into your salsa!

WHAT'S IN IT: Limes are an excellent source of vitamin C. A whole lime has just one gram of sugar and twenty milligrams of vitamin C. Lime zest contains limonoids (anticarcinogens) and essential oils. Conventionally grown limes may contain pesticide residues or wax: buy organically grown limes when possible. One average lime has twenty calories.

WHAT IT'S GOOD FOR: Fighting cancer and cholera. Of twenty-four citrus juices analyzed, limes were the most effective in stopping T-cell leukemia cells from proliferating. Also, the limonoids in limes inhibit the growth of human breast cancer cells. Adding lime juice to food prevented food-borne transmission of cholera in West Africa.

OLIVES

Olives are probably the oldest cultivated fruit; they most likely originated in Crete about seven thousand years ago.

WATER-COOLER FACT: Olives are mentioned in Homer's *Odyssey*.

WHAT'S IN IT: Olives are a very good source of monounsaturated fat, and a good source of iron, vitamin E, and dietary fiber. One cup of olives has 155 calories. Plain olives, not pitted or stuffed, have the highest polyphenol and antioxidant content, and one ounce of green olives has four grams of fat, which is mostly unsaturated.

WHAT IT'S GOOD FOR: Protecting you from heart disease and other diseases of the arteries: stroke, impotence, and premature wrinkling. When free radicals cause the oxidation of cholesterol, the oxidized cholesterol damages blood vessels, inflames arteries, and can eventually lead to a heart attack or a stroke. The antioxidants in olives prevent the oxidation of cholesterol and arterial damage.

OLIVE OIL

Popeye was so right to love Olive Oyl. Here's a guy who loved spinach and Olive Oyl—no wonder he had all those muscles! Homer called it liquid gold, and it was probably the first commercially produced food.

WATER-COOLER FACT: Olive oil is a fruit juice and contains oleocanthal, a compound with the same pain-relieving mechanism as ibuprofen (such as Motrin and Advil). Fifty grams—not quite two ounces—of olive oil supplies enough oleocanthal to produce an effect of about 10 percent of a dose of ibuprofen. Oleocanthal stings a little in the back of the throat.

WHAT'S IN IT: Olive oil is a concentrated source of monounsaturated fat, vitamin E, vitamin K, beta-carotene, and lutein. Darker olive oils and virgin olive oils have more blood clot–fighting polyphenols than clear or light olive oils. One tablespoon has 120 calories and fourteen grams of fat, like all oils. Extra-virgin olive oil, the least refined olive oil, smokes at about 410° F, and free radicals are created at this very hot temperature.

WHAT IT'S GOOD FOR: Helping you regulate your blood pressure. A study of 155 men showed that those who did not usually eat a Mediterranean diet who ate five teaspoons of olive oil a day reduced their systolic blood pressure by 3 percent. Also, olive oil can help protect you from breast cancer. Women who eat more than two teaspoons of olive oil a day have a 73 percent reduced risk of breast cancer compared with women who eat little or no olive oil.

POMEGRANATES

When the French named the hand grenade after the seed-scattering properties of the pomegranate, and then called the military group that tossed those grenades "grenadiers," they must have known what a powerful weapon the pomegranate is in the battle for tasty health.

WATER-COOLER FACT: Pomegranates first grew in ancient Persia; Thomas Jefferson planted some at Monticello in 1771.

WHAT'S IN IT: A rich source of folic acid, potassium, fiber- and vitamin C, pomegranates are also very high in polyphenols. One medium pomegranate has 105 calories.

WHAT IT'S GOOD FOR: Reducing your risk for heart disease and slowing the progression of prostate cancer. It also keeps your bad cholesterol down: drinking forty grams (about 1.5 ounces) a day of concentrated pomegranate juice reduces LDL. In a small study, people with thickened carotid arteries who drank eight ounces of pomegranate juice daily for a year reduced their systolic blood

❋ LITTLE BITES

Infusing olive oil with rosemary will minimize the oxidation of olive oil's helpful phytosterols.

❋ LITTLE BITES

Buy 100 percent pomegranate juice. Pomegranate juice is made with the entire fruit, including the rind, and therefore the polyphenols from the rind are retained in the juice.

pressure by 21 percent. Men with recurrent prostate cancer who drank eight ounces of pomegranate juice each day had slower disease progression and less cell growth than those who did not have the juice.

Delicious Dairy

CHEESE, LOWER FAT

Everybody wants to be the big cheese. That term was coined to describe people rich enough to purchase an entire wheel of cheese at one time. Today, however, I'd recommend choosing a smaller piece of a variety of great lower-fat cheeses.

WATER-COOLER FACT: It takes ten pounds of milk to make one pound of cheese.

WHAT'S IN IT: Cheese contains high-quality protein, principally casein, which has all the essential amino acids. One ounce of part-skim, low-moisture mozzarella contains three grams of fat, seventy-nine calories, and 207 milligrams of calcium. Low-fat cottage cheese is very high in protein but is also only a modest source of calcium because in the manufacturing process, 50 percent to 75 percent of the calcium is removed when the whey is drained. Most lower-fat nondairy cheeses are lactose-free.

WHAT IT'S GOOD FOR: Keeping your bones healthy and perhaps reducing the risk of metabolic syndrome, a disease in which overweight and sedentary people have high blood pressure and are at risk of diabetes, heart attack, and stroke. Ounce for ounce, cheese has almost six times the calcium of milk. Greater intakes of calcium, vitamin D, and lower-fat dairy products are significantly associated with a lower prevalence of metabolic syndrome in three major studies of over fifteen thousand men and women.

KEFIR

First of all, it's pronounced "KEE-fur" and was originally made from fermented camels' milk . . . Yuck! Thankfully, someone figured out how to make it from cows' milk. It's an enzyme-rich, thick, creamy drink filled with healthy microbes that get your digestive tract running smoothly.

✳ **LITTLE BITES**

Lactose intolerant? Have hard, aged cheeses. They have the least lactose, and some have almost none.

✛ **DOCTOR IT UP!**

Allow cheese to warm to room temperature to liberate its flavors.

WATER-COOLER FACT: Yogurt often has just two strains of bacteria. Kefir, a drinkable, cultured, enzyme-rich relative of yogurt, often contains ten strains—five times as many live and active cultures, which are the bacteria that are good for your digestion.

WHAT'S IN IT: Kefir is a good source of calcium, potassium, and protein. It's also rich in probiotics, which are healthy bacteria that help fight infection and bad bacteria. It can be made from dairy and nondairy milk.

WHAT IT'S GOOD FOR: Keeping your stomach in good shape. Stress, infection, and antibiotics may disrupt the balance of healthy bacteria in the intestine, and probiotics help to maintain the balance. Specific strains of *Lactobacilli* and other helpful bacteria found in kefir reduce the severity and duration of acute diarrhea. Kefir's probiotics may also alleviate or reduce symptoms of inflammatory bowel disease, irritable bowel syndrome, antibiotic-associated diarrhea, lactose intolerance, and ulcerative colitis.

PARMIGIANO-REGGIANO

It's not just because I'm Italian American that Parmigiano-Reggiano is one of my favorite foods. It takes at least twelve months to make this nutty, aromatic wonder, and the average Italian Parmigiano is aged twenty-four months. Could it add that much to your healthy life span if taken orally, regularly, and as directed by this ChefMD? It's lower in sodium than most other hard cheeses, and fluffs up in volume, so you (tastefully) fool your eye.

WATER-COOLER FACT: In a study involving over sixty thousand women, those who ate at least four servings a day of dairy foods had a 41 percent lower risk of colorectal cancer than those eating less than one serving: the biggest benefit came from eating cheese such as Parmigiano-Reggiano. One ounce grated fluffs up to a half cup of snowy goodness.

WHAT'S IN IT: Parmigiano-Reggiano is a concentrated source of milk's nutrients. A one-hundred-gram (3.3-ounce) piece of Parmigiano-Reggiano has 392 calories, 1,160 milligrams of calcium, one hundred milligrams of potassium, twenty-eight grams of fat, as well as vitamins A, B1, B2, B6, and B12. It has a protein content of 36 percent. It has very little lactose and is very rich in glutamate.

✳ **LITTLE BITES**

Studies have found that probiotics, such as those found in kefir, may improve the bioavailability of B vitamins, calcium, iron, zinc, copper, magnesium, and phosphorus.

✳ **LITTLE BITES**

Conjugated linoleic acid (CLA) and sphingomyelin—beneficial compounds found in milk fat—are higher in the summer than in the winter. Since Parmigiano-Reggiano cheese is made from milk produced between May and November, it is a concentrated source of both CLA and sphingomyelin, both of which are thought to help fight cancer!

WHAT IT'S GOOD FOR: Increasing female fertility. An eight-year study of more than eighteen thousand women suggests that full-fat dairy foods such as Parmigiano-Reggiano may increase fertility. Women who ate at least one serving of high-fat dairy products a day were 27 percent less likely to experience ovulation-related fertility problems than those who ate less than one serving of dairy per day.

YOGURT

Yogurt's creamy and thick texture is the basis of its original Turkish name—Yoghurmak, which means "to thicken."

WATER-COOLER FACT: Ounce for ounce, yogurt has more calcium and folic acid than milk.

WHAT'S IN IT: Yogurt is a very good source of phosphorus, vitamin B2, and iodine. One eight-ounce cup of plain low-fat yogurt has approximately 155 calories and four hundred milligrams of calcium. A fermented food, some yogurt contains lactic acid–producing healthy bacteria, or probiotics.

WHAT IT'S GOOD FOR: Helping you live longer, fight off infection, reduce inflammation, and keep your stomach healthy. An Italian study found that elderly people who ate yogurt or drank milk three times a week or more had a 38 percent decreased risk of death. Yogurt was given daily to eleven subjects with antibiotic-resistant bacteria; all eleven cleared antibiotic-resistant bacteria out of their systems in four weeks. Only one of the twelve subjects who were not given the yogurt got rid of their bacteria. Yogurt taken orally or vaginally by pregnant women in early pregnancy reduced vaginitis during pregnancy by 81 percent. A one-month Finnish study of patients with Crohn's disease and ulcerative colitis found that eating yogurt with probiotics reduced inflammation; a yogurt without probiotics did not. Full-fat yogurt improves female fertility; low-fat and frozen yogurts worsen it.

Nutritious Nuts

ALMONDS

The Romans showered newlyweds with almonds as a fertility charm. Do you think that's how a certain part of the male body got named?

WATER-COOLER FACT: An ounce of almonds (twenty-three average almonds) contains 3.3 grams of fiber—the most of any nut.

WHAT'S IN IT: Almonds are a very good source of vitamin E, and a good source of magnesium and riboflavin. A one-ounce serving has 164 calories and fourteen grams of fat.

WHAT IT'S GOOD FOR: Reducing your triglycerides and cholesterol, and preventing gallstones. Twenty-two people replaced half of their dietary fat with almonds. Their blood triglyceride levels decreased by 14 percent, their total cholesterol decreased by 4 percent, their LDL cholesterol by 6 percent, and their HDL cholesterol increased by 6 percent. Also, men who frequently ate nuts such as almonds had a 30 percent less risk of gallstones than men who rarely or never ate them.

PECANS

The pecan is truly an American nut. The tree is native to North America, and both George Washington and Thomas Jefferson counted it among their favorite foods.

WATER-COOLER FACT: Shaking unshelled pecans is a way to find out how fresh they are—if they rattle, they're no longer fresh.

WHAT'S IN IT: Pecans are 53 percent fat by weight, but less than 10 percent of that is saturated fat. Pecans also contain potassium, fiber, vitamin B1, and vitamin E. A quarter cup of pecans weighs less than an ounce and consists of about sixteen small pecan halves, 171 calories, and eighteen grams of fat.

WHAT IT'S GOOD FOR: Lowering your LDL "lousy" cholesterol, and reducing your risk for coronary heart disease. Pecans contain monounsaturated fat, which is linked to lowering LDL cholesterol levels. A trial involving twenty-three people with high cholesterol showed that eating seventy-two grams of pecans (almost three-quarters of a cup) a day decreased their total cholesterol by 7 percent, LDL by 10 percent, triglycerides by 11 percent, and increased HDL by 6 percent beyond that seen in people following the National Cholesterol Education Program's step 1 diet for reducing cholesterol. One ounce of nuts five days a week is the dose consistently shown to reduce the risk of heart disease.

※ **LITTLE BITES**

Roast almonds gently at 350°F to retain their delicate, healthy, polyunsaturated fats.

※ **LITTLE BITES**

Of all nuts, pecans have the most antioxidants.

Eating just four whole walnuts
a day can significantly increase
the amount of omega-3 polyunsaturated fatty acids in the blood.

WALNUTS

Nuts stored airtight will not absorb the flavors of other foods, and will stay fresher longer in the freezer or refrigerator.

WATER-COOLER FACT: An ounce and a half of walnuts eaten after a high-fat meal (eighty grams of fat, 35 percent saturated) reversed arterial stiffening within four hours . . . better than olive oil.

WHAT'S IN IT: Walnuts are an excellent source of omega-3 essential fatty acids. Walnuts also contain protein, potassium, folate, and fiber. One ounce of walnuts (about fourteen halves) has 185 calories, four grams of protein, and eighteen grams of fat. Walnuts reduce LDL oxidation and other measures of inflammation in the bloodstream.

WHAT IT'S GOOD FOR: Keeping your arteries flexible and your heart healthy. Omega-3s reduce the risk of cardiovascular disease by reducing inflammation in the blood vessels, especially the arteries. In one study, twenty-four subjects were fed a fatty diet followed by about twenty walnut halves. Subjects had their blood flow increase by 24 percent, had more elastic arteries, and a slower start to arterial inflammation.

Sensational Spices

Capsaicin, the chemical responsible
for making chilies hot, may have the
power to kill prostate cancer cells.
And the hotter the chili, the more
capsaicin.

CHILIES

Some like it hot. If you do, there are hot chilies. But there are also sweet and mild chilies, and all chilies are great culinary medicine.

WATER-COOLER FACT: Most of a chili's heat—by a factor of sixteen—is in the ribs that attach the seeds to the chili, not the seeds or the flesh. The burn from a chili can be cooled with continuous contact with something icy cold because the nerve receptors are cooled, or something crunchy like chips or celery, which sends the brain a different signal.

WHAT'S IN IT: Chilies are a very good source of vitamins A, C, and dietary fiber. They are also a good source of iron and potassium, and they are rich in antioxidants. Two teaspoons of dried chili pepper have twenty-six calories.

WHAT IT'S GOOD FOR: Helping you lose weight, in two ways. First, chilies can help you reach satiety faster. Twenty-four subjects who consumed 0.9 grams of hot red pepper (very hot: 80,000 Scoville units) before each meal ate fewer calories and less fat than those who took a placebo. Maybe their mouths hurt too much to eat more. Second, chilies can boost your metabolism. Thirteen subjects were fed one of four meals: high fat; high fat and ten grams of hot red pepper; high carbohydrate; and high carbohydrate and ten grams of hot red pepper. The addition of hot red pepper increased thermogenesis (the process by which the body generates heat by increasing the metabolic rate above normal), particularly after the high-fat meal. Hotter chilies seem to have more benefits, including the ability to clear insulin from the bloodstream.

✚ **DOCTOR IT UP!**

For extra flavor, toast dried chilies for five seconds over an open flame before seeding, soaking, and pureeing them for chili and sauces.

CHOCOLATE

Cocoa was considered a royal drink in ancient Mexico and was drunk out of gold goblets. Montezuma reportedly drank fifty or more goblets of it a day. Talk about a chocoholic!

WATER-COOLER FACT: Fermenting cocoa beans gives them their chocolate flavor. Cocoa powder that has not been "dutched" or chemically treated with alkali has more flavonoids than dutched cocoa powder, and is lighter in color.

WHAT'S IN IT: Chocolate is a very complex food, containing hundreds of chemicals, including caffeine, though much less caffeine than in coffee. Chocolate also contains magnesium and calcium. One hundred grams (about 3.3 ounces) of a Hershey's Special Dark chocolate bar has 531 calories.

WHAT IT'S GOOD FOR: Helping you control your blood pressure. Five studies showed that a polyphenol-rich cocoa dropped systolic blood pressure by 4.7 millimeters of mercury and diastolic by 2.8 millimeters of mercury. Barely one-quarter ounce daily of dark chocolate (thirty calories of Ritter Sport Halbbitter) dropped pressures by 2.9 and 1.9 millimeters of mercury after eighteen weeks. This reduces the risk of stroke by 8 percent, heart disease by 5 percent, and overall mortality by 4 percent.

❋ **LITTLE BITES**

Dark chocolate can help dilate your arteries because it improves nitric oxide bioavailability (body readiness). Nitric oxide is the naturally occurring chemical that helps your arteries expand when needed.

CINNAMON

Cinnamon is one of the oldest spices and has been used for millennia as a medicine.

WATER-COOLER FACT: Cinnamon's essential oils have been shown to have more antibacterial activity than Cool Mint Listerine.

WHAT'S IN IT: Cinnamon is a tree bark and an excellent source of manganese, which you need for forming skin, bone, and cartilage and regulating blood sugar. Cinnamon is also a very good source of fiber, iron, and calcium. One tablespoon of ground cinnamon has eighteen calories.

WHAT IT'S GOOD FOR: Possibly regulating blood sugar and blood pressure levels. Cinnamon may help protect you from diabetes—it improves the body's response to sugar by improving insulin sensitivity, and people with normal blood sugar have a slower than usual blood sugar rise after eating a dessert with cinnamon, like rice pudding. Less than a teaspoon of cinnamon daily lowered blood sugar by 7 percent in one study. The calcium and fiber in cinnamon bind bile salts, which helps to lower cholesterol levels. Cinnamon extract has also been found in the laboratory to inhibit the growth of cancerous tumor cells and act as an antimicrobial and antioxidant.

✳ **LITTLE BITES**

Among twenty-six spices, cloves are the most powerful antioxidant, and exhibit the strongest free radical scavenging activity.

CLOVES

Breath mint, anyone? Over two thousand years ago the Chinese chewed cloves as a natural breath freshener to avoid offending the emperor. To avoid offending your Inner ChefMD, eat more cloves.

WATER-COOLER FACT: Cloves begin as bright red flower buds of an evergreen, and dry to dark brown.

WHAT'S IN IT: Cloves are an excellent source of manganese; a very good source of fiber, vitamins C and K, and omega-3 fatty acids; and a good source of magnesium and calcium. Two teaspoons of ground cloves have fourteen calories.

WHAT IT'S GOOD FOR: Keeping your blood sugar levels down. Thirty-six type 2 diabetics who ate up to three grams of cloves for thirty days showed a decrease in their blood sugar from an average of

225 milligrams per deciliter to an average of 150 milligrams per deciliter. They also had decreased triglycerides, total cholesterol, and LDL levels.

CURRY POWDER AND TURMERIC

Fuzzy memory? Eat more curry. Upset stomach? Try curry powder. Cancer prevention? Again, have some curry—because curry contains turmeric, which was introduced to Europe in the thirteenth century, although it had been cultivated and harvested in India for at least twenty-five hundred years. Hopefully, it won't take you that long to try a ChefMD recipe.

WATER-COOLER FACT: Curry powders are as individual as the region they come from, but they all contain some turmeric. Curry powder fortified with iron effectively treated iron-deficiency anemia in an African research study.

WHAT'S IN IT: Curry powder is an excellent source of iron and manganese and a good source of vitamin B6, fiber, and potassium. Turmeric is anti-inflammatory, antimicrobial, and antioxidant, and it is about 3 percent curcumin, which is thought to be the active ingredient. Two teaspoons of either curry powder or turmeric have about sixteen calories.

WHAT IT'S GOOD FOR: Protecting you from Alzheimer's. Data from the Singapore National Mental Health Survey suggests that those who consume curry dishes between monthly and daily had a 49 percent reduced risk of cognitive impairment, and those who ate curry once every six months had a 38 percent reduced risk. Also, one gram of curcumin twice daily cut the relapse rate by 80 percent over six months in a study of eighty-two patients with stable ulcerative colitis. Oil improves curcumin's bioavailability.

GARLIC

Did you know that the Egyptians built the pyramids on a diet of bread, water, and garlic? It's a good thing that there are less strenuous things to do with garlic.

WATER-COOLER FACT: Garlic has been called the "stinking rose" for the aroma it can leave on your breath. Parsley has been traditionally believed to undo this effect, which is perhaps the reason parsley pairs with garlic and lemon zest to make the tangy garnish gremolata.

WHAT'S IN IT: Garlic is an excellent source of manganese and a very good source of vitamin B6 and vitamin C. It is also a good source of protein, vitamin B1, selenium, calcium, potassium, and iron. Three average cloves of garlic have thirteen calories.

WHAT IT'S GOOD FOR: Protecting you from a variety of cancers. People in southern Europe who ate the most garlic had a 26 percent reduced risk for colorectal cancer, a 10 percent reduced risk for breast cancer, a 22 percent reduced risk for ovarian cancer, and a 19 percent reduced risk for prostate cancer, compared with those who ate the least garlic. Also, the allicin found in garlic is a powerful antibacterial agent that is effective in killing bacteria in dilutions as weak as 1:128.

GINGER

As a kid, I liked Mary Ann better! But Ginger is my new favorite.

WATER-COOLER FACT: While commonly thought to be a root, ginger is actually the underground stem of the plant *Zingiber officinale,* which grows in moist, tropical soil.

WHAT'S IN IT: Ginger is a good source of potassium and vitamin B6. A one-ounce piece of ginger has twenty calories. Dried ginger has less gingerol and more shogaol, another anti-inflammatory.

WHAT IT'S GOOD FOR: Helping reduce nausea from many causes, reducing inflammation, and possibly lessening arthritis pain. Six well-designed scientific studies show that ginger reduces *hyperemesis gravidum,* a severe form of nausea and vomiting during pregnancy. And similar studies show ginger's effectiveness for postoperative nausea and vomiting. In one well-done study, ginger has been found to be more effective than the over-the-counter drug Dramamine for treating motion sickness. Ginger extract has been used by osteoarthritis patients to relieve pain.

HONEY

Honey, if you ain't eating honey, you're crazy! Even Hippocrates, the father of modern medicine, recommended honey because he thought it cured diseases.

WATER-COOLER FACT: The average worker bee makes half a teaspoon of honey in her lifetime.

WHAT'S IN IT: One ounce of honey has 128 calories. Honey is one of the few sweeteners that contain vitamins, minerals, amino acids, and antioxidants. It is a source of vitamins B2 and B6, iron, and manganese. One teaspoon has twenty-one calories.

WHAT IT'S GOOD FOR: Helping you recover from a burn or wound, and treating nighttime cough. Honey's low pH (3.2 to 4.5) prevents the growth of bacteria. In a study comparing the wound-healing effects of honey to silver sulfadiazine, topical use of honey showed an early abatement of acute inflammatory changes and better control of infection. A study of kids with colds showed less coughing and better sleep with up to two teaspoons thirty minutes before bed. Do not give honey to infants younger than twelve months old, because there is a risk of botulism.

OREGANO

In ancient Greek and Roman weddings, brides and grooms were crowned with oregano laurels. For a long, healthy marriage they should have been eating them instead of wearing them. In Greek, the word *oregano* means "mountain joy."

WATER-COOLER FACT: Gram for gram, oregano has four times more antioxidant activity than blueberries, twelve times more than oranges, thirty times more than potatoes, and forty-two times more than apples.

WHAT'S IN IT: Oregano is an excellent source of vitamin K; a very good source of iron, manganese, and dietary fiber; and a good source of calcium, magnesium, vitamins A and C, and omega-3 fatty acids. It is very high in antioxidants, such as rosmarinic acid, and the antibacterial oils thymol and carvacrol. Two teaspoons of dried, ground oregano have nine calories.

WHAT IT'S GOOD FOR: Guarding you against infection. In the lab, oregano's essential antibacterial oils thymol and carvacrol inhibit the growth of the bacterium *Staphylococcus aureus,* the most common cause of staph infections. An edible oregano oil fruit film kills more than 50 percent of *E. coli* bacteria in food.

ROSEMARY

Over two thousand years ago, Greek students were convinced that rosemary helped memory and placed sprigs of the herb in their hair while studying for exams. Today, some of the benefits believed to be true for thousands of years are being scientifically proven correct, including helping concentration.

WATER-COOLER FACT: When you smell rosemary, the scent triggers free radical scavenging activity in your body and decreases the level of the stress hormone cortisol in your body.

WHAT'S IN IT: Rosemary is a good source of iron, calcium, and fiber. It is also high in antioxidants such as carnosic acid and carnosol, which have been shown to inhibit the growth of human colon cancer cells in the lab. Two teaspoons of dried rosemary have seven calories.

WHAT IT'S GOOD FOR: Reducing the risk of intestinal and breast cancers from charred or overcooked meat. Dried rosemary powder has reduced heterocyclic amine formation by up to 77 percent in ground beef burgers grilled at temperatures up to 400° F. Rosemary appears also to protect the body by activating detoxifying enzymes in the liver, and protecting brain cells from oxidation.

Marvelous Meats, Fish, and Poultry

BEEF, LEAN AND GRASS-FED

USDA-certified 100 percent organic beef is free of antibiotics, chemicals, and added hormones. Grass-fed, it becomes even better and a small part of what to eat, especially at a feast.

WATER-COOLER FACT: Compared with a three-ounce serving of skinless chicken breast, a three-ounce serving of lean beef has just one more gram of saturated fat, eight times more vitamin B12, six times more zinc, and three times more iron.

WHAT'S IN IT: In all four-legged animals, the tenderloin runs along the middle of the spine and is the leanest and most tender (hence the name) part of the animal. Beef is a very good source of protein and vitamin B12, and it is a good source of vitamins B2, B6, and niacin. A four-ounce portion of broiled beef tenderloin has 240 calories and thirty-two grams of protein. The tenderloins of grass-fed cattle have higher levels of protein, conjugated linoleic acid, omega-3 fatty acids, and vitamins A and E than the tenderloins of corn-fed beef. Cattle are what they eat: pasture grass has up to fifteen times more alpha-linolenic acid (an omega-3) than feed lot grain mixes. Half of the fat in beef is monounsaturated; olive oil is 77 percent monounsaturated.

WHAT IT'S GOOD FOR: Replacing iron for people with iron-deficiency anemia. The downside: most men and postmenopausal women do not need additional iron in their diets, as it is an oxidant, so keep portions small.

BISON OR BUFFALO

Oh, give me a home, where the buffalo roam . . . because if you're going to eat meat, bison is among the most nutritious, leanest, tastiest, and lowest in saturated fat.

WATER-COOLER FACT: Bison are the largest land mammal in North America since the end of the Ice Age. Hunted almost to extinction in the late nineteenth century, their numbers have rebounded.

WHAT'S IN IT: Bison meat has less fat, fewer calories, and less cholesterol than beef, and it has more iron and vitamin B12. It is also more tender. A hundred-gram (3.3-ounce) serving of cooked lean bison has 143 calories, and grass-fed bison have higher levels of omega-3 fatty acids than corn-fed bison. It can be used in any recipe that calls for beef: cook medium-rare for the richest flavor.

WHAT IT'S GOOD FOR: Saving your immune system from chemicals. Its omega-3s are important in reducing risk for heart disease. Bison are not given growth hormones or antibiotics. For some people, it's steak without guilt.

SALMON

The salmon is a very smart fish. It swims around in the ocean for years and then when it's time to spawn, it finds its way back to the freshwater stream to where it was born. It's no wonder that eating salmon bestows many health and brain benefits.

WATER-COOLER FACT: The fatty acid EPA in salmon appears to protect skin against sunburn by reducing inflammation induced by the ultraviolet B rays of the sun.

✳ **LITTLE BITES**

Red meat contains heme iron, the type most readily absorbed by the body, as well as carnosine (an amino acid, also highly bioavailable), which may help people with autism.

✳ **LITTLE BITES**

Wine, tea, and coffee help stop iron absorption from plant and dairy foods.

WHAT'S IN IT: Salmon is an excellent source of omega-3 essential fatty acids EPA (eicosapentaenoic acid) and DHA (decosahexagenoic acid) and of vitamin D and selenium; a very good source of protein, niacin, and vitamin B12; and a good source of vitamin B6. A four-ounce portion of baked Chinook salmon has twenty-one hundred milligrams of omega-3s. Seven ounces of raw wild salmon has 281 calories.

WHAT IT'S GOOD FOR: Preventing sudden death, stroke, and keeping your brain healthy. The Nurses' Health Study reports that death from heart disease was 29 percent to 34 percent lower in women who consumed fish once a week than those who ate fish less than once a month. Eating baked or broiled but not fried fish once weekly lowers heart rate and decreases heart rate variability. Japanese researchers found that of over forty thousand men and women followed for ten years, those who ate fish eight times weekly versus just once had 56 percent lower heart attack risk. Also, salmon may help protect you from Alzheimer's. Of 815 home-care patients who participated in a study, those who ate fish once a week had a 60 percent lower risk of developing Alzheimer's.

SARDINES

Poor little sardines—stuffed in a can and usually destined to end up as a snack on top of a cracker. In the ChefMD eating plan, however, they reach the pinnacle of culinary pride as one of our fifty fabulous ChefMD recommended foods. The sardine finally gets the respect it deserves!

WATER-COOLER FACT: Buy canned sardines that are packed in oil, so you get all the omega-3. Buy fresh sardines whenever they are available.

WHAT'S IN IT: Sardines are an excellent source of vitamin B12; a very good source of selenium, vitamin D, omega-3 fatty acids, and protein; and a good source of calcium and vitamin B3. A 3.5-ounce serving of sardines in sardine oil contains about thirty-three hundred milligrams of omega-3 fatty acids. An ounce of sardines—about two canned fish—has fifty calories.

WHAT IT'S GOOD FOR: Protecting you from macular degeneration, the leading cause of blindness in the United States. People who consume omega-3-rich fish like sardines once a week reduce their early macular degeneration risk by 42 percent; those who eat fish three times a week reduce their risk by 75 percent. Sardines and other oily fish can also reduce triglyceride levels. Lactating mothers who eat three ounces of sardines twice weekly provide their infants with more omega-3 fatty acids in their breast milk, and omega-3s have been shown to aid infants' brain development and to protect their mental health and intelligence.

TURKEY

Ben Franklin was very disappointed when the bald eagle was chosen as the national bird because he really liked turkeys. Well, ChefMD is siding with ole Ben on this one. Turkey is a great choice in poultry for flavor and nutrition.

WATER-COOLER FACT: In Mexico, turkey with mole sauce *(mole de guajolote)* is so popular that it's considered by many to be the national dish.

WHAT'S IN IT: Like all poultry, turkey is an excellent source of the amino acid tryptophan, a very good source of lean protein and selenium, and a good source of vitamin B6.

WHAT IT'S GOOD FOR: Maintaining optimal health. Turkey is a good source of lean protein and is rich in selenium, which is involved in thyroid hormone metabolism, antioxidant defense systems, immune function, and DNA repair. Turkey is also rich in vitamin B3, which helps to control insulin and blood sugar.

Delectable Drinks

COFFEE

Coffeehouses first appeared in England in the 1650s and the word *tips* was coined: a sign reading TO INSURE PROMPT SERVICE (TIPS) was placed by a tin at a coffeehouse, and those who wanted to get their coffee faster threw in a coin.

WATER-COOLER FACT: Coffee has more fiber than orange juice.

WHAT'S IN IT: Coffee contains magnesium, potassium, and between 72 and 130 milligrams of caffeine per average brewed cup. Coffee is

---

✳ LITTLE BITES

Ounce for ounce, a turkey breast contains less fat, less cholesterol, more protein, and more iron than a chicken breast.

✚ DOCTOR IT UP!

You can cook turkey with the skin and remove it afterward; it protects the bird from drying out but does not add calories or fat.

a heavily sprayed crop: look for organics for fewer exposures. One cup of coffee has two calories.

WHAT IT'S GOOD FOR: Protecting men from Parkinson's disease and preventing colon cancer, breast cancer, and diabetes in women. A study of more than forty-seven thousand men who drank at least one cup of coffee a day showed they had a 40 percent less chance of developing Parkinson's disease than men who did not drink coffee. A study of ninety-six thousand men and women over twelve years found that three cups daily in women reduced the risk of colon cancer by half in women but not in men. Premenopausal women who drink four or more cups of coffee a day have a 40 percent less risk of breast cancer than those who do not drink coffee. Two or three cups of coffee daily in a study of eighty-eight thousand young and middle-aged women reduced the relative risk of diabetes by 42 percent over nondrinkers. The downside: coffee may exacerbate premenstrual syndrome.

TEA

Tea is powerful—and not just powerful medicine. In fact, it has even caused wars (the American Revolution, sparked in part by the Boston Tea Party—some party!). But tea is so good for us that perhaps after two-hundred-plus years, we all need to stop fighting and enjoy a "cuppa"—because four of five cups drunk in the United States are actually glasses of iced tea.

WATER-COOLER FACT: Black tea, oolong tea, green tea, and white tea all come from the same plant. White tea is produced from buds and young leaves that do not undergo fermentation. Leaves for green tea are slightly fermented before being dried, leaves for oolong tea are fermented for two to three days, and leaves for black tea are completely fermented. Each tea has unique benefits and flavors.

WHAT'S IN IT: Tea has no carbohydrates, fat, protein, or calories: its health benefits are attributed to catechins, which are the flavonoids present in fresh tea leaves. Because they are processed less than oolong and black teas, white and green teas generally contain greater catechin levels. But black teas contain more theaflavins and thearubigins. All are flavonoids.

WHAT IT'S GOOD FOR: Helping protect you from having a heart attack and stroke, and perhaps delaying cancer onset. An analysis of seventeen studies found that drinking twenty-four ounces of tea a day was associated with an 11 percent reduced risk of heart attack. A six-year study suggests that drinking more than three cups of green tea a day is associated with a lower risk of heart attack. Forty ounces of tea daily delayed cancer onset by 7.4 years in women and 3.2 years in men, over a ten-year span. Thirty-two ounces of black tea daily for four months dilated the blood vessels of men with heart disease. The effect was visible within two hours of drinking just sixteen ounces.

VEGETABLE JUICE

Are you like a kid when it comes to vegetables? Still hiding brussels sprouts in your napkin and trying to feed your green beans to the dog? If so, take heart. There's a delicious, quick, and easy way to get your veggies—vegetable juice!

WATER-COOLER FACT: Vegetable juice is one of the most alkalinizing foods: it provides buffering minerals important in protecting your bones from osteoporosis.

WHAT'S IN IT: This will vary, if you make your own, depending on what vegetables you use. Be sure to include some leafy greens, such as swiss chard, kale, or spinach. They will help protect you from heart disease. An eight-ounce glass of a commercial vegetable juice such as low-sodium V8 has fifty calories, 169 milligrams of sodium, and nine grams of sugar. If you are watching your salt intake, you might try a low-sodium variety such as Knudsen Very Veggie Low Sodium vegetable juice, which has 35 milligrams of sodium and 760 milligrams of potassium; look for the organic version.

WHAT IT'S GOOD FOR: Protecting you from Alzheimer's and against DNA damage. A ten-year study of almost two thousand people showed that those who drank fruit and vegetable juices at least three times a week had a 76 percent reduced risk of Alzheimer's disease compared with people who drank fruit and vegetable juices less than once a week. In another study of eleven male football players, those who drank about 5.5 ounces of vegetable juice three times daily had dramatically decreased levels of oxidative DNA damage by day four compared with those who drank mineral water over the same period.

※ LITTLE BITES

Homemade vegetable juice made in a juicer has more protein than commercial juice.

Organic wines have significantly higher levels of polyphenols than nonorganic wines.

WINE

My toast at the end of my television segments is *"C'ent anni! May you live one hundred years!"* Being a home winemaker and a wine lover, I truly believe that drinking wine might really help you live a hundred years!

WATER-COOLER FACT: Nearly all grape juice and wine is white: it is the grape skins that give red and rosé wines their color.

WHAT'S IN IT: Five ounces of red wine has 125 calories and hundreds of micrograms of resveratrol, the touted longevity compound found in grape skin. Resveratrol is produced by the vine in response to stress, including fungal infection. Wine has much higher concentrations of resveratrol than grapes or grape juice, because juice is fermented by yeast (a fungus) to become wine. Food with protein appears to improve the bioavailability of polyphenols in red wine, and the polyphenol quercetin improves the bioavailability of resveratrol. Red wine has more polyphenols than white.

WHAT IT'S GOOD FOR: In proper dosages, reducing risk for heart disease, mortality, and the risk of stroke. Moderate wine drinking (one to two drinks a day for women, and two drinks a day for men who are not at risk for liver disease or addiction) reduces the risk of heart disease by up to 30 percent, of type 2 diabetes, and of total and ischemic stroke. Red wine raises HDL (healthy) cholesterol, as does all alcohol, and red wine makes LDL (lousy) cholesterol more resistant to oxidation. Resveratrol suppresses the proliferation of many cancer cells, and quercetin suppresses leukemia cell growth. However, drinking more than the recommended amount increases the risk of cirrhosis, heart failure, high blood pressure, hemorrhagic stroke, nearly all cancers, and sudden death.

THE RIGHT STORAGE FOR YOUR MEDICINE CHEST

- GREAT GRAINS: Store in airtight opaque containers in a cool, dark place.
- BENEFICIAL BEANS: Store as you would grains.
- VITAL VEGETABLES: As a general rule they are perishable and should be kept in the refrigerator. Tomatoes are an exception.

- **FLAVORFUL FRUITS:** Cooling them will help them last longer. But keep some in a bowl on the counter, where you'll see them and be more likely to eat them.
- **DELICIOUS DAIRY:** Keep in the refrigerator.
- **NUTRITIOUS NUTS:** Keep in an airtight container in the freezer or refrigerator, to prevent spoilage.
- **SENSATIONAL SPICES:** Store in an airtight container at room temperature. Dried herbs and spices will keep longer than fresh.
- **MARVELOUS MEATS, FISH, AND POULTRY:** These should always be kept well chilled and often freeze well, especially when fresh.
- **DELECTABLE DRINKS:** Keep coffee beans in the freezer to preserve freshness.

CHAPTER 5

Recipes and Meals: WHAT TO EAT AND HOW TO MAKE IT, FOR EVERY MEAL (INCLUDING DESSERT)

Cooking is primarily fun . . . the more [people] know what they are doing, the more fun it is.

—JAMES BEARD

Learning how to cook can save your life. It's much easier than most people think, especially for fruits and vegetables. The recipes in this collection are some of the best, tastiest, and easiest I know. By following them, you will be letting your Inner Chef get to work for you, and at the same time, feed the doctor inside.

Eating should be both pleasurable and guiltless. Through these fifty recipes, I'll show you how to accomplish both.

To be included in the book, each recipe had to help you:

- Absorb more of the best of what you're eating
- Avoid anti-nutrients—no trans fats and no high-fructose corn syrup in any product
- Enjoy eating—each recipe is highly rated for aroma, color, texture, taste, and appearance
- Get in and out of the kitchen quickly—thirty minutes or less for most
- Feel satisfied after eating
- Use at least one of the fifty ChefMD foods in chapter 4
- Use organics when it makes a difference to your health.

All ChefMD recipes let you incorporate blasts of flavor into dishes with very few calories—barely 250 per serving on average. If you try every recipe in the book (and I hope you will), you will get about 27 percent of your calories from fat, 7 percent from saturated fat, 48 percent from carbs, and twenty-two grams of fiber per thousand calories, too.

Enjoy!

ChefMD Essentials

To make shopping simple, I offer ChefMD essentials: some of my favorite brand-name products that come in jars, boxes, and cans. It's easy in our hectic world to compromise taste and nutrition for convenience. But these mostly widely available pantry products have all three, proving that minimally processed can mean delicious and nutritious. Almost all are in large grocery stores and national health food stores, including Whole Foods, Wild Oats, and Trader Joe's, some exclusively.

Plus, I offer fourteen days of nearly no-cook menu plans—ten minutes or less per meal—for those days when fast is the only thing you have time for. I've used many of the ChefMD essentials in these menu plans, and highlight them for you here so you always have the basis for easy, exciting ChefMD meals readily at hand.

Neither I nor ChefMD has a financial relationship with any of these companies. These recommendations are made purely on the basis of the foods' flavor, nutrition, and convenience.

Açai. Sambazon Pure Açai Smoothie Pack comes in individual hundred-gram packs, providing a convenient way to incorporate this antioxidant-rich, chocolate-scented berry into smoothies and drinks. Each pack contains frozen açai puree: no sugars or preservatives are added.

Agave nectar. New to the modern culinary scene, agave nectar tastes of honey meeting maple syrup. Unlike other sweeteners, agave nectar has a low glycemic index, which helps raise blood sugar and insulin levels slowly. **Madhava Agave Nectar** comes in a light grade, which has a mild flavor, and amber and dark, both of which are more intense and molasses-like.

Barley. When dinner needs to be on the table in a snap, who has time to simmer barley on the stove for forty-five minutes? I like **Mother's Quick Cooking Barley:** it's nationally distributed, chewy and convenient, and great for risottos, soups, and stews. You will find the same nuttiness you do in traditional barley.

Barbecue sauce. Trader Joe's All Natural is smoky-sweet with just the right amount of kick, without artificial flavors or preservatives. Yum.

Beans. Both **Westbrae Natural** and **Eden** produce a variety of canned organic beans, from buttery and creamy cannellini beans to nutty and toasty garbanzo beans. The thick, starchy liquid adds body to soups and stews, which works for the no-salt-added varieties. To add a creamier texture to dips and tacos, look for **Bearitos Fat-Free Traditional Refried Beans** or **Fat-Free Black Bean Refried Beans**, which are vegetarian and lard-free.

Brown rice. Whole grains, such as brown rice, usually require a longer cooking time than white rice to soften the nutrient-rich bran layer. Enjoy the convenience of fully cooked brown rice, such as **Uncle Ben's Ready Whole Grain Rice** in an 8.8-ounce package, for an easy weekday meal. A quick ninety seconds in the microwave produces warm fluffy kernels of whole grain goodness. **Trader Joe's** has a fully cooked Brown Rice, in a 10.5-ounce package.

Canned tomatoes. When tomatoes aren't in season, canned tomatoes are a great alternative to using hard, mealy, gassed-red tomatoes from overseas. **Muir Glen** produces an extensive line of organic tomato products, including diced, whole, crushed, fire-roasted, no-salt-added, paste, sauce, and ketchup. The fire-roasted variety, in particular, possesses a smoky flavor rarely canned: they're almost as good as doing it yourself.

Cereal. Kashi GOLEAN Crunch! cereal is produced from a blend of seven whole grains and sesame and contains no refined sweeteners, additives, or preservatives. These crunchy honey-kissed clusters add ten grams of fiber (especially bran), seven grams of protein, and very few calories to your morning meal. In fact, it makes a great morning meal!

Chicken broth. Indispensable. Quality boxed stock delivers a slow-cooked flavor without simmering a huge pot on the stove all day long. Both **Trader Joe's** and **Pacific Natural Foods Organic Low-Sodium Free Range Chicken Broth** are produced from organic, free-range chickens. These two brands are a terrific find for soups, stews, and whole grains.

Chicken sausage. As an alternative to the traditional pork or beef-based sausages, fully cooked chicken sausages provide the same flavors and texture without the added fat and calories. **Sausages by Amy** are made without preservatives, MSG, nitrites, or nitrates and contain up-to-the-moment mix-ins such as cranberries, maple sugar, and chipotle peppers. **Trader Joe's** also produces a line of fully cooked chicken sausages in flavors such as sweet Italian and sun-dried tomato. **Applegate Farms** brand is the only national organic brand I have found.

Chocolate milk. Sure, it's a treat: creamy and smooth, chocolate milk will often satisfy any chocoholic's cravings. **Horizon Organic Chocolate Low-fat Milk** combines organic milk, organic sugar, and organic cocoa to produce a delightfully sweet and creamy indulgence—with no added corn syrup, unlike most others. As a dairy-free alternative, choose shelf-stable boxes of chocolate soy milk such as **Silk** brand.

Cottage cheese. Cabot Vermont Style No-Fat Cottage Cheese and **Horizon Organic Low-Fat Cottage Cheese** are available in most major grocery stores. Both of these brands will surprise you by delivering flavor and creaminess usually only found in full-fat products.

Crabmeat. Picking crabmeat from a whole crab can be a messy and time-consuming experience; enjoy the convenience of fully cooked, pasteurized canned crabmeat. Look for "lump" or "jumbo lump" crabmeat, which contains larger chunks of sweet, delicate morsels than "claw" or "special" meat. **Byrd's Crabmeat** or **Jack's Catch** brand crabmeat are available in many grocery stores. Both brands contain fresh crabmeat that has not been frozen and has a fresh, slightly briny flavor.

Frozen berries. Since frozen berries are frozen at the peak of harvest, they retain much of their sweet, juicy, burst-in-your-mouth flavor. **Cascadian Farm** offers frozen organic blueberries, strawberries, raspberries, and blackberries.

Ginger. A family-operated company, **the Ginger People,** offers an extensive line of exciting ginger products ranging from ginger chews to ginger beer. Organic crystallized ginger combines the spiciness of soft, tender ginger with the sweetness of organic cane sugar. Ginger-spiked cooking sauces, which come in flavors such as

Sweet Ginger Chili and Ginger Peanut, can be slathered on anything that cries out for a spicy ginger kick.

Greek yogurt. Can a creamy and silky texture be obtained from nonfat dairy? **Fage** produces a thick, authentic Greek-style yogurt that has a more velvety texture than traditional yogurt. Its creaminess is low calorie, too, so it's a good substitute for sour cream or even cream cheese, if drained. Comes in total (whole milk), 2%, and 0%.

Kefir. As the major U.S. manufacturer of kefir, a creamy enzyme-rich yogurt-like drink, **Lifeway** produces a range of kefir products, including milk, yogurt, and kefir cheese, which is a lot like thick sour cream and truly addictive. Kefir comes in several flavors, such as pomegranate, strawberry, and blueberry, in low-fat and nonfat varieties.

Lentils. Canned lentils are fully cooked and need only be rinsed and drained. A major manufacturer and distributor of whole grain products, **Bob's Red Mill** offers three varieties of dried lentils, which can be found in most major grocery stores. My favorite are the red lentils, which have a peppery flavor, gorgeous color, and cook in less time than the green or brown lentils. **Arrowhead Mills** also produces these lovely gems. And a real wonder: **Trader Joe's** sometimes has precooked, refrigerated, ready-to-eat cooked lentils in the refrigerated section; they're low in sodium, too.

Marinade. Mrs. Dash Mesquite Grille 10-Minute Marinade blends fourteen herbs and spices with a hint of apple to dress up any food that covets a coating of mouth-puckering bliss. Sweet, spicy, and smoky all at once, with no added salt, no MSG, and very few calories.

Mushrooms. Pennsylvania Exotics sliced mixed exotic mushrooms, found in the produce section, are prepped and ready to be washed and used in a stir-fry. The blend contains shiitake, crimini, and oyster mushrooms. **Frieda's** is another high-quality brand.

Oats. When you don't have the time to prepare traditional steel-cut oatmeal, which can steal precious morning minutes, and you want the taste of Irish oatmeal, turn to quick-cooking steel-cut oats. **McCann's Quick Cooking Irish Oatmeal** requires just minutes to transform into a steaming bowl of soul-warming goodness. **Trader**

Joe's Instant Steel Cut Oatmeal is cooked and frozen: microwave it for three minutes, and you're done. Steel-cut oats are nuttier, chewier, and denser than old-fashioned rolled oats, and this instant variety gets you there quicker, with a little sacrifice in texture and nuttiness, but none in flavor or nutrition. I like mine with crystallized ginger and cinnamon.

Old Bay seasoning. Old Bay seasoning has been a mainstay pairing with seafood for the past sixty years, using the same formula of various herbs and spices. The lengthy ingredient list (celery salt, mustard, red pepper, bay leaves, cloves, allspice, ginger, mace, cardamom, cinnamon, and paprika) combines magically to seem familiar yet special. There's nothing like it. Most supermarkets carry it. Penzeys.com has an equivalent as well as other carefully chosen, high-quality spices.

Pancake mix. Pancake mix contains premeasured dry ingredients that take the hassle out of baking. **Bob's Red Mill Buckwheat Pancake and Waffle Mix** is made with organic stone-ground wholegrain wheat and buckwheat flours and raw sugar. This is a rare and earthy mix.

Pasta. Ronzoni Healthy Harvest pasta contains a whole-wheat blend that cooks up lighter than most whole-wheat pastas; **Barilla PLUS** multigrain pastas feature barley and oats, which supply soluble fiber; egg whites and legumes, which offer protein; and flax, which provides heart-healthy omega-3 fatty acids. **Trader Joe's** also offers a 100 percent whole-wheat pasta line: look for the awesome multigrain with added flax. In the refrigerator section, **Buitoni** produces 100 percent whole-wheat three-cheese tortellini and whole-wheat four-cheese ravioli, which require only a brief simmer before dinner.

Salsa. Frontera captures the robust flavors of Mexico in its festive line of salsas, which come in mild, medium, and hot in myriad flavors ranging from Roasted Red Pepper and Garlic Salsa to Tangy Two-Chile Salsa. They are all low calorie, easy to use, distinctively different, and amazingly good.

Sardines. Brunswick sardines are available packed in spring water, olive oil, or tomato and basil and contain no added preservatives, chemicals, or MSG. And they're inexpensive and not fishy-smelling or -tasting.

Soup. Unlike the canned varieties, which are high in sodium and commonly condensed, boxed soups possess a fresh, from-scratch flavor and require just minutes to prepare. **Pacific Natural Foods** produces an extensive line of terrific organic soups: Organic Roasted Red Pepper and Tomato with fresh roasted garlic and vine-ripened tomatoes, and Creamy Butternut Squash are both great. Both varieties are also available in light varieties with 50 percent less sodium. **Imagine** and **Trader Joe's** also make organic creamy soups, which are dairy-free.

Soy-based mayonnaise. **Nasoya Nayonaise** provides the same creaminess and richness without the extra calories, saturated fat, and sometimes trans fat. The neutral flavor acts as a blank canvas for a host of mix-ins, such as herbs, chipotle peppers, tapenade, and sundried tomato paste.

Soyrizo. Chorizo is a pork-based sausage spiced with herbs and seasonings, but is commonly high in saturated fat and may not be produced from organically raised pigs. **Melissa's Soyrizo,** a meatless alternative produced from soybeans, crumbles and browns just like chorizo, but without the saturated fat and with much of the flavor.

Tea. **Tazo** produces a full line of flavorful black and green teas available in whole leaf, filter bags, and bottled teas. Some are certified organic. There are many other wonderful brands, too, such as **Good Earth** and **Foojoy.**

Teriyaki sauce. **Soy Vay Veri Veri Teriyaki** is a savory, richly meaty sauce for Asian-inspired dishes and stir-fries. Ingredients include preservative-free soy sauce, sugar (not the usual high-fructose corn syrup), and lots of aromatics. Unlike other bottled sauces, Veri Veri Teriyaki sauce contains no additional salt or preservatives.

Tofu. **Mori-Nu, Vitasoy, Trader Joe's,** and **White Wave** tofu are produced from non-GMO soybeans and contain no preservatives, and several are organic. Even more convenient are precooked, pre-seasoned tofu products, such as ready-to-eat **White Wave** baked tofu, a certified kosher and vegan food with flavors ranging from Sesame Peanut Thai Style to Zesty Lemon Pepper. Use it instead of chicken in salads, and even on pizza.

Tomato sauce. Classico produces a line of well-balanced, slightly sweet chunky tomato sauces that combine fresh ingredients and seasonings to deliver a made-from-scratch, slow-cooked home-made flavor. Traditional flavors include Tomato & Basil and Roasted Garlic; for the more adventurous palate, try Cabernet Marinara with Herbs. They're low calorie, have no saturated fat, and are not high in sodium. Add a little red wine vinegar if you like.

Tortilla chips. Guiltless Gourmet Tortilla Chips have nearly the same hearty, roasted corn flavor and satisfying crunch as traditional deep-fried chips. Try the Spicy Black Bean and Smoked Cheddar or Blue Corn flavors. They're great in chilaquiles.

Vegetable juice. A tomato-based vegetable cocktail, such as **V8 100% Vegetable Juice,** acts as an instant base for soups and stews and is perfect for plumping up whole-wheat couscous and cooking other quick-cooking grains. Both tart and sweet, V8 contains a blend of eight vegetable juices with no added sugars unlike many juices and mixes, and just sixty calories in eight ounces. Spicy V8 has an excellent kick, and low-sodium V8 delivers, too.

Whole grains. Bob's Red Mill produces quinoa, which possesses a delightfully crunchy texture, and barley, which is both chewy and nutty. So does **Natural Ovens.** They both have excellent gluten-free whole-grain bread and cake mixes as well. Other whole grains include spelt berries, wheat berries, farro, and gluten-free grains: amaranth, sorghum, millet, wild rice, and the Egyptian grain teff. Enjoy!

Breakfast/Brunch

CHOCOLATE BLACKBERRY BREAKFAST SMOOTHIE

Preparation time: 5 minutes • Cooking time: 0 minutes
Yield: 4 1-cup servings • 152 calories per serving, 18% from fat

INGREDIENTS

2 cups organic soy chocolate milk, such as Organic Valley or Trader Joe's brand
1 cup organic silken tofu, drained, such as Mori Nu brand
2 cups frozen organic blackberries, such as Cascadian Farm brand
1/8 teaspoon ground cloves

Nutritional Analysis per Serving	
Total Fat	3.1 g
Fat Calories	27.8
Cholesterol	0 mg
Saturated Fat	0.6 g
Polyunsaturated Fat	1.6 g
Monounsaturated Fat	0.7 g
Fiber	4.0 g
Carbohydrates	26.0 g
Sugar	14.9 g
Protein	6.2 g
Sodium	54.8 mg
Calcium	78.3 mg
Magnesium	57.6 mg
Zinc	0.8 mg
Selenium	0.3 mcg
Potassium	356.0 mg

PREPARATION

Combine the chocolate milk and tofu in a blender container. Cover and blend until fairly smooth, about 30 seconds. Add the blackberries and cloves; cover and blend until thickened, about 30 seconds to 1 minute.

SUBSTITUTIONS

Organic chocolate milk, such as Horizon brand, may replace the soy chocolate milk. Organic soft tofu may replace the silken tofu.

TIPS

Frozen blackberries give this quick shake a thick texture and gorgeous purple color. One or two teaspoons of organic agave nectar or dark honey may be added for a slightly sweeter flavor.

CREAMY GOAT CHEESE PESTO OMELET

Preparation time: 5 minutes • Cooking time: 10 minutes
Yield: 2 servings • 371 calories per serving, 33% from fat

INGREDIENTS

1/2 cup frozen shelled edamame (organic preferred)
4 large organic egg whites
1/2 cup organic fat-free cottage cheese, such as Horizon or Friendship brand
1/4 cup crumbled goat cheese
1 1/2 tablespoons prepared basil pesto
1 tablespoon chopped fresh basil
4 slices whole-wheat bread, toasted
Organic fruit preserves (optional)

PREPARATION

Heat a large nonstick skillet over medium heat until hot. Coat lightly with cooking spray; add the edamame and cook until beginning to brown, 2 to 3 minutes.

In a medium bowl, beat together the egg whites and cottage cheese; add to the skillet and stir in the edamame. Cook without stirring for 2 minutes or until set on bottom. Gently lift the edges of the omelet with a spatula to allow the uncooked portion of eggs to flow to the edges and set. Continue cooking for 2 minutes or until the center is almost set. Combine the goat cheese and pesto; spoon the mixture down the center of the omelet. Using a large spatula, fold half of the omelet over the filling. Reduce heat to low; cook for 2 minutes or until the cheese melts and the center is set. Use the large spatula to cut the omelet in half; transfer to serving dishes and top with basil. Serve with toast, and, if desired, preserves.

SUBSTITUTIONS

Feta cheese may replace the goat cheese, and peas may replace the edamame.

TIP

Try different types of pesto in this dish: sundried tomato, cilantro, even arugula.

Nutritional Analysis per Serving	
Total Fat	14.2 g
Fat Calories	127.5
Cholesterol	18.0 mg
Saturated Fat	4.4 g
Polyunsaturated Fat	0.1 g
Monounsaturated Fat	1.0 g
Fiber	5.7 g
Carbohydrates	33.0 g
Sugar	6.5 g
Protein	30.5 g
Sodium	614.3 mg
Calcium	131.6 mg
Magnesium	32.8 mg
Zinc	0.8 mg
Selenium	20.0 mcg
Potassium	309.9 mg

QUICK STEEL-CUT OATS WITH APPLES, GINGER, AND WALNUTS

Preparation time: 10 minutes • Cooking time: 8 minutes
Yield: 4 servings • 254 calories per serving, 31% from fat

INGREDIENTS

3 cups water
3 green tea tea bags, such as Tazo brand
1 cup quick-cooking steel-cut oats, such as McCann's brand
1/8 teaspoon salt
1 cup packaged unpeeled, diced fresh organic apple wedges
1/3 cup chopped walnuts, toasted
2 tablespoons finely chopped crystallized ginger
4 teaspoons organic agave nectar, such as Madhava brand

PREPARATION

Bring the water to a boil in a medium saucepan. Add the tea bags; turn off heat and let steep for 4 minutes. Discard the tea bags. Add the oats and salt to saucepan. Bring to a boil stirring once; then reduce heat to low. Cover; simmer 6 to 7 minutes or until thick, stirring once. Remove from heat; stir in the apples, walnuts, and ginger.

Nutritional Analysis per Serving	
Total Fat	9.2 g
Fat Calories	82.5
Cholesterol	0 mg
Saturated Fat	1.0 g
Polyunsaturated Fat	5.5 g
Monounsaturated Fat	1.7 g
Fiber	5.1 g
Carbohydrates	39.7 g
Sugar	10.0 g
Protein	7.1 g
Sodium	75.0 mg
Calcium	32.7 mg
Magnesium	124.9 mg
Zinc	1.6 mg
Selenium	0.5 mcg
Potassium	238.4 mg

Transfer to serving bowls; drizzle 1 teaspoon agave nectar over each serving.

SUBSTITUTIONS

One cup of diced fresh apple may replace the packaged diced fresh apple wedges, and ½ teaspoon ground ginger may replace the crystallized ginger, though the oatmeal will be less sweet.

TIP

Brewing the green tea right in the saucepan you will be using for the oats saves cleaning another container or teapot.

Nutritional Analysis per Serving	
Total Fat	6.0 g
Fat Calories	54.4
Cholesterol	116.2 mg
Saturated Fat	2.5 g
Polyunsaturated Fat	0.7 g
Monounsaturated Fat	1.0 g
Fiber	2.4 g
Carbohydrates	25.9 g
Sugar	4.2 g
Protein	12.0 g
Sodium	652.4 mg
Calcium	202.9 mg
Magnesium	52.1 mg
Zinc	0.7 mg
Selenium	11.2 mcg
Potassium	332.2 mg

SKILLET CHILAQUILES WITH CACTUS PADDLES, EGGS, AND KALE

Preparation time: 15 minutes • Cooking time: 10 minutes
Yield: 4 servings • 209 calories per serving, 26% from fat

INGREDIENTS

4 large organic egg whites
2 large organic eggs
1 1/2 cups chipotle salsa
1 cup bottled or canned nopales strips (cactus paddles), drained and rinsed
2 1/2 cups stone-ground baked tortilla chips, such as Guiltless Gourmet brand
2 cups packed finely chopped kale leaves (without stems)
1/2 cup crumbled queso añejo

PREPARATION

In a medium bowl, beat together the egg whites and eggs with a fork; set aside. Heat the salsa in a large nonstick skillet over medium-high heat until sizzling, about 1 minute. Stir in the nopales, then chips, stirring until the chips are coated with salsa. Stir in the eggs. Sprinkle the kale evenly over all. Reduce heat to medium; simmer uncovered 8 minutes or until eggs are set and kale is steamed to crisp-tender. Transfer mixture to serving plates; top with cheese.

SUBSTITUTIONS

Roasted garlic or another favorite salsa may replace the chipotle salsa and moist queso fresco may replace the drier queso añejo (both are Mexican cheeses found in most supermarkets). Fresh nopales can be found in some produce sections pre-diced or in strips: fresh substitutes well for the more widely available bottled nopales.

TIPS

One 15-ounce jar or can of nopales, drained, will equal 1 cup fresh. Nopales strips are often salty and are best rinsed in cold water and drained. If you can find it, use dinosaur (lancinato) kale: it cooks more quickly and is more tender than most kale varieties.

TANGY AND COOL BUTTERMILK AND AVOCADO BREAKFAST SMOOTHIE

Preparation time: 5 minutes • Cooking time: 0 minutes
Yield: 4 1-cup servings • 145 calories per serving, 29% from fat

INGREDIENTS

1 cup organic fat-free cottage cheese, such as Horizon or Friendship brand
2 cups 1% low-fat buttermilk
1/2 ripe avocado, peeled, seeded, and diced
1 tablespoon organic agave nectar, such as Madhava brand
4 ice cubes or 1/2 cup crushed ice

PREPARATION

Place the cottage cheese and ½ cup of the buttermilk in a blender container. Cover and blend until fairly smooth, about 30 seconds. Scrape down the sides of the blender; add the avocado. Cover and blend until fairly smooth, about 30 seconds more. Add the remaining 1½ cups of the buttermilk and the agave nectar; cover and blend 10 seconds. Add the ice; cover and blend until the smoothie is thick and ice has melted.

Nutritional Analysis per Serving	
Total Fat	4.9 g
Fat Calories	44.4
Cholesterol	10.0 mg
Saturated Fat	1.3 g
Polyunsaturated Fat	0.5 g
Monounsaturated Fat	2.5 g
Fiber	1.7 g
Carbohydrates	15.1 g
Sugar	12.4 g
Protein	11.5 g
Sodium	341.8 mg
Calcium	178.0 mg
Magnesium	7.3 mg
Zinc	0.2 mg
Selenium	0.1 mcg
Potassium	121.9 mg

Organic 1% milk may replace the buttermilk.

TIP

Haas avocados have the highest oil content and are best here, but other varieties, especially Fuerte, will also work well.

Nutritional Analysis per Serving	
Total Fat	10.7 g
Fat Calories	96.5
Cholesterol	2.5 mg
Saturated Fat	1.1 g
Polyunsaturated Fat	2.4 g
Monounsaturated Fat	4.3 g
Fiber	6.8 g
Carbohydrates	46.3 g
Sugar	11.8 g
Protein	10.3 g
Sodium	46.5 mg
Calcium	138.7 mg
Magnesium	36.4 mg
Zinc	1.1 mg
Selenium	2.2 mcg
Potassium	269.4 mg

WARM AND NUTTY CINNAMON QUINOA CEREAL

Preparation time: 5 minutes • Cooking time: 20 minutes
Yield: 4 servings • 310 calories per serving, 30% from fat

INGREDIENTS

1 cup organic 1% low-fat milk
1 cup water
1 cup organic quinoa, such as Trader Joe's or Bob's Red Mill brand
2 cups fresh blackberries (organic preferred)
1/2 teaspoon ground cinnamon
1/3 cup chopped pecans, toasted
4 teaspoons organic agave nectar, such as Madhava brand

PREPARATION

Combine the milk, water, and quinoa in a medium saucepan. Bring to a boil over high heat. Reduce the heat to medium-low; cover and simmer for 15 minutes or until most of the liquid is absorbed. Turn off heat; let stand covered for 5 minutes. Stir in the blackberries and cinnamon; transfer to four bowls and top with the pecans. Drizzle 1 teaspoon agave nectar over each serving.

SUBSTITUTIONS

Low-fat soy milk may replace the low-fat milk, blueberries may replace the blackberries, dark honey may replace the agave nectar, and walnuts may replace the pecans.

TIP

While the quinoa cooks, roast the pecans in a 350°F toaster oven for 5 to 6 minutes or in a dry skillet over medium heat for about 3 minutes.

Lunch

BROCCOLI, CHEESE, AND KALAMATA OLIVE PIZZA

Preparation time: 20 minutes • *Cooking time: 10 minutes*
Yield: 4 servings (2 slices each) • *328 calories per serving, 27% from fat*

INGREDIENTS

1 pound broccoli (with stems), finely chopped

1/2 cup thinly sliced mixed bell peppers (organic preferred)

1/2 cup thinly sliced red onion

Salt and freshly ground black pepper (optional)

1/4 cup unsalted tomato paste

1 10-ounce fully cooked whole-wheat pizza crust, such as Boboli brand

2 plum tomatoes, thinly sliced

14 kalamata olives, pitted and thinly sliced (about 1/4 cup)

2 1-ounce sticks part-skim mozzarella string cheese, pulled into shreds

3 tablespoons grated Parmigiano-Reggiano cheese

1/4 cup chopped fresh basil

Nutritional Analysis per Serving	
Total Fat	10.8 g
Fat Calories	96.7
Cholesterol	10.9 mg
Saturated Fat	4.7 g
Polyunsaturated Fat	0.6 g
Monounsaturated Fat	3.4 g
Fiber	9.9 g
Carbohydrates	47.3 g
Sugar	5.9 g
Protein	19.0 g
Sodium	745.4 mg
Calcium	317.5 mg
Magnesium	44.2 mg
Zinc	0.8 mg
Selenium	5.0 mcg
Potassium	654.2 mg

PREPARATION

Preheat the oven to 450°F. Heat a large nonstick skillet over medium-high heat until hot; coat with cooking spray. Add the broccoli, peppers, and onion; stir-fry 3 to 4 minutes or until the broccoli is crisp-tender and the peppers and onion are soft. Season to taste with salt and pepper, if desired.

Spread the tomato paste thinly over the pizza crust. Arrange the sliced tomatoes over the crust; top with broccoli mixture, olives, and strands of string cheese. Bake the pizza directly on the oven rack for about 10 minutes or until the crust is golden brown. Transfer to a cutting board; top with the Parmigiano-Reggiano cheese and basil. Cut into eight wedges.

SUBSTITUTIONS

Organic pizza sauce may replace the tomato paste. Part-skim cheddar string cheese may replace the part-skim mozzarella cheese.

TIPS

Baking the pizza directly on the oven rack produces a crispier crust. Use a large flat cookie sheet or a pizza peel to slide the pizza in and out of the oven.

Nutritional Analysis per Serving	
Total Fat	8.5 g
Fat Calories	76.3
Cholesterol	7.6 mg
Saturated Fat	2.5 g
Polyunsaturated Fat	1.0 g
Monounsaturated Fat	3.4 g
Fiber	5.4 g
Carbohydrates	32.3 g
Sugar	7.1 g
Protein	11.9 g
Sodium	725.9 mg
Calcium	305.9 mg
Magnesium	56.2 mg
Zinc	1.7 mg
Selenium	41.4 mcg
Potassium	464.2 mg

KALAMATA OLIVE AND MUSHROOM MUFFULETTA SANDWICHES

Preparation time: 15 minutes • Cooking time: 0 minutes
Yield: 4 servings • 239 calories per serving, 30% from fat

INGREDIENTS

8 ounces crimini (brown) mushrooms, sliced
1/2 cup hot or mild giardiniera (pickled vegetables), undrained
16 kalamata olives, pitted and halved
2 1-ounce sticks part-skim mozzarella string cheese, pulled into shreds
1 cup coarsely chopped watercress (organic preferred)
4 whole-wheat English muffins, split and toasted

PREPARATION

In a medium bowl, combine the mushrooms, giardiniera, olives, cheese, and watercress; mix well. Serve the mixture in muffins as a sandwich or open-faced.

SUBSTITUTIONS

Smoked mozzarella string cheese sticks or ½ cup shredded part-skim mozzarella cheese may replace the string cheese, and arugula may replace the watercress.

TIPS

Leaving some of the pickling juices clinging to the giardiniera takes the place of the oil and lemon juice used in traditional muffuletta sandwiches. Try a combination of hot and mild giardiniera for medium heat.

PASTA E FAGIOLI (PASTA AND BEAN) SOUP

Preparation time: 10 minutes • Cooking time: 15 minutes
Yield: 4 1½-cup servings • 308 calories per serving, 26% from fat

INGREDIENTS

1 small fennel bulb, untrimmed
1 teaspoon olive oil

4 garlic cloves, peeled and minced

2 cups organic low-sodium vegetable broth

1/2 cup whole-wheat medium-size pasta, such as wagon wheels or rotini

1 1/2 cups reduced-sodium spicy vegetable juice

1 14.5-ounce can organic fire-roasted diced or crushed tomatoes, such as Muir Glen brand, undrained

1 15- or 16-ounce can organic no-salt-added navy beans, drained

1/2 cup frozen peas

1/4 teaspoon crushed red pepper flakes (optional)

1/2 cup crumbled feta cheese

Nutritional Analysis per Serving	
Total Fat	9.1 g
Fat Calories	81.9
Cholesterol	25.0 mg
Saturated Fat	4.5 g
Polyunsaturated Fat	0.4 g
Monounsaturated Fat	2.1 g
Fiber	10.6 g
Carbohydrates	42.9 g
Sugar	10.3 g
Protein	14.5 g
Sodium	768.0 mg
Calcium	249.2 mg
Magnesium	73.0 mg
Zinc	2.4 mg
Selenium	5.4 mcg
Potassium	854.7 mg

PREPARATION

Cut off and reserve 2 tablespoons of the feathery fennel fronds for garnish. Chop enough of the fennel bulb to yield 1 cup. Heat the oil in a large saucepan over medium heat. Add the chopped fennel; cook for 4 minutes, stirring occasionally. Stir in the garlic; cook for 1 minute. Add the broth and pasta, then bring to a boil over high heat. Reduce heat and simmer uncovered for 5 minutes.

Stir in the vegetable juice, diced tomatoes, beans, peas, and if desired, pepper flakes. Return to a simmer; cook for 10 minutes or until pasta and fennel are tender, stirring occasionally. Ladle into shallow bowls; top with fennel fronds and feta cheese.

SUBSTITUTIONS

Chicken broth may replace the vegetable broth. Cannellini or great northern beans may replace the navy beans, and goat cheese may replace the feta cheese.

TIP

The soup will keep covered and chilled up to four days. Add additional broth if the soup becomes too thick after refrigeration.

Nutritional Analysis per Serving	
Total fat	9.8 g
Fat Calories	88.4
Cholesterol	0 mg
Saturated Fat	0.6 g
Polyunsaturated Fat	0.2g
Monounsaturated Fat	0.1 g
Fiber	7.6 g
Carbohydrates	30.5 g
Sugar	8.5 g
Protein	11.8 g
Sodium	863.8 mg
Calcium	188.4 mg
Magnesium	48.0 mg
Zinc	0.6 mg
Selenium	1.1 mcg
Potassium	685.7 mg

PORTUGUESE CALDO VERDE

Preparation time: 5 minutes • Cooking time: 30 minutes
Yield: 4 1½-cup servings • 239 calories per serving, 37% from fat

INGREDIENTS

8 ounces soy (meatless) chorizo, removed from its casing and crumbled
3/4 cup chopped yellow onion
3 cups low-sodium chicken broth
1 14.5-ounce can organic no-salt-added diced tomatoes, such as Muir Glen
*   brand, undrained*
2 cups sweet potatoes, scrubbed and cut into 3/4-inch chunks
3 cups packed coarsely chopped kale or swiss chard

PREPARATION

Cook the chorizo with the onion in a large saucepan over medium heat for 3 minutes, stirring frequently. Add the broth, tomatoes, and sweet potatoes; bring to a boil. Reduce heat; cover and simmer for 10 minutes or until vegetables are tender. Stir in kale; cover and continue to simmer for 10 minutes.

SUBSTITUTIONS

Vegetable broth may replace the chicken broth and peeled and diced butternut squash may replace the sweet potatoes (increase cooking time by 5 minutes if using butternut squash).

TIPS

Look for soy chorizo (such as Melissa brand Soyrizo) in the produce section of most supermarkets.

ROASTED RED PEPPER, WINE, AND RED LENTIL SOUP

Preparation time: 10 minutes • *Cooking time: 30 minutes*
Yield: 4 1½-cup servings • *261 calories per serving, 18% from fat*

INGREDIENTS

1 tablespoon olive oil
2 large organic carrots, thinly sliced
1 medium yellow onion, chopped
1 1/2 teaspoons Jamaican jerk seasoning
3/4 cup red lentils, such as Bob's Red Mill brand
1 cup dry white wine, such as Chenin Blanc or Chablis
1 cup water
2 cups packaged roasted red pepper soup, such as Pacific or Imagine brand
1/2 cup 2% Greek-style strained yogurt, such as Fage brand

Nutritional Analysis per Serving	
Total Fat	5.3 g
Fat Calories	47.5
Cholesterol	6.7 mg
Saturated Fat	1.5 g
Polyunsaturated Fat	1.1 g
Monounsaturated Fat	2.1 g
Fiber	3.2 g
Carbohydrates	30.8 g
Sugar	11.5 g
Protein	12.0 g
Sodium	504.0 mg
Calcium	128.2 mg
Magnesium	7.1 mg
Zinc	0.1 mg
Selenium	0.2 mcg
Potassium	155.4 mg

PREPARATION

Heat the oil in a large saucepan over medium-high heat. Add the carrots, onion, and jerk seasonings; cook for 2 minutes, stirring frequently. Stir in the lentils to coat with oil. Stir in the wine and water; bring to a boil. Reduce heat; simmer uncovered for 10 minutes. Stir in soup; return to a boil. Cover; simmer for 15 minutes or until the lentils and vegetables are tender. Ladle into shallow bowls; top with yogurt.

SUBSTITUTIONS

Sweet onion (such as Vidalia) may replace the yellow onion, and fat-free yogurt may replace the 2%.

TIPS

Organic roasted red pepper and tomato soup may be found in Whole Foods markets and many better supermarkets.

Nutritional Analysis per Serving	
Total Fat	6.9 g
Fat Calories	62.0
Cholesterol	192.9 mg
Saturated Fat	1.3 g
Polyunsaturated Fat	0.3 g
Monounsaturated Fat	0.2 g
Fiber	5.5 g
Carbohydrates	39.0 g
Sugar	2.9 g
Protein	22.8 g
Sodium	453.8 mg
Calcium	144.6 mg
Magnesium	57.9 mg
Zinc	1.4 mg
Selenium	20.5 mcg
Potassium	354.4 mg

SHRIMP AND EGG BURRITOS WITH WHITE BEANS AND CORN

Preparation time: 10 minutes • Cooking time: 5 minutes
Yield: 4 servings • 314 calories per serving, 20% from fat

INGREDIENTS

2 large organic eggs
2 large organic egg whites
2 tablespoons organic low-fat sour cream
1 cup organic no-salt-added canned navy beans, drained
1 cup frozen corn kernels
6 ounces cooked shrimp, chopped (about 1 1/4 cups)
1/2 cup tomatillo salsa or salsa verde, such as Frontera brand
4 8-inch whole-wheat flour tortillas, warmed
1/4 cup chopped cilantro

PREPARATION

In a medium bowl, beat together the eggs, egg whites, and sour cream with a fork. Heat a large nonstick skillet over medium-high heat; coat with cooking spray. Add the egg mixture; cook, stirring occasionally until eggs are soft-set, for 2 to 3 minutes. Transfer to a plate; set aside.

Add the beans, corn, shrimp, and salsa to the same skillet; mix well and heat through. Return the eggs to skillet and heat through, breaking the eggs into chunks. Spoon the mixture down the center of the tortillas; top with cilantro. Fold in the sides of the tortillas over the filling; roll up, burrito-fashion.

SUBSTITUTIONS

Bay shrimp may replace the chopped cooked shrimp, cannellini or great northern beans may replace the navy beans, and jalapeño salsa may replace the tomatillo salsa. If fresh corn is in season, cut the kernels from two large ears to replace the frozen corn.

TIPS

To warm the tortillas, stack and wrap them in a clean dish towel, moistened with a tablespoon of water. Cook on high power in the microwave oven for 30 to 40 seconds.

SPICY AND RICH SAUSAGE AND KIDNEY BEAN CHILI

Preparation time: 5 minutes • *Cooking time: 20 minutes*
Yield: 4 1¼-cup servings • *262 calories per serving, 24% from fat*

INGREDIENTS

- 1 large white onion, chopped
- 2 teaspoons olive oil
- 4 links fully cooked chipotle chicken sausage (organic preferred), cut into 1/4-inch slices (about 9 ounces)
- 1 14.5-ounce can organic no-salt-added diced tomatoes, such as Muir Glen brand, undrained
- 1/2 cup habañero-flavored salsa
- 1/2 cup brewed coffee
- 2 teaspoons dried oregano (preferably Mexican), crushed
- 1 15-ounce can organic no-salt-added kidney beans, undrained
- Optional toppings: diced ripe avocado, chopped cilantro, lime wedges

Nutritional Analysis per Serving	
Total Fat	7.2 g
Fat Calories	64.4
Cholesterol	39.9 mg
Saturated Fat	1.7 g
Polyunsaturated Fat	0.8 g
Monounsaturated Fat	1.4 g
Fiber	9.9 g
Carbohydrates	30.4 g
Sugar	6.3 g
Protein	20.1 g
Sodium	613.2 mg
Calcium	122.6 mg
Magnesium	55.4 mg
Zinc	0.9 mg
Selenium	1.3 mcg
Potassium	632.5 mg

PREPARATION

Set aside ½ cup of the onion for garnish. Cook the remaining onion in oil in a large saucepan over medium-high heat for 2 minutes. Add the chicken sausage; cook and stir for 1 minute. Add the tomatoes, salsa, coffee, and oregano; bring to a boil. Reduce heat; simmer uncovered for 10 minutes. Add the beans; return to a boil and simmer for 5 minutes. Ladle the chili into shallow bowls; top with the reserved onion and garnish as desired.

SUBSTITUTIONS

Andouille or other spicy chicken sausage may replace the chipotle chicken sausage. Jalapeño or other full-flavored salsa may replace the habañero salsa. Ordinary Greek or Italian leaf oregano can substitute for the Mexican oregano: the former are slightly sharper and less aromatic.

TIPS

For extra heat and tropical flavor, add a whole habañero chili pepper along with the canned tomatoes; remove from the chili before serving. Using the liquid from the canned kidney beans gives the chili a nicely thickened sauce.

TERIYAKI TOFU, VEGETABLES, AND BUCKWHEAT NOODLES

Nutritional Analysis per Serving	
Total Fat	13.4 g
Fat Calories	120.7
Cholesterol	0 mg
Saturated Fat	2.0 g
Polyunsaturated Fat	2.6 g
Monounsaturated Fat	2.4 g
Fiber	10.4 g
Carbohydrates	46.6 g
Sugar	9.4 g
Protein	23.5 g
Sodium	683.5 mg
Calcium	165.2 mg
Magnesium	54.5 mg
Zinc	0.9 mg
Selenium	10.0 mcg
Potassium	628.7 mg

Preparation time: 15 minutes • Cooking time: 15 minutes
Yield: 4 servings • 391 calories per serving, 30% from fat

IINGREDIENTS

4 ounces buckwheat (soba) noodles, uncooked
14 ounces organic extra-firm tofu, drained and cut into 3/4-inch cubes
3 tablespoons bottled teriyaki sauce, such as Soy Vay brand
4 teaspoons dark sesame oil
8 ounces halved small (or quartered medium) brussels sprouts
1 4-ounce package sliced exotic mushrooms, such as Pennsylvania Exotics brand
1 large red bell pepper, cored and diced (organic preferred)
1 10-ounce package frozen baby lima beans
1/2 cup organic low-sodium vegetable broth
2 teaspoons sesame seeds, toasted

PREPARATION

Cook the noodles according to package directions, reducing cooking time by 1 minute. Meanwhile, combine the tofu and teriyaki sauce; set aside.

Heat 2 teaspoons of the oil in a large, deep sauté pan or skillet over medium-high heat. Add the brussels sprouts, mushrooms, and bell pepper; stir-fry for 3 minutes. Add the lima beans; stir-fry for 3 minutes. Add the broth; bring to a simmer and cook for 3 minutes or until vegetables are crisp-tender. Stir in the tofu mixture; heat through. Stir in the drained noodles; cook for 1 minute. Transfer to four shallow bowls; drizzle with the remaining 2 teaspoons sesame oil and top with the sesame seeds.

SUBSTITUTIONS

Two cups of frozen shelled edamame may replace the frozen lima beans. Seasoned baked tofu may replace the extra-firm tofu, and sliced crimini mushrooms (sometimes called baby bellas) may replace the sliced exotic mixed mushrooms.

TIPS

Extra-firm tofu or baked tofu may come in Asian or Thai flavors—any will work well in this recipe. Orgran brand buckwheat noodles are gluten-free and are Australian instead of Japanese.

TOASTED WALNUT AND CREAMY WHITE BEAN PITAS

Preparation time: 15 minutes • Cooking time: 0 minutes
Yield: 4 servings • 334 calories per serving, 22% from fat

INGREDIENTS

1 small garlic clove, peeled
1 15-ounce can organic no-salt-added navy, great northern, or cannellini
    beans, drained
2 teaspoons walnut oil
2 teaspoons lemon juice
1 teaspoon chopped fresh rosemary
1/4 teaspoon salt
1/4 teaspoon freshly ground black pepper
4 6-inch whole-wheat pita bread rounds
3 cups coarsely chopped watercress (organic preferred)
1 cup organic grape or cherry tomatoes, halved
3 tablespoons chopped walnuts, toasted

Nutritional Analysis per Serving	
Total Fat	8.5 g
Fat Calories	76.5
Cholesterol	0 mg
Saturated Fat	0.8 g
Polyunsaturated Fat	4.7 g
Monounsaturated Fat	1.3 g
Fiber	12.8 g
Carbohydrates	55.7 g
Sugar	2.6 g
Protein	12.5 g
Sodium	537.8 mg
Calcium	115.2 mg
Magnesium	105.8 mg
Zinc	3.2 mg
Selenium	28.7 mcg
Potassium	549.1 mg

PREPARATION

With the motor running, drop the garlic clove through the tube of a food processor; process until minced. Add the beans, walnut oil, lemon juice, rosemary, salt, and pepper; process with on/off pulses until smooth, scraping down the sides of the work bowl once.

Cut each pita bread round in half crosswise; open into pockets. Combine the watercress, cherry tomatoes, and walnuts; stuff the pockets with half of the mixture. Spoon the bean mixture into pockets; top with the remaining watercress mixture.

SUBSTITUTIONS

Extra-virgin olive oil may replace the walnut oil. Arugula may replace the watercress. Pecans may replace the walnuts, and white balsamic vinegar may replace the lemon juice.

TIP

Toast the walnuts in a toaster oven at 350° F for about 5 minutes or until fragrant.

Dinner

Nutritional Analysis per Serving	
Total Fat	6.7 g
Fat Calories	60.7
Cholesterol	61.0 mg
Saturated Fat	2.1 g
Polyunsaturated Fat	0.4 g
Monounsaturated Fat	1.6 g
Fiber	3.0 g
Carbohydrates	11.5 g
Sugar	7.3 g
Protein	24.0 g
Sodium	709.0 mg
Calcium	68.8 mg
Magnesium	50.9 mg
Zinc	4.2 mg
Selenium	30.3 mcg
Potassium	719.2 mg

BISON STEAK AND BROCCOLI SALAD

Preparation time: 10 minutes • *Cooking time: 10 minutes*
Yield: 4 servings • *202 calories per serving, 30% from fat*

INGREDIENTS

1/3 cup bottled teriyaki sauce, such as Soy Vay brand

2 teaspoons dark sesame oil

2 teaspoons peeled, finely grated fresh ginger

1 pound organic well-trimmed boneless bison sirloin steak, thawed if frozen

2 cups broccoli florets

1 tablespoon rice vinegar

6 cups packed mesclun or spring mix salad greens (organic preferred)

1 cup broccoli sprouts

PREPARATION

Combine the teriyaki sauce, sesame oil, and ginger in a large bowl. Spoon 2 tablespoons of the mixture over both sides of the steak; let stand for 5 minutes. Meanwhile, place the broccoli in a microwave-safe bowl. Cover with waxed paper; cook on high power for 2 to 3 minutes or until crisp-tender. Add to the bowl with the teriyaki mixture; toss well and set aside.

Grill the steak over medium-hot coals or over medium-high heat on a gas grill or broil in the oven for 3 to 4 minutes per side for rare depending on the thickness of steak (do not overcook or the meat will be tough). Transfer the steak to a carving board; let stand 5 minutes.

Add the vinegar to the broccoli mixture; toss. Add the salad greens; toss well and transfer to four serving plates. Carve the steak crosswise into thin slices and arrange over the salads. Top with the broccoli sprouts.

SUBSTITUTIONS

A well-trimmed, grass-fed boneless beef top sirloin steak may replace the bison. Sherry vinegar may replace the rice vinegar.

Bison may be found at Whole Foods or Trader Joe's grocery stores, on the Web at WildIdeaBuffalo.com and RockyMountainBuffalo .com, or special-ordered from better supermarkets.

BUTTERNUT BARLEY RISOTTO WITH GOAT CHEESE AND TOASTED ALMONDS

Preparation time: 10 minutes • Cooking time: 18 minutes
Yield: 4 servings • 247 calories per serving, 27% from fat

INGREDIENTS

3 cups water

3 green tea tea bags, such as Tazo brand

1 cup quick-cooking pearled barley, such as Mother's brand

3 cups 1/2-inch diced butternut squash (about 12 ounces)

2 teaspoons Madras curry powder, or other spicy Indian curry powder

3/4 teaspoon salt

1/2 cup crumbled goat cheese

1/4 cup sliced unblanched almonds, toasted

PREPARATION

Bring the water to a boil in a medium saucepan over high heat (or in a 1-quart Pyrex measuring cup in the microwave oven). Add the tea bags; turn off the heat and let steep for 5 minutes. Remove and discard the tea bags.

Toast the barley in a dry sauté pan or deep skillet over medium-high heat for 2 to 3 minutes, stirring occasionally. Add the squash, 1 cup of the tea, the curry, and the salt. Simmer, stirring frequently, until the tea is absorbed, 3 to 4 minutes. Add additional tea by half cupfuls, simmering until the tea is absorbed before adding additional liquid. This should take 12 to 14 minutes. When the barley and squash are tender and all tea has been incorporated, remove from heat. (The barley should be on the wet side to make a creamy sauce; if it is dry, stir in a little hot water.) Stir in the goat cheese until melted and creamy. Transfer to serving plates; top with almonds.

Nutritional Analysis per Serving	
Total Fat	7.8 g
Fat Calories	70.4
Cholesterol	11.2 mg
Saturated Fat	3.2 g
Polyunsaturated Fat	0.9 g
Monounsaturated Fat	2.9 g
Fiber	7.2 g
Carbohydrates	39.4 g
Sugar	2.3 g
Protein	9.0 g
Sodium	513.1 mg
Calcium	99.9 mg
Magnesium	50.2 mg
Zinc	0.4 mg
Selenium	1.2 mcg
Potassium	433.3 mg

SUBSTITUTIONS

Turmeric may replace the curry powder, and feta cheese may replace the goat cheese (but it will not melt completely).

TIP

Look for packages of peeled, cut-up butternut squash in the fresh produce section of better supermarkets. The cubes are large and will need to be cut into half-inch pieces.

Nutritional Analysis per Serving	
Total Fat	10.5 g
Fat Calories	94.4
Cholesterol	89.6 mg
Saturated Fat	1.6 g
Polyunsaturated Fat	4.2 g
Monounsaturated Fat	3.4 g
Fiber	2.0 g
Carbohydrates	20.2 g
Sugar	14.3 g
Protein	32.6 g
Sodium	363.5 mg
Calcium	34.6 mg
Magnesium	55.0 mg
Zinc	1.2 mg
Selenium	59.2 mcg
Potassium	877.9 mg

CEDAR-PLANKED ROASTED SALMON WITH CANDIED GINGER AND BERRY SALSA

Preparation time: 15 minutes • Cooking time: 12 minutes
Yield: 4 servings • 309 calories per serving, 31% from fat

INGREDIENTS

3 tablespoons organic seedless raspberry preserves
2 tablespoons fresh lime juice
1/2 cup each: fresh blueberries, raspberries, and sliced strawberries (organic preferred)
2 tablespoons finely chopped red onion
1 tablespoon finely chopped crystallized ginger
4 5-ounce fresh Alaskan king salmon fillets, skin on
1/2 teaspoon sea salt

PREPARATION

Cover a cedar plank in cold water for at least 15 minutes. Preheat the oven to 450°F. Combine the preserves and lime juice in a medium bowl; mix well. Transfer 2 tablespoons of the mixture to a small bowl. Add the berries, onion, and ginger to remaining mixture in the bowl; toss and set aside.

Drain the cedar plank. Place the salmon, skin sides down, on the plank. Sprinkle with salt and spread the reserved preserve mixture evenly over the salmon. Roast in oven for 10 to 12 minutes or until salmon is opaque in center. Transfer the salmon to serving plates; top with ginger and berry salsa.

One 10-ounce package frozen mixed organic berries, such as Whole Foods 365 or Cascadian Farm brand, thawed and well drained, may replace the fresh berries.

TIP

Purchase cedar planks (about 12 × 6 inches and about ½ inch thick) at your local hardware store, Whole Foods markets, or better cookware shops. They are usually sold four to a package for about $15. (The plank will become dark and give off a lovely fragrance as it perfumes the fish while it bakes and may be reused if not too charred.) A less expensive option is to visit your local lumber store and ask for an untreated 8-foot cedar plank (around $12) cut into eight 1-foot sections.

CHEESE RAVIOLI WITH TOFU AND BABY PEAS

Preparation time: 5 minutes • Cooking time: 15 minutes
Yield: 4 servings • 307 calories per serving, 31% from fat

INGREDIENTS

1 1/2 cups low-sodium chicken broth

2 teaspoons chili garlic sauce or puree

1 9-ounce package refrigerated whole-wheat cheese-filled ravioli

2 cups low-sodium vegetable juice

1 cup frozen peas

8 ounces organic firm tofu, drained and cut into 3/4-inch cubes

2 tablespoons chopped fresh basil

Nutritional Analysis per Serving	
Total Fat	10.4 g
Fat Calories	93.9
Cholesterol	42.5 mg
Saturated Fat	4.2 g
Polyunsaturated Fat	0.01 g
Monounsaturated Fat	0 g
Fiber	6.3 g
Carbohydrates	35.6 g
Sugar	5.8 g
Protein	17.8 g
Sodium	821.1 mg
Calcium	175.6 mg
Magnesium	1.1 mg
Zinc	0.01 mg
Selenium	0 mcg
Potassium	456.1 mg

PREPARATION

Combine the chicken broth and chili garlic sauce in a large saucepan; bring to a boil over high heat. Stir the ravioli into the broth mixture. Reduce heat; cover and simmer for 6 to 8 minutes or until the ravioli are tender. Pour in the vegetable juice; bring to a simmer. Stir in pcas; simmer until heated through, about 2 minutes. Stir in the tofu; heat through. Ladle into shallow bowls; top with basil.

Vegetable broth may replace the chicken broth, and flavored tofu (such as White Wave Mediterranean–flavored tofu) may replace the regular tofu. Flat leaf parsley may replace the basil. Whole-wheat tortellini may replace the ravioli.

TIPS

Look for whole-wheat ravioli, such as Buitoni brand, in the refrigerated section of the supermarket.

CIOPPINO

Preparation time: 10 minutes • Cooking time: 15 minutes
Yield: 4 1½-cup servings • 256 calories per serving, 21% from fat

Nutritional Analysis per Serving	
Total Fat	5.8 g
Fat Calories	52.3
Cholesterol	41.9 mg
Saturated Fat	0.9 g
Polyunsaturated Fat	1.0 g
Monounsaturated Fat	3.3 g
Fiber	2.5 g
Carbohydrates	18.4 g
Sugar	8.8 g
Protein	24.9 g
Sodium	697.9 mg
Calcium	92.3 mg
Magnesium	84.2 mg
Zinc	0.9 mg
Selenium	33.9 mcg
Potassium	559.8 mg

INGREDIENTS

1 tablespoon olive oil

1 cup chopped sweet yellow onion

4 garlic cloves, peeled and minced

2 14.5-ounce cans organic fire-roasted diced tomatoes, such as Muir Glen brand, drained

1 cup low-sodium chicken broth

1/2 cup fruity red wine, such as Syrah

2 teaspoons Old Bay seasoning

1/4 teaspoon crushed red pepper flakes (optional)

8 ounces each: Pacific halibut fillet, skinned and cut into 1-inch chunks, and bay scallops

2 tablespoons chopped fresh flat-leaf parsley

PREPARATION

Heat the oil in a large deep skillet over medium-high heat. Add the onion; cook for 5 minutes, stirring occasionally. Add the garlic and cook 1 minute longer. Add the tomatoes, broth, wine, and seasonings; bring to a boil. Reduce heat; simmer uncovered for 8 minutes, stirring occasionally.

Stir in the halibut and scallops; cook until opaque, about 5 minutes. Ladle into shallow bowls; top with parsley.

Merlot may replace the Syrah; crumbled bay leaves and dried thyme may replace the Old Bay seasoning; mahimahi may replace the halibut, and uncooked shrimp may replace the scallops.

TIP

Look for Old Bay seasoning in the spice aisle of the supermarket.

CUMIN-CRUSTED SALMON OVER SILKY SWEET POTATOES

Preparation time: 15 minutes • Cooking time: 15 minutes
Yield: 4 servings • 406 calories per serving, 35% from fat

Nutritional Analysis per Serving	
Total Fat	15.9 g
Fat Calories	142.7
Cholesterol	69.2 mg
Saturated Fat	2.6 g
Polyunsaturated Fat	2.8 g
Monounsaturated Fat	5.4 g
Fiber	5.8 g
Carbohydrates	39.9 g
Sugar	7.4 g
Protein	27.2 g
Sodium	636.7 mg
Calcium	116.9 mg
Magnesium	99.0 mg
Zinc	1.6 mg
Selenium	36.5 mcg
Potassium	1,057.7 mg

INGREDIENTS

2 large or 3 medium sweet potatoes, scrubbed and cut into 3/4-inch chunks
(about 1 1/2 pounds)
2 teaspoons cumin seeds
2 teaspoons ground cardamom
3/4 teaspoon salt
4 5-ounce fresh Alaskan king salmon fillets, skin on
1/2 cup packaged sweet potato soup
2 tablespoons pepitas (pumpkin seeds), toasted

PREPARATION

Preheat the oven to 425° F. Steam or microwave the sweet potatoes in a medium bowl until very tender (8 to 10 minutes for steamed, 4 to 5 minutes for microwaved).

Sprinkle the cumin seeds, cardamom, and ¼ teaspoon of the salt over the meaty sides of the salmon. Heat a large oven-proof non-stick skillet over medium-high heat until hot. Coat with cooking spray. Add the salmon, seasoned sides down; cook for 3 minutes or until browned. Turn the fillets over; place the skillet in the oven, and bake for 8 to 10 minutes or until the salmon is opaque in the center.

Add the soup and the remaining ½ teaspoon salt to the hot cooked sweet potatoes. Mash with a potato masher to desired consistency. Transfer to serving plates; top with the salmon and pepitas.

Butternut squash soup may replace the sweet potato soup, and toasted sliced almonds may replace the pepitas.

TIP

For a spicier flavor, add 1 teaspoon chipotle hot pepper sauce, such as Tabasco brand, or ¼ teaspoon cayenne pepper to the sweet potatoes.

Nutritional Analysis per Serving	
Total Fat	7.1 g
Fat Calories	63.6
Cholesterol	35.4 mg
Saturated Fat	1.1
Polyunsaturated Fat	1.6 g
Monounsaturated Fat	1.6 g
Fiber	5.5 g
Carbohydrates	34.7 g
Sugar	4.7 g
Protein	33.8 g
Sodium	512.7 mg
Calcium	69.5 mg
Magnesium	16.7 mg
Zinc	0.6 mg
Selenium	2.5 mcg
Potassium	218.6 mg

CURRIED TURKEY TENDERLOIN WITH PENNE AND ROASTED ASPARAGUS

Preparation time: 15 minutes • Cooking time: 12 minutes
Yield: 4 servings • 330 calories per serving, 19% from fat

INGREDIENTS

6 ounces multigrain penne, such as Barilla PLUS brand (about 2 cups)
12 ounces organic turkey tenderloin, cut into 1-inch chunks
2 teaspoons Madras curry powder
3 cups asparagus spears, cut into 1-inch pieces
3 teaspoons dark sesame oil
1/2 cup 2% Greek-style strained yogurt, such as Fage brand
3/4 teaspoon sea salt
Toasted sesame seeds (optional)

PREPARATION

Preheat the oven to 450°F. Cook the penne according to the package directions. Meanwhile, toss the turkey chunks with the curry powder in a large bowl. Add the asparagus and 1 teaspoon of the oil; toss well. Spread the mixture into a single layer on a 15 × 10-inch jelly roll pan. Bake for 10 minutes or until the turkey is no longer pink in the center and the asparagus is crisp-tender.

Drain the penne and return to same pot. Add the yogurt and toss well. Add the turkey mixture; toss again. Transfer to serving plates; top with sea salt and the remaining 2 teaspoons of the oil. Garnish as desired.

Kosher salt may replace the sea salt, drained low-fat yogurt may replace the 2% yogurt, and turmeric may replace the curry powder.

TIP

Sprinkling the salt and drizzling the last 2 teaspoons of the sesame oil over the dish gives more of a fresh pop in flavor than simply stirring these ingredients in during cooking.

GINGER PEANUT GRILLED CHICKEN WITH SWEET POTATOES AND SUGAR SNAP PEAS

Preparation time: 15 minutes • Cooking time: 10 minutes
Yield: 4 servings • 324 calories per serving, 13% from fat

INGREDIENTS

1/2 cup ginger peanut dipping and cooking sauce, such as the Ginger People brand
4 4-ounce boneless, skinless chicken breast halves
1 large or 2 small sweet potatoes, scrubbed and cut into 3/4-inch chunks (about 1 pound)
8 ounces fresh sugar snap peas
3/4 teaspoon sea salt
1/4 cup chopped fresh cilantro

Nutritional Analysis per Serving	
Total Fat	4.4 g
Fat Calories	39.7
Cholesterol	65.8 mg
Saturated Fat	1.4 g
Polyunsaturated Fat	0.3 g
Monounsaturated Fat	0.3 g
Fiber	4.9 g
Carbohydrates	37.6 g
Sugar	9.1 g
Protein	31.3 g
Sodium	671.7 mg
Calcium	91.0 mg
Magnesium	32.1 mg
Zinc	0.9 mg
Selenium	20.2 mcg
Potassium	591.1 mg

PREPARATION

Prepare the charcoal or gas grill, or preheat the broiler. Place ¼ cup of the ginger peanut sauce in a large bowl; set aside. Spread the remaining sauce evenly over both sides of the chicken.

Place the sweet potatoes in a steamer over simmering water for 4 minutes. Add the peas; steam 2 to 3 minutes longer or until the vegetables are tender. Transfer 2 tablespoons of the steaming water to bowl with the ginger peanut sauce; mix well. Add the vegetables to bowl; toss with the sauce.

Meanwhile, grill the chicken over medium heat on a covered grill or broil 4 to 5 inches from a heat source for 4 minutes per side or until the chicken is cooked through. Transfer the vegetables to serving plates; top with the chicken. Rub the salt between your fingers, sprinkling it over the dish, and top with cilantro.

SUBSTITUTIONS

Kosher salt may replace sea salt, and chopped basil or tarragon may replace the cilantro.

TIP

Look for the Ginger People brand ginger peanut dipping and cooking sauce by the marinades in the supermarket.

Nutritional Analysis per Serving	
Total Fat	8.6 g
Fat Calories	77.2
Cholesterol	83.6 mg
Saturated Fat	1.6 g
Polyunsaturated Fat	3.3 g
Monounsaturated Fat	3.1 g
Fiber	3.6 g
Carbohydrates	15.0 g
Sugar	10.5 g
Protein	31.3 g
Sodium	511.1 mg
Calcium	153.3 mg
Magnesium	59.7 mg
Zinc	1.7 mg
Selenium	18.5 mcg
Potassium	952.2 mg

GRILLED CITRUS TROUT OVER CRUNCHY MEDITERRANEAN SLAW

Preparation time: 15 minutes • Cooking time: 8 minutes
Yield: 4 servings • 264 calories per serving, 29% from fat

INGREDIENTS

2 large oranges, peeled
3 tablespoons reduced-sodium soy sauce
1 tablespoon dark sesame oil
4 6- to 8-ounce fresh whole rainbow trout, dressed and deboned
3 cups packaged coleslaw mix

PREPARATION

Prepare a charcoal or gas grill, or preheat your oven's broiler. Coarsely chop the oranges, saving their juice. Measure 2 tablespoons of the juice (squeeze the chopped oranges gently to extract juice if necessary) into a large bowl. Add the soy sauce and sesame oil; mix well. Remove 2 tablespoons of the mixture for brushing over the trout. Open the trout like a book. Brush 1 tablespoon of the reserved mixture over the open, skinless trout.

Grill the trout, covered, with skin sides down, on an oiled grill, or broil 5 inches from the heat source in a broiler for 3 minutes. Brush the remaining reserved tablespoon of the soy sauce mixture over the fish. Continue grilling or broiling for 3 to 4 minutes or until the trout is opaque in its center.

Add the chopped oranges and coleslaw mix to the soy sauce mixture in a large bowl. Toss well and transfer to four serving plates. Serve with the trout.

SUBSTITUTION

Salmon may replace the rainbow trout.

TIP

Ask your fish retailer to dress the fish, which means removing the heads and tails from each whole trout, and to debone them.

HEALTHY REAL HAMBURGERS

Preparation time: 10 minutes • Cooking time: 10 minutes
Yield: 4 servings • 296 calories per serving, 32% from fat

INGREDIENTS

    2 teaspoons olive oil
    2 garlic cloves, peeled
    1/2 teaspoon each: salt and freshly ground black pepper
    1 teaspoon dried oregano (Mexican preferred), crushed
    1 pound well-trimmed grass-fed (preferably organic) beef chuck steak,
        ground
    4 whole-wheat hamburger buns, split
    1/2 ripe avocado, peeled, seeded, and cut into 8 slices
    4 organic romaine lettuce leaves
    4 slices organic tomato
    Optional garnishes: salsa, spicy brown mustard, ketchup, giardiniera, or
        pepperoncini peppers

Nutritional Analysis per Serving	
Total Fat	10.9 g
Fat Calories	98.0
Cholesterol	60.0 mg
Saturated Fat	2.9 g
Polyunsaturated Fat	1.9 g
Monounsaturated Fat	5.0 g
Fiber	5.6 g
Carbohydrates	26.5 g
Sugar	4.7 g
Protein	26.8 g
Sodium	565.3 mg
Calcium	62.7 mg
Magnesium	46.9 mg
Zinc	5.6 mg
Selenium	21.6 mcg
Potassium	299.0 mg

PREPARATION

Using a folded paper towel, oil a grill or grill pan with the olive oil. Coarsely chop the garlic on a chopping board. Sprinkle the salt over the garlic; use the side of the knife to "cream" the garlic into a paste. Sprinkle on the pepper and oregano and mash them into the paste. Combine the mixture with the ground chuck, mixing lightly. Form the mixture into four ½-inch-thick patties.

Place the burgers on the grill or grill pan over medium-high heat. Grill covered 5 minutes. Turn the patties; continue grilling covered 3 to 4 minutes for medium doneness. Place buns cut sides down on grill during the last minute of cooking to lightly toast them. Serve the patties in buns, with avocado slices, lettuce, tomato, and optional garnishes.

SUBSTITUTIONS

Texturized vegetable protein (made from soy) can substitute for one-quarter of the beef; it will reduce saturated fat and any heterocyclic amines. Ground grass-fed, preferably organically raised beef tenderloin can substitute for a quarter of the ground chuck, but the patties will cook more quickly and be slightly dry.

TIPS

Choose a chuck steak that has the visible fat from around its edges trimmed off. Have your meat retailer grind the steak for you. To grind it yourself, cut the steak into chunks and process with on/off pulses until finely chopped in a large food processor. Do not overmix the meat when forming into patties as that can make the burgers tough.

Nutritional Analysis per Serving	
Total Fat	1.4 g
Fat Calories	12.8
Cholesterol	65.8 mg
Saturated Fat	0.4 g
Polyunsaturated Fat	0.3 g
Monounsaturated Fat	0.3 g
Fiber	0.1 g
Carbohydrates	4.9 g
Sugar	4.0 g
Protein	26.3 g
Sodium	433.9 mg
Calcium	13.9 mg
Magnesium	32.4 mg
Zinc	0.9 mg
Selenium	20.3 mcg
Potassium	297.6 mg

HONEYED CHINESE CHICKEN BREASTS

Preparation time: 10 minutes • Cooking time: 10 minutes
Yield: 4 servings • 143 calories per serving, 9% from fat

INGREDIENTS

3 tablespoons oyster sauce

2 teaspoons peeled, minced fresh ginger

1 teaspoon chili garlic sauce or puree

4 boneless, skinless chicken breast halves (about 4 ounces each)

1 tablespoon dark honey

1 tablespoon reduced-sodium soy sauce

PREPARATION

Prepare a charcoal or gas grill or preheat your oven's broiler. Combine the oyster sauce, ginger, and chili garlic sauce; mix well. Transfer 1 tablespoon of the mixture to a small bowl; set aside.

Spread the remaining mixture over both sides of the chicken; let stand 5 to 10 minutes.

Grill or broil the chicken for 4 to 5 minutes per side or until the chicken is cooked through. Add the honey and soy sauce to the reserved oyster sauce mixture; mix well. Serve as a dipping sauce for the chicken.

SUBSTITUTION

Bottled minced ginger may replace the fresh.

TIP

When honey is added to a marinade, there is a chance it will burn during grilling. Adding honey to the reserved marinade for a dipping sauce is a sweet solution to the problem.

PARMIGIANO CAESAR SALAD WITH SHRIMP

Preparation time: 20 minutes • Cooking time: 0 minutes
Yield: 4 servings • 197 calories per serving, 34% from fat

INGREDIENTS

2 slices whole-wheat bread
1 1/2 tablespoons each: fresh lemon juice and walnut oil
1 tablespoon Worcestershire sauce
1 garlic clove, peeled and minced
1/2 teaspoon anchovy paste (optional)
8 ounces cooked medium shrimp
8 cups packed torn organic romaine lettuce (about 12 ounces)
2 tablespoons grated or finely shredded Parmigiano-Reggiano cheese

Nutritional Analysis per Serving	
Total Fat	7.5 g
Fat Calories	67.7
Cholesterol	112.8 mg
Saturated Fat	1.1 g
Polyunsaturated Fat	3.7 g
Monounsaturated Fat	1.5 g
Fiber	3.5 g
Carbohydrates	16.4 g
Sugar	4.9 g
Protein	16.3 g
Sodium	436.4 mg
Calcium	143.6 mg
Magnesium	37.4 mg
Zinc	1.3 mg
Selenium	23.4 mcg
Potassium	428.8 mg

PREPARATION

Preheat the oven to 450° F. Lightly coat a cookie or baking sheet with olive oil cooking spray. For the croutons, cut the bread into ½-inch squares and coat with the cooking spray. Bake for 7 to 8 minutes or until crisp; set aside.

Meanwhile, combine the lemon juice, walnut oil, Worcestershire sauce, garlic, and if desired, anchovy paste in a large bowl. Remove 1 tablespoon of the dressing and toss it with shrimp in a small bowl. Let the shrimp stand at least 5 minutes or refrigerate for up to 1 hour.

Add the lettuce and croutons to the dressing in the large bowl; toss well and transfer to four serving plates. Top the salads with shrimp and sprinkle with cheese.

SUBSTITUTION

Shredded, cooked skinless chicken breast may replace the shrimp.

TIPS

Look for whole-wheat flour or wheat berries as the first ingredient on the package of whole-wheat bread (or multigrain bread). Avoid packages that state wheat flour or enriched wheat flour as the first ingredient: *enriched* simply means that a few stolen vitamins are added back. While preparing salad, chill serving bowls or plates in the freezer or refrigerator.

Nutritional Analysis per Serving	
Total Fat	4.2 g
Fat Calories	37.9
Cholesterol	10.0 mg
Saturated Fat	1.8 g
Polyunsaturated Fat	0.04 g
Monounsaturated Fat	0.02 g
Fiber	10.1 g
Carbohydrates	51.2 g
Sugar	7.7 g
Protein	12.5 g
Sodium	883.2 mg
Calcium	158.4 mg
Magnesium	5.4 mg
Zinc	0.1 mg
Selenium	0.01 mcg
Potassium	115.7 mg

PINTO BEAN AND CHEESE ENCHILADAS WITH ROASTED TOMATO SALSA

Preparation time: 20 minutes • Cooking time: 6 minutes
Yield: 4 servings • 298 calories per serving, 13% from fat

INGREDIENTS

1 15-ounce can fat-free refried pinto beans
1 large ripe tomato, chopped
1/4 cup plus 2 tablespoons chopped fresh cilantro
1 teaspoon ground cumin
1 12-ounce jar roasted tomato salsa (about 1 3/4 cups)
8 6- to 7-inch corn tortillas, warmed to soften
1/2 cup reduced-fat shredded Mexican cheese blend
Optional garnishes: diced avocado, low-fat sour cream

PREPARATION

Preheat the broiler. In a microwave-safe glass bowl, combine the beans, tomato, ¼ cup of the cilantro, cumin, and ½ cup of the salsa; mix well. Cover the bowl with waxed paper; cook in the microwave oven on high power until heated through, about 2 minutes.

Spoon ¼ cup of the salsa over bottom of 13 × 9-inch baking pan or Pyrex dish. Spoon about ⅓ cup of the hot bean mixture down the center of each tortilla; roll up and place seam side down in the baking pan. Spread the remaining cup of salsa evenly over tortillas. Broil 5 to 6 inches from heat until heated through, 5 to 6 minutes. Sprinkle the cheese and remaining 2 tablespoons cilantro over enchiladas. Broil 30 seconds or until the cheese is melted. Garnish with avocado and sour cream if desired.

SUBSTITUTIONS

Whole-wheat flour tortillas may replace the corn tortillas and, because they are pliable, do not have to be warmed before filling. Adding optional garnishes of a half of a ripe avocado (diced), and ¼ cup reduced-fat sour cream to the recipe will increase the calories for each serving to 358 and calories from fat to 23%.

TIPS

Look for Bearitos brand fat-free green chili organic refried beans in most supermarkets. Trader Joe's Lite Shredded 3 Cheese Blend "made from cows not treated with rBST" is a good choice for cheese.

Nutritional Analysis per Serving	
Total Fat	4.9 g
Fat Calories	43.7
Cholesterol	49.3 mg
Saturated Fat	0.8 g
Polyunsaturated Fat	0.7 g
Monounsaturated Fat	2.7 g
Fiber	5.4 g
Carbohydrates	24.1 g
Sugar	4.7 g
Protein	22.5 g
Sodium	694.9 mg
Calcium	53.0 mg
Magnesium	35.9 mg
Zinc	1.0 mg
Selenium	15.8 mcg
Potassium	532.6 mg

RED POZOLE WITH SHREDDED CHICKEN AND AVOCADO

Preparation time: 10 minutes • Cooking time: 15 minutes
Yield: 4 1⅓-cup servings • 241 calories per serving, 19% from fat

INGREDIENTS

2 teaspoons olive oil

1 cup thinly sliced organic carrots

5 garlic cloves, peeled and minced

1 1/2 cups roasted red pepper and garlic salsa, such as Frontera brand

1 3/4 cups no-salt-added beef broth

1 15-ounce can golden or white hominy, drained

1 teaspoon dried oregano (Mexican preferred), crushed

2 cups shredded or diced skinless cooked chicken breast

1/2 ripe avocado, peeled, seeded, and diced

Optional garnishes: lime wedges and chopped fresh oregano, cilantro, or the
    Mexican herb epazote

PREPARATION

Heat the oil in a large saucepan over medium-high heat. Add the carrots; cook for 2 minutes, stirring occasionally. Add the garlic; cook for 1 minute. Add the salsa; cook and stir for 1 minute. Add the broth, hominy, and oregano; bring to a boil. Reduce heat; simmer uncovered for 8 minutes or until carrots are tender. Stir in the chicken; heat through about a minute. Ladle into shallow bowls; top with avocado and garnish as desired.

SUBSTITUTION

Italian oregano may replace the Mexican oregano for slightly sweeter, less sharp flavor. Roasted tomato salsa may replace the roasted red pepper salsa.

TIPS

A rotisserie-roasted chicken is perfect for this recipe. Remove the skin and bones and shred the breast meat. Reserve the rest of the chicken for another meal. Using a high-quality salsa, such as Frontera brand, gives this quick-cooking dish the best flavor.

ROASTED TURKEY TENDERLOIN STUFFED WITH CRANBERRIES AND PECANS

Preparation time: 15 minutes • Cooking time: 15 minutes
Yield: 4 servings • 303 calories per serving, 34% from fat

Nutritional Analysis per Serving	
Total Fat	11.9 g
Fat Calories	107.2
Cholesterol	45.0 mg
Saturated Fat	1.1 g
Polyunsaturated Fat	1.9 g
Monounsaturated Fat	4.7 g
Fiber	2.9 g
Carbohydrates	21.0 g
Sugar	10.4 g
Protein	30.5 g
Sodium	197.1 mg
Calcium	47.5 mg
Magnesium	10.0 mg
Zinc	0.4 mg
Selenium	0.3 mcg
Potassium	75.1 mg

INGREDIENTS

2 8-ounce organically raised turkey tenderloins
1/4 cup mesquite marinade, such as Mrs. Dash brand
2 teaspoons olive oil
1/4 cup finely chopped red onion
1/3 cup low-sodium chicken broth
1/3 cup dried sweetened cranberries
2 slices honey whole-wheat bread, cubed and toasted
1/4 cup chopped pecans, toasted

PREPARATION

Preheat the oven to 450° F. To butterfly the tenderloins, cut each tenderloin in half lengthwise almost through to the other side; open them like a book. Use a meat mallet to pound the tenderloins to half-inch thickness. Turn the tenderloins over; brush the marinade evenly over the surface. Transfer the tenderloins, marinated sides down, to a foil-lined 15 × 10-inch jelly roll pan or baking sheet with sides; set aside while preparing the stuffing.

Heat the oil in a large nonstick skillet over medium-high heat. Add the onion; cook for 2 minutes. Add the broth and cranberries; simmer for 2 minutes or until the cranberries are plumped. Add the toasted bread cubes and pecans; mix well. Spoon the mixture onto half of each opened tenderloin. Close the other side of the tenderloin, covering the stuffing. Use a rubber spatula to scrape any marinade from the foil back over the top of the tenderloins. Bake for 15 minutes or until the turkey is cooked through (internal temperature reaches 165° F.). Slice each of the two tenderloins crosswise in half; transfer to four serving plates.

SUBSTITUTIONS

Golden raisins or sultanas may replace the dried cranberries. A thick barbecue sauce may replace the mesquite marinade.

Lining the jelly roll pan with foil will substantially reduce cleanup time. Mrs. Dash makes a great mesquite marinade.

ROASTED WINTER VEGETABLES WITH CRANBERRY-STUDDED QUINOA

Preparation time: 10 minutes • Cooking time: 20 minutes
Yield: 4 servings • 359 calories per serving, 31% from fat

Nutritional Analysis per Serving	
Total Fat	13.0 g
Fat Calories	117.3
Cholesterol	12.6 mg
Saturated Fat	3.5 g
Polyunsaturated Fat	0.9 g
Monounsaturated Fat	3.4 g
Fiber	6.6 g
Carbohydrates	47.8 g
Sugar	16.6 g
Protein	17.9 g
Sodium	359.7 mg
Calcium	192.2 mg
Magnesium	28.2 mg
Zinc	1.0 mg
Selenium	3.5 mcg
Potassium	527.8 mg

INGREDIENTS

1 1/2 cups low-sodium chicken broth

3/4 cup organic quinoa, such as Trader Joe's or Bob's Red Mill brand

1/4 cup dried sweetened cranberries

3 cups cauliflower florets (about 10 ounces)

8 ounces small brussels sprouts, halved lengthwise

1 tablespoon olive oil

1/2 teaspoon freshly ground black pepper

1/4 cup organic barbecue sauce

8 ounces organic extra-firm tofu, drained and cut into 3/4-inch cubes

1/2 cup crumbled feta cheese

PREPARATION

Preheat the oven to 450° F. Bring the broth to a boil in a medium saucepan. Stir in the quinoa and cranberries. Reduce the heat; cover and simmer for 15 minutes or until most of liquid is absorbed. Turn off the heat; let stand covered for 5 minutes.

Meanwhile, arrange the cauliflower and brussels sprouts on a 15 × 10-inch jelly roll pan or baking sheet with sides. Drizzle the oil and sprinkle the pepper over vegetables; toss well to coat. Bake for 12 to 14 minutes or until the vegetables are browned on the bottom and crisp-tender. Transfer to a large bowl. Add the barbecue sauce; toss well. Add the tofu; toss lightly. Spoon the cooked quinoa mixture onto four serving plates. Top with the vegetable mixture and feta cheese.

SUBSTITUTIONS

Dried cherries may replace the cranberries, and small baby carrots may replace the cauliflower.

Look for organic quinoa at Trader Joe's and better markets or Bob's Red Mill brand in the health aisle of many supermarkets.

ROSEMARY GRILLED CHICKEN AND SUMMER VEGETABLES

Preparation time: 10 minutes • *Cooking time: 25 minutes*
Yield: 4 servings • *312 calories per serving, 35% from fat*

INGREDIENTS

2 tablespoons chopped fresh rosemary

3 garlic cloves, peeled and minced

4 organic chicken thighs (about 1 1/2 pounds)

Salt and freshly ground black pepper (optional)

1/4 cup spicy vegetable juice

1 tablespoon extra-virgin olive oil

4 1/2-inch-thick slices eggplant (from the large end)

2 medium zucchini squash, halved lengthwise (about 1/2 pound)

2 large plum tomatoes, halved lengthwise

1 15-ounce can organic no-salt-added chickpeas
    (garbanzo beans), drained

1/3 cup crumbled feta cheese

Nutritional Analysis per Serving	
Total Fat	12.2 g
Fat Calories	110.1
Cholesterol	57.9 mg
Saturated Fat	3.5 g
Polyunsaturated Fat	2.0 g
Monounsaturated Fat	5.0 g
Fiber	7.5 g
Carbohydrates	27.6 g
Sugar	3.8 g
Protein	23.8 g
Sodium	222.6 mg
Calcium	122.9 mg
Magnesium	79.4 mg
Zinc	3.3 mg
Selenium	11.2 mcg
Potassium	826.4 mg

PREPARATION

Prepare a charcoal or gas grill to medium heat. Combine 1 tablespoon of the rosemary and a third of the minced garlic in a large bowl; set aside. Loosen the skin from the thighs with your fingers. Press the remaining tablespoon of rosemary and the rest of the minced garlic under the skin; massage the skin to distribute the mixture evenly. Season the skinless sides of the chicken thighs with salt and pepper if desired. Place the chicken skin-side up on the grill. Grill covered for 10 minutes.

Combine the vegetable juice and oil; transfer 2 tablespoons of this mixture to the large bowl with reserved rosemary mixture. Brush the remaining mixture over both sides of the vegetables and add them to the grill. Turn the chicken over. Continue grilling covered for 5 minutes. Turn the vegetables; continue grilling covered for 5 minutes or until the vegetables are tender. Leave the chicken on the grill for 5 more minutes or until cooked through. Meanwhile, transfer vegetables to a carving board; cut into bite-size chunks. Add the cut vegetables to the bowl with the rosemary mixture. Add the chickpeas and toss well. Season with salt and pepper if desired; transfer to four serving plates. Remove the chicken from the grill and discard the skin from the thighs. Place the thighs over the vegetable mixture and sprinkle feta cheese over all.

SUBSTITUTIONS

Cannellini beans may replace the chickpeas, and yellow summer squash may replace the zucchini.

TIP

Check the vegetables, and as each is cooked, remove from the grill. The tomatoes will cook in less time than the zucchini.

Nutritional Analysis per Serving	
Total Fat	6.1 g
Fat Calories	54.5
Cholesterol	129.3 mg
Saturated Fat	0.9 g
Polyunsaturated Fat	1.9 g
Monounsaturated Fat	2.5 g
Fiber	8.0 g
Carbohydrates	44.8 g
Sugar	5.9 g
Protein	30.5 g
Sodium	387.0 mg
Calcium	113.6 mg
Magnesium	133.1 mg
Zinc	3.2 mg
Selenium	43.7 mcg
Potassium	760.0 mg

SAFFRON SCALLOP, SHRIMP, AND CHICKPEA PAELLA

Preparation time: 5 minutes • Cooking time: 15 minutes
Yield: 4 servings • 355 calories per serving, 15% from fat

INGREDIENTS

2 teaspoons olive oil

8 large sea scallops, patted dry (about 8 ounces)

12 large uncooked shrimp, peeled and deveined, thawed if frozen (about 8 ounces)

3 garlic cloves, peeled and minced

1 14.5-ounce can organic fire-roasted diced or crushed tomatoes, such as Glen Muir brand, undrained

1/2 teaspoon saffron threads, crushed

1/2 teaspoon hot pepper sauce, such as Tabasco brand

1 8.8-ounce package fully cooked brown rice, such as Uncle Ben's brand

1 15-ounce can organic no-salt-added chickpeas (garbanzo beans), drained

PREPARATION

Heat a large deep nonstick skillet over medium-high heat until hot. Spread 1 teaspoon of the oil over the sea scallops. Place the oiled sides down in a single layer in hot pan; sear for 1 to 2 minutes per side or just until opaque in center. Transfer to a bowl; set aside. Reduce the heat under the skillet to medium. Add the remaining teaspoon of oil, the shrimp, and the garlic to the skillet; cook for 3 to 4 minutes or until the shrimp are opaque. Add to the bowl with the scallops.

Add the tomatoes, saffron, and hot pepper sauce to the same skillet; mix well. Add the rice and chickpeas; simmer 5 minutes. Stir in the scallops and shrimp with any accumulated juices to the skillet; heat through, about 1 minute.

SUBSTITUTION

Either 1 pound sea scallops or 1 pound shrimp may replace the combination of scallops and shrimp.

TIP

Look for small vials of saffron threads imported from Spain in the spice section of the supermarket. A half-gram package holds ½ teaspoon of saffron.

SARDINE AND ARUGULA SALAD WITH RATATOUILLE

Preparation time: 10 minutes • Cooking time: 15 minutes
Yield: 4 servings • 209 calories per serving, 34% from fat

INGREDIENTS

3 cups 1/2-inch diced eggplant (about 8 ounces)

1 small red onion, chopped

2 teaspoons extra-virgin olive oil

1 14-ounce can quartered artichoke hearts in water, drained

1 14.5-ounce can organic fire-roasted diced tomatoes, such as Muir Glen brand, undrained

1 tablespoon chopped fresh thyme leaves

4 cups packed baby arugula (about 4 ounces, organic preferred)

2 3.75-ounce tins sardines in olive oil, such as Brunswick brand

4 teaspoons fresh lemon juice

1/4 teaspoon crushed red pepper flakes

Nutritional Analysis per Serving	
Total Fat	8.0 g
Fat Calories	71.7
Cholesterol	65.3 mg
Saturated Fat	1.1 g
Polyunsaturated Fat	2.7 g
Monounsaturated Fat	3.6 g
Fiber	4.0 g
Carbohydrates	18.2 g
Sugar	6.6 g
Protein	16.1 g
Sodium	690.5 mg
Calcium	252.3 mg
Magnesium	44.3 mg
Zinc	0.9 mg
Selenium	24.7 mcg
Potassium	484.7 mg

PREPARATION

Heat a large nonstick skillet over medium-high heat. Add the eggplant; cook until browned, 3 to 4 minutes, stirring occasionally. Stir in the onion, then the oil; cook for 1 minute, stirring occasionally. Reduce heat to medium-low; add the artichoke hearts and tomatoes. Simmer uncovered for 10 minutes or until vegetables are tender and sauce thickens. Stir in the thyme.

Arrange the arugula over one side of each of four large dinner plates. Drain the sardines and arrange them over the arugula. Sprinkle the lemon juice and pepper flakes over the salads. Spoon the ratatouille alongside the salads.

SUBSTITUTIONS

For a spicier flavor, organic fire-roasted tomatoes with green chilies may replace the fire-roasted tomatoes. A teaspoon of dried thyme may replace the fresh thyme (add the dried thyme with the tomatoes).

TIP

The soft bones in the sardines provide a good source of calcium, but tins of boneless, skinless sardines are also available.

Nutritional Analysis per Serving	
Total Fat	11.4 g
Fat Calories	102.8
Cholesterol	43.9 mg
Saturated Fat	3.8 g
Polyunsaturated Fat	1.3 g
Monounsaturated Fat	1.9 g
Fiber	11.8 g
Carbohydrates	53.9 g
Sugar	14.7 g
Protein	20.4 g
Sodium	862.9 mg
Calcium	223.4 mg
Magnesium	43.6 mg
Zinc	0.5 mg
Selenium	13.0 mcg
Potassium	308.1 mg

SICILIAN PASTA WITH SWISS CHARD, GOAT CHEESE, AND BASIL

Preparation time: 10 minutes • Cooking time: 15 minutes
Yield: 4 1¼-cup servings • 143 calories per serving, 31% from fat

INGREDIENTS

8 ounces whole-wheat penne pasta, uncooked (about 2 cups)

4 cups packed coarsely chopped swiss chard (with stems)

2 cups tomato basil spaghetti sauce, such as Classico brand

1/4 teaspoon crushed red pepper flakes

1 3 3/4-ounce can sardines in oil, drained

1/2 cup crumbled goat cheese

1/4 cup julienned fresh basil leaves

Cook the pasta according to the package directions, adding the swiss chard to the pasta cooking water during the last 3 minutes of cooking. Drain in a colander.

Add the spaghetti sauce and the pepper flakes to the same pot; cook over medium-high heat until hot. Drain the sardines, break them into chunks, and stir them into the sauce. Stir in the drained pasta mixture. Toss well and transfer to four serving plates. Top with goat cheese and basil.

SUBSTITUTIONS

Kale may replace the swiss chard, feta cheese may replace the goat cheese, and Italian parsley may replace the basil.

TIPS

If it seems hard to switch from regular pasta to whole wheat, start by trying a whole-wheat pasta blend, such as Ronzoni Healthy Harvest Blend or Barilla PLUS. Good whole-wheat pastas include Trader Joe's and Whole Foods' 365 Organic Everyday Value. When purchasing spaghetti sauce, look for the brand lowest in sodium and saturated fat; taste it; and then adapt it to your own taste with seasonings, oil, and vinegar.

STIR-FRIED GIANT SHRIMP, BABY BOK CHOY, AND PORTOBELLOS

Preparation time: 15 minutes • *Cooking time: 10 minutes*
Yield: 4 servings • *285 calories per serving, 17% from fat*

INGREDIENTS

2 teaspoons dark sesame oil

8 ounces baby bok choy heads, quartered lengthwise (about 3 cups)

8 ounces portobello mushrooms, sliced

16 colossal uncooked shrimp, peeled and deveined (about 1 pound)

1/2 teaspoon five-spice powder

3 tablespoons oyster sauce

1 8.8-ounce package fully cooked brown rice, such as Uncle Ben's brand

Optional garnishes: chopped fresh cilantro, thinly sliced green onions (both white and green parts)

Nutritional Analysis per Serving	
Total Fat	5.3 g
Fat Calories	47.6
Cholesterol	172.4 mg
Saturated Fat	0.9 g
Polyunsaturated Fat	2.1 g
Monounsaturated Fat	1.6 g
Fiber	2.8 g
Carbohydrates	29.4 g
Sugar	2.0 g
Protein	28.9 g
Sodium	703.5 mg
Calcium	85.3 mg
Magnesium	89.0 mg
Zinc	2.5 mg
Selenium	67.4 mcg
Potassium	588.5 mg

PREPARATION

Heat the oil in a large nonstick skillet over medium-high heat. Add the bok choy; stir-fry for 2 minutes. Add the mushrooms; stir-fry for 3 minutes. Toss the shrimp with the five-spice powder; add to the skillet and stir-fry 3 minutes or until the shrimp are opaque. Add the oyster sauce; stir-fry for 1 to 2 minutes or until the sauce thickens.

Heat the rice in microwave oven according to package directions; transfer to the serving plates and top with the shrimp mixture. Garnish as desired.

SUBSTITUTIONS

Hoisin sauce may replace the oyster sauce for a sweeter flavor and 3 cups sliced bok choy from a large head may replace the baby bok choy. Crimini mushrooms (brown mushrooms sometimes labeled as "baby portobellos") may replace the portobellos.

TIPS

"Colossal" is the industry name for extra-large shrimp, which are usually 10 to 16 count per pound. Five-spice powder and oyster sauce are found in the ethnic foods aisle of the supermarket. If you can find Morton & Basset brand five-spice powder, try its blend: it is salt-free, has no MSG or preservatives, and is not irradiated.

WARM BEEF TENDERLOIN SALAD WITH MANGO AND AVOCADO

Preparation time: 10 minutes • Cooking time: 10 minutes
Yield: 4 servings • 283 calories per serving, 34% from fat

INGREDIENTS

1/4 cup finely chopped shallots
3/4 cup mango nectar
1/2 teaspoon each: salt and freshly ground black pepper
2 grass-fed beef tenderloin steaks (about 8 ounces each)
6 cups packed arugula (organic preferred)
1 ripe mango, peeled, seeded, and sliced
1/2 ripe avocado, peeled, seeded, and thinly sliced

PREPARATION

Combine the shallots and mango nectar in a small saucepan. Bring to a boil over high heat. Reduce the heat; simmer uncovered until reduced to about ⅓ cup, 6 to 8 minutes. Remove from heat; set aside.

Meanwhile, sprinkle salt and pepper over steaks. Heat a large nonstick skillet over medium-high heat until hot. Add the steaks; sear for 3 minutes. Turn the steaks over and reduce the heat to medium. Continue cooking for 3 to 4 minutes for medium-rare steak or longer to desired doneness. Transfer steaks to a carving board; let stand 5 minutes.

Arrange the arugula on four serving plates. Arrange the mango and avocado slices attractively over arugula. Carve the steaks crosswise into thin strips and arrange over the salads. Drizzle the mango mixture over salads.

SUBSTITUTIONS

Sweet onion, such as Vidalia, may replace the shallots, and watercress may replace the arugula. Papaya can substitute for the mango.

TIP

Look for organically raised, grass-fed beef at many better supermarkets.

Nutritional Analysis per Serving	
Total Fat	10.7 g
Fat Calories	96.6
Cholesterol	66.7 mg
Saturated Fat	3.1 g
Polyunsaturated Fat	0.8 g
Monounsaturated Fat	5.2 g
Fiber	3.6 g
Carbohydrates	21.8 g
Sugar	16.1 g
Protein	26.0 g
Sodium	355.3 mg
Calcium	85.4 mg
Magnesium	51.3 mg
Zinc	4.8 mg
Selenium	28.6 mcg
Potassium	682.9 mg

Nutritional Analysis per Serving	
Total Fat	10.5 g
Fat Calories	94.6
Cholesterol	16.0 mg
Saturated Fat	4.4 g
Polyunsaturated Fat	0.9 g
Monounsaturated Fat	0.5 g
Fiber	5.8 g
Carbohydrates	26.4 g
Sugar	6.5 g
Protein	13.2 g
Sodium	563.4 mg
Calcium	292.4 mg
Magnesium	49.3 mg
Zinc	2.4 mg
Selenium	18.0 mcg
Potassium	470.2 mg

CHERRY TOMATO AND MOZZARELLA MORSEL SALAD

Preparation time: 15 minutes • Cooking time: 0 minutes
Yield: 4 servings • 240 calories per serving, 37% from fat

INGREDIENTS

3 cups each: packed torn organic romaine lettuce and torn curly endive or
*   frisée*
1 cup halved cherry tomatoes
8 ounces bocconcini (small) fresh mozzarella cheese balls, drained
1/2 cup giardiniera (pickled vegetables), hot or mild or a combination, as de-
*   sired, drained*
1/4 cup olive and sun-dried tomato tapenade, such as Olivier brand
1/4 cup chopped fresh flat-leaf parsley
Freshly ground black pepper
4 whole-wheat dinner rolls, warmed

PREPARATION

Combine the lettuces, tomatoes, cheese, and giardiniera in a large bowl. Top with the tapenade and parsley. Toss well and transfer to serving plates. Add freshly ground black pepper to taste. Serve with warm rolls.

SUBSTITUTIONS

Black or kalamata olive tapenade may replace the olive and sun-dried tomato tapenade. Both are found in the condiment or olive section of the supermarket. Perlini (pearl-size) mozzarella or diced fresh mozzarella may take the place of bocconcini.

TIP

Tubs of fresh mozzarella cheese balls can be found in the deli or specialty cheese section of the supermarket.

GARLICKY POTATO SALAD WITH SPINACH AND LEMON

Preparation time: 15 minutes • Cooking time: 0 minutes
Yield: 4 servings • 155 calories per serving, 28% from fat

INGREDIENTS

3 cups packed organic baby spinach leaves

2 garlic cloves, peeled and minced

1/3 cup low-fat soy mayonnaise or sandwich spread

1/4 teaspoon each: salt and freshly ground black pepper

1 teaspoon grated lemon peel

2 14.5-ounce cans sliced new potatoes, chilled, rinsed, and well drained (organic preferred)

2 tablespoons chopped dill weed (optional)

Nutritional Analysis per Serving	
Total Fat	5.0 g
Fat Calories	45.0
Cholesterol	0 mg
Saturated Fat	0.8 g
Polyunsaturated Fat	2.8 g
Monounsaturated Fat	1.4 g
Fiber	4.8 g
Carbohydrates	25.4 g
Sugar	1.0 g
Protein	3.4 g
Sodium	626.6 mg
Calcium	24.6 mg
Magnesium	23.2 mg
Zinc	0.5 mg
Selenium	1.5 mcg
Potassium	374.1 mg

PREPARATION

Combine the spinach and garlic in a large glass microwave-safe bowl. Cook uncovered on high power for 1 minute or until spinach wilts. Transfer to a paper towel and pat dry. Wipe out the bowl if wet. Add the mayonnaise, salt, pepper, and lemon peel to bowl; mix well. Add the potatoes; toss lightly. Add the spinach and garlic mixture; mix well. Stir in the dill, if desired. Chill until serving time.

SUBSTITUTION

Nonfat Greek yogurt such as Fage brand may substitute for the mayo. Slicing and simmering or steaming baby new potatoes takes just a few minutes and is almost as quick (and much more flavorful) than opening a can.

TIP

The potato salad will keep covered and chilled up to three days and is a good source of resistant starch.

Nutritional Analysis per Serving	
Total Fat	2.6 g
Fat Calories	23.6
Cholesterol	0 mg
Saturated Fat	0.4 g
Polyunsaturated Fat	0.4 g
Monounsaturated Fat	1.7 g
Fiber	3.9 g
Carbohydrates	13.2 g
Sugar	7.8 g
Protein	1.2 g
Sodium	471.0 mg
Calcium	34.4 mg
Magnesium	16.0 mg
Zinc	0.2 mg
Selenium	0.6 mcg
Potassium	224.7 mg

SAUERKRAUT WITH ONION, APPLE, AND TOASTED CARAWAY

Preparation time: 5 minutes • Cooking time: 15 minutes
Yield: 4 servings • 74 calories per serving, 29% from fat

INGREDIENTS

1 teaspoon caraway seeds
2 teaspoons extra-virgin olive oil
1 medium sweet onion, thinly sliced
1 large organic apple, cored and julienned or diced
2 cups drained sauerkraut, rinsed and drained again

PREPARATION

Toast the caraway seeds in a large nonstick skillet over medium-high heat until fragrant, 1 to 2 minutes. Remove from the skillet; set aside. Add the oil and onion to the skillet; cover and cook for 2 to 3 minutes or until onion is tender. Reduce heat; cook uncovered, stirring frequently until the onion is tender and golden brown, about 10 minutes. Stir in the apple; heat through. Stir in the sauerkraut and reserved caraway seeds; heat through.

SUBSTITUTION

Walnut or canola oil may replace the olive oil.

TIPS

This hearty side dish may be served warm or at room temperature. Gala and Fuji are good choices for the apple. To get the apple its cleanest, spritz it lightly with a three-to-one water-to-vinegar solution and rinse. In a hurry? Use packaged organic apple slices.

SPICY GAZPACHO WITH CRAB

Preparation time: 25 minutes • Cooking time: 0 minutes • Chilling time: 2 hours

Yield: 4 1¼-cup servings • 104 calories per serving, 35% from fat

Nutritional Analysis per Serving	
Total Fat	4.2 g
Fat Calories	37.9
Cholesterol	30.9 mg
Saturated Fat	0.5 g
Polyunsaturated Fat	0.6 g
Monounsaturated Fat	2.5 g
Fiber	1.5 g
Carbohydrates	6.9 g
Sugar	3.6 g
Protein	10.5 g
Sodium	432.8 mg
Calcium	51.4 mg
Magnesium	15.0 mg
Zinc	0.3 mg
Selenium	1.5 mcg
Potassium	349.5 mg

INGREDIENTS

1 cup each: 1/4-inch diced unpeeled cucumber, yellow or orange bell pepper, seeded ripe tomato (organic preferred)

1/4 cup minced red onion

1 cup organic tomato juice

1/2 cup bottled clam juice

2 tablespoons cider vinegar

1 tablespoon extra-virgin olive oil

1/2 teaspoon hot pepper sauce, such as Tabasco brand

1 cup canned drained crabmeat, such as Byrd or Jack's Catch brands (about 6 ounces)

Salt and freshly ground black pepper (optional)

Optional garnishes: chopped fresh basil, finely diced avocado

PREPARATION

In a large bowl, combine the cucumber, bell pepper, tomato, onion, tomato juice, clam juice, vinegar, oil, and hot pepper sauce; mix well. Transfer 1½ cups (about half) of the mixture to a blender or food processor. Puree until fairly smooth; return to the bowl. Stir in the crabmeat; season to taste with salt and pepper, if desired. Refrigerate for at least 2 hours or up to 8 hours before serving. Garnish as desired.

SUBSTITUTIONS

Ripe yellow tomato may replace the red tomato, and red bell pepper may replace the yellow or orange pepper.

TIPS

Lump crabmeat is more expensive than claw meat; either works well in this soup. This cold soup is the perfect appetizer in the months when tomatoes and fresh picked vegetables are at their peak.

Nutritional Analysis per Serving	
Total Fat	10.0 g
Fat Calories	90.2
Cholesterol	0 mg
Saturated Fat	1.5 g
Polyunsaturated Fat	1.3 g
Monounsaturated Fat	6.6 g
Fiber	7.1 g
Carbohydrates	14.3 g
Sugar	4.0 g
Protein	3.2 g
Sodium	432.3 mg
Calcium	43.2 mg
Magnesium	29.9 mg
Zinc	0.6 mg
Selenium	1.4 mcg
Potassium	464.6 mg

FRESH TOMATILLO GUACAMOLE

Preparation time: 15 minutes • Cooking time: 0 minutes
Yield: 6 servings (¼ cup guacamole, ½ cup broccoli, and ½ cup carrots per serving) • 147 calories per serving, 56% from fat

INGREDIENTS

2 ripe medium Haas avocados, peeled, seeded, and diced
1/4 cup finely chopped husked fresh tomatillo
2 teaspoons seeded and minced serrano chili pepper
3/4 teaspoon dried oregano (Mexican preferred), crushed
2 garlic cloves, peeled and minced
1 teaspoon salt
1 tablespoon chopped fresh cilantro
3 cups broccoli florets, blanched
3 cups small baby carrots (organic preferred)

PREPARATION

Gently combine the avocados, tomatillo, chili pepper, oregano, garlic, and salt. Mash to desired consistency with a fork. Garnish with cilantro. Serve with broccoli and carrots for dipping.

SUBSTITUTIONS

A jalapeño chili pepper may replace the serrano. Sliced jicama, cucumber, and radish may replace the broccoli and carrots.

TIPS

In the summertime, look for purple tomatillos from farmers' markets and from some Whole Foods and local markets. The guacamole may be chilled up to 1 hour before serving. Place plastic wrap directly over the surface to keep the guacamole from browning or sprinkle the top with fresh lime juice. Crushing the oregano before adding it to the recipe brings out the herb's flavor.

Desserts

AÇAI BERRY AND BANANA DESSERT SOUP

Preparation time: 5 minutes   •   Cooking time: 0 minutes
Yield: 2 1¼-cup servings   •   247 calories per serving, 15% from fat

INGREDIENTS

1 ripe medium banana, peeled and broken into chunks
1 cup low-fat pomegranate-flavored kefir, such as Lifeway brand
1 3.5-ounce packet frozen açai berry puree, such as Sambazon Pure Açai
    Smoothie Pack, partially thawed (about 1/2 cup)
1 cup nonfat coffee frozen yogurt
1/4 cup pomegranate seeds
2 tablespoons chopped fresh mint

PREPARATION

Add the banana, kefir, and açai berry puree to a blender container. Cover; blend until fairly smooth. Add the frozen yogurt; blend until it is thick and smooth. Pour into two chilled shallow soup bowls; top with the pomegranate seeds and mint.

SUBSTITUTIONS

Vanilla frozen yogurt may replace the coffee frozen yogurt, strawberry kefir may replace the pomegranate kefir, and chocolate-covered espresso beans may replace the pomegranate seeds.

TIP

Look for packaged açai berry puree (four individual packets per package) in the freezer section at Whole Foods markets, health food stores, and some supermarkets.

Nutritional Analysis per Serving	
Total Fat	4.2 g
Fat Calories	37.4
Cholesterol	9.0 mg
Saturated Fat	1.1 g
Polyunsaturated Fat	0.6 g
Monounsaturated Fat	2.0 g
Fiber	3.0 g
Carbohydrates	41.8 g
Sugar	32.1 g
Protein	12.6 g
Sodium	135.9 mg
Calcium	190.7 mg
Magnesium	5.8 mg
Zinc	0.1 mg
Selenium	0.2 mcg
Potassium	401.9 mg

Nutritional	Analysis
Total Fat	0.7 g
Fat Calories	6.3
Cholesterol	0.8 mg
Saturated Fat	0.2 g
Polyunsaturated Fat	0.2 g
Monounsaturated Fat	0.1 g
Fiber	4.4 g
Carbohydrates	23.8 g
Sugar	18.1 g
Protein	2.4 g
Sodium	13.1 mg
Calcium	32.1 mg
Magnesium	19.3 mg
Zinc	0.3 mg
Selenium	0.6 mcg
Potassium	251.1 mg

BLACKBERRY, KIWI, AND MANGO FRUIT SALAD

Preparation time: 10 minutes • Cooking time: 0 minutes
Yield: 4 ½-cup servings • 102 calories per serving, 6% from fat

INGREDIENTS

1 tablespoon dark honey
Dash of ground cloves
1/3 cup low-fat berry-flavored kefir, such as Lifeway brand
1 pint fresh blackberries (organic preferred)
2 kiwifruit, peeled and diced
1 ripe mango, peeled and diced
2 teaspoons chopped fresh basil

PREPARATION

Combine the honey and cloves in a medium bowl. Gradually whisk in the kefir, mixing well. Add the blackberries, kiwifruit, and mango; toss lightly. Transfer to serving dishes; top with the basil.

SUBSTITUTIONS

If fresh blackberries are not available, use frozen, partially thawed blackberries. If fresh mango is not available, look for bottled peeled sliced mango in the produce section of your supermarket. Use 1¼ cups diced drained bottled mango to replace the fresh. Chopped mint may replace the basil.

TIPS

If the mango is not ripe, place in a paper bag and store at room temperature for a day or two: It will soften slightly and ripen. To easily dice a fresh mango, stand it on the blossom end and cut down past the narrow pit on either side forming two halves. The flesh around the seed of a ripe mango is yellow. Cut crosswise and lengthwise ½-inch slices (tic-tac-toe fashion) through the mango flesh all the way to the skin, forming ½-inch squares. Hold the scored portion with both hands and bend the peel backward. Cut cubes away from the skin with a tablespoon into a bowl.

CINNAMON ORANGE DREAMSICLE

Preparation time: 5 minutes • Cooking time: 0 minutes
Yield: 3 1-cup servings • 117 calories per serving, 16% from fat

INGREDIENTS

1 teaspoon grated orange peel
2 large oranges, peeled and quartered
2 cups low-fat soy milk
2 tablespoons ground flax meal
1/4 teaspoon ground cinnamon
1 tablespoon dark honey (optional)
4 ice cubes or 1/2 cup crushed ice

PREPARATION

Combine the orange peel, oranges, soy milk, flax meal, cinnamon, and honey in a blender container. Cover; blend 1 minute or until fairly smooth. Add the ice; blend until thick and smooth.

SUBSTITUTION

Fat-free or 1% milk may replace the low-fat soy milk.

TIP

Grate the peel from one of the oranges before peeling the orange for the drink.

Nutritional Analysis per Serving	
Total Fat	2.3 g
Fat Calories	20.4
Cholesterol	0 mg
Saturated Fat	0.1 g
Polyunsaturated Fat	0.4 g
Monounsaturated Fat	0.2 g
Fiber	5.2 g
Carbohydrates	21.6 g
Sugar	13.2 g
Protein	5.0 g
Sodium	31.3 mg
Calcium	145.0 mg
Magnesium	12.5 mg
Zinc	0.3 mg
Selenium	2.2 mcg
Potassium	331.9 mg

MAPLE SYRUP TRIPLE BERRY PARFAIT

Preparation time: 15 minutes • Cooking time: 0 minutes
Yield: 4 servings • 215 calories per serving, 14% from fat

INGREDIENTS

1 17.6-ounce tub 2% Greek-style strained yogurt, such as Fage brand
2 tablespoons pure maple syrup, preferably Grade B and dark
1/8 teaspoon ground cinnamon
2 cups sliced strawberries (organic preferred)
1 cup each: blueberries and raspberries (organic preferred)
1 cup naturally sweetened multigrain cereal clusters, such as Kashi GOLEAN brand

Nutritional Analysis per Serving	
Total Fat	3.6 g
Fat Calories	32.7
Cholesterol	6.2 mg
Saturated Fat	1.9 g
Polyunsaturated Fat	0.2 g
Monounsaturated Fat	0.1 g
Fiber	4.6 g
Carbohydrates	36.7 g
Sugar	21.9 g
Protein	13.9 g
Sodium	66.4 mg
Calcium	131.6 mg
Magnesium	14.5 mg
Zinc	0.6 mg
Selenium	0.4 mcg
Potassium	251.2 mg

PREPARATION

In a small bowl, combine the yogurt, syrup, and cinnamon. In another small bowl, combine the strawberries, blueberries, and raspberries. Spoon half of the berries into four large goblets or clear dessert dishes. Top with half of the yogurt mixture and half of the cereal. Repeat, layering once with remaining berries, yogurt, and cereal. Serve immediately or refrigerate up to 4 hours before serving.

SUBSTITUTIONS

Nonfat yogurt may replace the 2% yogurt, and blackberries may replace the raspberries or blueberries. Agave nectar may replace the maple syrup.

TIP

Look for tubs of Greek-style strained yogurt, such as Fage brand, in many better supermarkets.

Nutritional Analysis per Serving	
Total Fat	6.3 g
Fat Calories	56.6
Cholesterol	0.8 mg
Saturated Fat	0.7 g
Polyunsaturated Fat	1.7 g
Monounsaturated Fat	3.1 g
Fiber	7.4 g
Carbohydrates	31.0 g
Sugar	19.1 g
Protein	3.5 g
Sodium	16.4 mg
Calcium	75.3 mg
Magnesium	28.0 mg
Zinc	0.5 mg
Selenium	1.4 mcg
Potassium	519.2 mg

PAPAYA FILLED WITH GINGERED BLUEBERRIES

Preparation time: 10 minutes • Cooking time: 0 minutes
Yield: 4 servings • 102 calories per serving, 6% from fat

INGREDIENTS

1/4 cup low-fat berry-flavored kefir, such as Lifeway brand
1 tablespoon finely chopped crystallized ginger
1/8 teaspoon ground cinnamon
2 cups blueberries (organic preferred)
2 ripe medium papayas
1/4 cup chopped pecans, toasted

PREPARATION

Combine the kefir, ginger, and cinnamon in a small bowl. Add the blueberries; toss lightly. Cut the papayas in half lengthwise; scoop out and discard the seeds. Fill the papaya hollows with blueberry mixture; top with pecans.

If fresh blueberries are not available, use frozen, partially thawed blueberries. Or substitute fresh raspberries or blackberries. Toasted sliced almonds may replace the pecans.

TIP

Serve with soup spoons to eliminate the need to peel the papaya first. Use the spoon to scoop into the ripe papaya, leaving the skin behind.

STEEL-CUT OAT PUDDING WITH DARK CHOCOLATE AND LIME

Preparation time: 10 minutes • Cooking time: 10 minutes
Yield: 4 servings • 183 calories per serving, 32% from fat

INGREDIENTS

1 1/4 cups low-fat soy milk
3/4 cup canned lite coconut milk
1/3 cup quick-cooking steel-cut oats, such as McCann's brand
2 tablespoons muscovado sugar
2 tablespoons fresh lime juice
1 ounce dark chocolate, chopped
3/4 teaspoon finely grated lime peel

Nutritional Analysis per Serving	
Total Fat	6.7 g
Fat Calories	60.7
Cholesterol	0.5 mg
Saturated Fat	4.8 g
Polyunsaturated Fat	0.3 g
Monounsaturated Fat	0.2 g
Fiber	2.7 g
Carbohydrates	26.5 g
Sugar	11.1 g
Protein	5.1 g
Sodium	69.3 mg
Calcium	94.0 mg
Magnesium	2.5 mg
Zinc	0.2 mg
Selenium	1.5 mcg
Potassium	131.6 mg

PREPARATION

In a medium saucepan, combine the soy milk, coconut milk, and oats. Bring to a simmer over medium-high heat, stirring frequently. Reduce heat to low; simmer, stirring constantly, for 7 minutes (mixture will be thin). Remove from heat; stir in the sugar and lime juice. Let stand in the saucepan uncovered for 10 minutes or until slightly thickened. Transfer to bowls; top with the chocolate and lime peel. Serve warm, at room temperature, or chilled.

SUBSTITUTIONS

Turbinado sugar (a minimally refined sugar) may replace the muscovado (an unrefined dark sugar) and fat-free or 1% milk may replace the soy. Dark chocolate is optimally 70 percent or higher in cocoa.

TIPS

Look for muscovado sugar at Whole Foods markets and health food stores. Organic turbinado raw cane sugar is found in many supermarkets. Seek out artisan chocolate makers in the United States who are doing amazing work such as veregoods.com and Jacques Torres in New York City, Vosges chocolate in Chicago, DeVries chocolate in Denver, and Fiori in Seattle. We love chocolate.

Nutritional Analysis per Serving	
Total Fat	2.3 g
Fat Calories	20.7
Cholesterol	3.3 mg
Saturated Fat	0.5 g
Polyunsaturated Fat	0.1 g
Monounsaturated Fat	0.01 g
Fiber	4.4 g
Carbohydrates	30.5 g
Sugar	22.9 g
Protein	6.4 g
Sodium	53.7 mg
Calcium	46.1 mg
Magnesium	11.0 mg
Zinc	0.1 mg
Selenium	0.7 mcg
Potassium	147.6 mg

STRAWBERRY POMEGRANATE BLENDER BLASTER

Preparation time: 5 minutes • Cooking time: 0 minutes
Yield: 3 1-cup servings • 161 calories per serving, 12% from fat

INGREDIENTS

2 cups frozen unsweetened strawberries (about 8 ounces, organic preferred)
1 cup unsweetened pomegranate juice
1 cup low-fat pomegranate-flavored kefir, such as Lifeway brand
2 tablespoons ground flax meal
1/4 teaspoon vanilla extract
1/8 teaspoon ground nutmeg

PREPARATION

Add the strawberries and pomegranate juice to a blender. Cover and blend until fairly smooth, about 30 seconds. Add the kefir, flax meal, vanilla, and nutmeg; cover again and blend until smooth, about 30 seconds more.

SUBSTITUTION

Low-fat strawberry or mixed berry kefir may replace the pomegranate kefir.

TIPS

Flax meal, such as Bob's Red Mill brand, can be found in health food stores and many supermarkets. Bottles of unsweetened pomegranate juice are usually located in the produce section of the supermarket.

WALNUT-SCENTED DESSERT PANCAKES WITH BANANAS AND AGAVE NECTAR

Preparation time: 15 minutes • Cooking time: 5 minutes
Yield: 4 servings • 246 calories per serving, 32% from fat

INGREDIENTS

1/2 cup buckwheat pancake mix, such as Bob's Red Mill brand
1/2 cup low-fat soy milk
1/4 cup golden raisins
1 large organic egg white
3 teaspoons walnut oil
1/4 cup chopped walnuts, toasted
2 small ripe bananas, peeled and sliced
2 tablespoons agave nectar, warmed

Nutritional Analysis per Serving	
Total Fat	8.9 g
Fat Calories	80.0
Cholesterol	1.3 mg
Saturated Fat	0.9 g
Polyunsaturated Fat	5.8 g
Monounsaturated Fat	1.5 g
Fiber	3.3 g
Carbohydrates	37.4 g
Sugar	22.4 g
Protein	6.0 g
Sodium	217.0 mg
Calcium	77.8 mg
Magnesium	24.2 mg
Zinc	0.3 mg
Selenium	3.8 mcg
Potassium	298.2 mg

PREPARATION

Combine the pancake mix, soy milk, raisins, egg white, and 2 teaspoons of the oil, mixing just until large lumps disappear. (Do not overmix or the pancakes will be tough.) Fold in the walnuts; let stand for 2 minutes.

Heat a large nonstick griddle over medium heat until hot. Coat with cooking spray. Drop the batter by level tablespoonfuls onto the hot griddle. Turn when the pancakes bubble and the bottoms are golden brown; continue to cook until the second sides are golden brown, about 1 minute.

Meanwhile, heat a large nonstick skillet over medium-high heat until hot. Add the remaining teaspoon of oil, then the banana slices. Cook until the slices are browned, turning once, about 30 seconds per side. Transfer the pancakes to four warmed serving plates; top with the bananas and drizzle nectar over all.

SUBSTITUTIONS

Whole-wheat pancake and waffle mix may replace the buckwheat pancake mix. Vanilla soy milk or 1% milk may replace the plain soy milk, and pure maple syrup may replace the agave nectar.

TIPS

An electric skillet set at 375° F may replace the griddle. Keep the pancakes warm as they are made on serving plates in a 200° F oven.

Fourteen-Day Menu Plan

What if you don't have time to cook? No worries! We've created an easy, off-the-shelf way of eating with some of the most flavorful foods widely available . . . nearly everywhere. Why not use ready-to-go pre-prepared foods when you can? They're easy, fast, and still great for your doctor inside. Here are fourteen days of menus to get you started: simple, fast meals with less than ten minutes of cooking each, and packed with flavor and goodness that will make you sing with happiness.

All of the suggested meals may be prepared in less than ten minutes, and most in less than five minutes. An asterisk (*) after an ingredient means preferred brands are included in ChefMD Essentials (page 89).

DAY 1

BREAKFAST

Orange juice with calcium, vitamin D, and extra pulp, such as Tropicana

Toasted multigrain or whole-wheat plus flax bread spread with natural peanut or almond butter and topped with thinly sliced whole apple

Brewed coffee or tea

LUNCH

Bowl of heated butternut squash soup, such as Imagine or Trader Joe's*, topped with a dollop of Greek yogurt, such as Fage*

An unpeeled ripe peach or nectarine

Wasa, RyKrisp, or other high-fiber flatbread crackers

Low-fat soy milk or skim milk

SNACK

Handful of sultanas or golden raisins

DINNER

Prepared, marinated grilled chicken breast (deli or takeout) topped with Classico* tomato basil pasta sauce, served with sautéed salad-bar mushrooms and green pepper strips

Salad-bar or prewashed mesclun salad greens with crumbled feta or goat cheese and toasted almonds drizzled with balsamic vinegar and a little extra-virgin olive oil

Whole-grain dinner roll
Glass of dry red wine or sparkling water with bitters

DESSERT
Dark chocolate chips, eaten one at a time
Espresso or cappuccino

DAY 2

BREAKFAST
High-fiber, low-sugar cereal, such as Kashi* or granola with
low-fat soy or skim milk and fresh or partially thawed blueberries
Berry or pomegranate kefir, such as Lifeway*
Brewed coffee or tea

LUNCH
Mesclun salad greens topped with chopped raw vegetables from
the salad bar with a squeeze of juice from a lemon or lime wedge
and drizzled with a little walnut or extra-virgin olive oil
Four or five good-quality olives and a half pint of thick Greek
yogurt, such as Fage*, drizzled with dark honey
Whole-wheat bread sticks
Iced coffee or tea

SNACK
Sliced ripe papaya sprinkled with lime juice and chili powder

DINNER
Smoked trout or peppered mackerel fish fillet, such as Ducktrap
brand
Whole-wheat couscous hydrated in vegetable juice cocktail,
such as V8*, with canned drained chickpeas and cumin seeds
Steamed broccoli touched by extra-virgin olive oil and a squeeze
of lemon
Glass of red wine or sparkling water with a lime

DESSERT
Low-fat creamy fudge bar, such as So Delicious

DAY 3

BREAKFAST
Bowl of quick-cooking steel-cut oatmeal, such as McCann's or
Quaker*, with dried apricot or papaya pieces, and hazelnuts

Low-fat soy or skim milk
Brewed coffee or tea

LUNCH
Bowl of heated cream of mushroom soup, such as Imagine or Trader Joe's*, with leftover chopped cooked chicken stirred in, sprinkled with a little freshly grated Parmigiano-Reggiano cheese
RyKrisp, Wasa, or other whole-grain crackers
Sliced cucumbers sprinkled with seasoned rice vinegar and fresh basil
Iced coffee or tea

SNACK
Small handful of toasted pecans

DINNER
Grilled or broiled large portobello mushroom cap brushed with barbecue sauce, in a toasted whole-wheat hamburger bun with a slice of part skim mozzarella cheese, romaine lettuce, and sliced tomato
Deli roasted vegetable salad in olive oil
Glass of fruity red wine or sparkling water with orange slice

DESSERT
Açai Berry and Banana Dessert Soup (page 139)

DAY 4
BREAKFAST
Raisin bran with chopped dates or figs and low-fat soy or skim milk
Pink grapefruit half with a light drizzle of agave nectar, such as Madhava*
Brewed coffee or tea

LUNCH
Large scoop of fat-free organic cottage cheese, such as Cabot or Horizon*, on dinner-size salad of mesclun greens with cherry tomato halves, drizzled with tapenade or olive relish
Handful of baked corn tortilla chips, such as Guiltless Gourmet*
Seedless grapes
Iced coffee or tea

SNACK
Small piece of good-quality dark chocolate

DINNER
Take-out sushi
Sautéed baby spinach with ginger coins with a splash of teriyaki
sauce, such as Soy Vay*
Cooked buckwheat (soba) noodles
Asian pear or ripe Bosc pear
Brewed green tea, such as Tazo*

DESSERT
Strawberry Pomegranate Blender Blaster (page 144)

DAY 5

BREAKFAST
Low-sodium tomato juice with lime and Tabasco
Toasted whole-grain English muffin with almond butter and a
slice of swiss cheese
Blackberries or sliced strawberries sprinkled with cinnamon
Brewed coffee or tea

LUNCH
Bowl of heated roasted tomato soup, such as Imagine or Trader
Joe's*, garnished with diced ripe tomato, chopped fresh basil or
Italian parsley, and whole-wheat croutons
Mesclun salad greens drizzled with balsamic vinegar and a small
amount of extra-virgin olive oil
Low-fat soy or skim milk

SNACK
Bing cherries or two plums

DINNER
Ready-to-eat cooked shrimp and salad bar cut-up vegetables
stir-fried with curry powder and a little vegetable broth
Ready-to-eat brown rice warmed with spicy vegetable juice
cocktail with golden raisins
Garnishes of chopped cilantro, peach or mango chutney, or
Greek-style yogurt, such as Fage*
Brewed jasmine tea

DESSERT
Papaya Filled with Gingered Blueberries (page 142)

DAY 6

BREAKFAST
Egg white omelet with low-fat shredded cheese
Slice of whole-wheat or multigrain toast with all fruit raspberry preserves
Brewed coffee or tea

LUNCH
Veggie burger cooked according to package directions spread with barbecue sauce on a whole-wheat hamburger bun with baby spinach or arugula and a slice of ripe tomato
A ripe unpeeled peach or nectarine
Iced tea

SNACK
Small handful of slivered toasted almonds

DINNER
Progresso canned lentil soup with shredded skinless rotisserie chicken, heated and topped with a diced slice of multigrain toast for croutons
Salad of sliced ripe tomatoes and crumbled goat cheese on romaine lettuce topped with chopped fresh basil and a light drizzle of balsamic vinegar glaze or syrup
Glass of white wine or iced tea

DESSERT
Low-fat vanilla frozen yogurt sprinkled with chopped crystallized ginger, such as the Ginger People*

DAY 7

BREAKFAST
Chocolate Blackberry Breakfast Smoothie (page 95)
Low-sugar high-fiber power bar or low-sugar granola bar
Brewed coffee or tea

LUNCH
Bowl of heated butternut squash soup, such as Imagine or Trader Joe's*, with sliced fully cooked spicy chicken sausage, cinnamon, and chopped deli grilled or roasted vegetables
Baked whole-wheat pita chips
Wedge of watermelon or cantaloupe

Sparkling water with a splash of pomegranate or fruit juice

SNACK
Multigrain crackers spread with natural peanut or almond butter

DINNER
Microwaved frozen cooked shrimp and take-out deli coleslaw (vinaigrette, not creamy) wrapped in warm corn tortillas with salsa, such as Frontera*, and chopped cilantro

Heated (microwave or in a covered saucepan) fat-free refried beans, such as Bearitos*

Sliced fresh pineapple (from a container of cored fresh pineapple in the produce section)

Lime seltzer

DESSERT
Candied ginger covered in dark chocolate
Espresso or coffee

DAY 8

BREAKFAST
Small cantaloupe half filled with seedless red grapes topped with low-fat, unsweetened, Greek-style yogurt and low-fat lightly sweetened muesli

Brewed coffee or tea

LUNCH
Deli grilled or roasted vegetables over watercress or arugula topped with chopped fresh dill or basil, crumbled feta or goat cheese, and toasted walnuts or pecans drizzled with a little extra-virgin olive oil and freshly ground black pepper

Whole-grain dinner roll
Iced tea

SNACK
Low-fat, high-fiber trail mix

DINNER
Sea scallops sprinkled with Old Bay seasoning* and pan-seared in a hot skillet two minutes per side

Microwaved fully cooked brown rice, such as Uncle Ben's or Trader Joe's*

Steamed or microwaved green beans or sugar snap peas
Iced tea or sparkling water with a splash of fruit juice or lime

DESSERT
Cinnamon Orange Dreamsicle (page 141)

DAY 9

BREAKFAST
Greek-style strained yogurt, such as Fage*, topped with fresh raspberries, toasted sliced almonds, and a drizzle of agave nectar, such as Madhava*
Brewed coffee or tea

LUNCH
Deli or take-out bulgur or tabouli salad
Baked whole-wheat pita chips
Wedge of good Greek feta cheese
Four or five kalamata olives
Cranberry juice cocktail mixed with sparkling water and a squeeze of lime

SNACK
Whole-wheat pretzels with coarse-grained mustard

DINNER
Salmon burgers (fresh from Whole Foods or frozen from Trader Joe's) cooked and served on a bed of microwaved wild rice (pre-cooked in a pouch from Trader Joe's)
Steamed or microwaved fresh broccoli florets, such as Manny's, from the produce section
Whole-grain dinner roll
Glass of red or white wine or iced tea

DESSERT
Dark chocolate–covered strawberries from the supermarket bakery department or specialty store

DAY 10

BREAKFAST
Wedge of honeydew melon
Bowl of high-fiber cereal with low-fat soy or skim milk
Brewed coffee or tea

LUNCH

Chopped skinless rotisserie or leftover grilled chicken breast mixed with Nasoya Nayonnaise*, arugula or watercress sprigs, dried cranberries, and toasted pecans served open faced on a toasted multigrain English muffin

An unpeeled apple or pear

Iced tea or coffee

SNACK

Baby carrots dipped in honey mustard

DINNER

Bowl of heated low-fat bean chili, topped with crumbled queso fresco cheese and chopped cilantro

Diced ripe avocado topped with salsa*

Handful of baked tortilla chips*

Ice cold tea

DESSERT

Scoop of low-fat vanilla frozen yogurt topped with sliced strawberries and dark chocolate chips

Coffee or espresso

DAY 11

BREAKFAST

Scrambled egg whites and one egg with salsa and lite shredded three-cheese blend rolled in a warm whole-wheat flour tortilla

Low-fat fruit-flavored kefir, such as Lifeway*

LUNCH

Sandwich of drained canned salmon in water, diced avocado, and arugula or spinach tossed with balsamic vinegar and a little olive oil in whole-wheat pita pocket bread

Seedless grapes

Iced coffee or tea

SNACK

Cut-up mixed fresh fruit from the produce section

DINNER

Sliced baked Asian-flavored tofu* served over microwaved brown rice* drizzled with teriyaki sauce, such as Soy Vay*

Steamed green beans sprinkled with sesame oil

Whole-grain dinner roll
Brewed green tea, such as Tazo*

DESSERT
Mango or papaya sorbet on a ring of fresh pineapple, topped with chopped crystallized ginger and curry powder

DAY 12
BREAKFAST
Smoked salmon on a toasted, halved, hollowed-out whole-wheat bagel spread lightly with a mixture of prepared horseradish and Nasoya Nayonnaise* topped with a thin slice of red onion and drained capers
Low-sodium tomato juice spiked with Tabasco
Brewed coffee

LUNCH
Heated, drained, canned no-salt-added organic pinto beans, such as Eden*, mixed with salsa, such as Frontera*, diced avocado, crumbled queso fresco or queso añejo, and chopped cilantro or green onions folded into a warm whole-wheat tortilla.
Lemonade with a splash of unsweetened pomegranate juice

SNACK
Dried cranberries and a tangerine or clementine

DINNER
Grilled or broiled skinless salmon fillet on a bed of mesclun salad greens with diced ripe bottled papaya or mango and avocado drizzled with a good-quality olive oil vinaigrette
Whole-grain dinner roll
Glass of white wine or iced tea

DESSERT
An unpeeled peach or nectarine sliced thin and crowned with two very small scoops of low-fat butter pecan ice cream

DAY 13
BREAKFAST
Low-fat vanilla yogurt with sliced strawberries or blueberries sprinkled with low-sugar granola or high-fiber, low-sugar cereal

Glass of low-fat chocolate milk or soy milk, such as Horizon
Brewed coffee or tea

LUNCH

Bowl of heated low-fat tomato or butternut squash soup, such as Imagine or Trader Joe's*
Purchased hummus spread on whole-wheat pita bread
Seedless grapes
Iced coffee or tea

SNACK

Four or five green olives and a stick of part-skim mozzarella or 2 percent cheddar string cheese

DINNER

Small take-out or deli grilled chicken breast half with brown rice, heated and topped with a dollop of cranberry chutney
Microwaved or steamed sugar snap peas
Small tossed green salad with a good-quality olive oil dressing
Fruity white wine or iced tea

DESSERT

Organic cinnamon applesauce

DAY 14

BREAKFAST

Tangy and Cool Buttermilk and Avocado Breakfast Smoothie (page 99)
Cut-up mixed fresh fruit from the salad bar
Brewed coffee or tea

LUNCH

Multigrain or whole-wheat bread sandwich with all-fruit strawberry preserves and natural peanut butter
Carrot sticks and celery sticks from the supermarket salad bar
Small banana or packaged fresh apple wedges from the produce section
Handful of Terra Exotic Vegetable Chips
Low-fat soy or skim milk

SNACK

Small handful of pepitas (pumpkin seeds) sprinkled with a little chili powder

DINNER

Deli or take-out poached salmon served with teriyaki sauce, such as Soy Vay*, for dipping

Steamed or microwaved fresh asparagus with a drizzle of sesame oil and toasted sesame seeds

Microwaved small sweet potato

Glass of red wine or sparkling water

DESSERT

Lemon sorbet with fresh blueberries or raspberries drizzled with a little almond or orange liqueur

Part Three

Living the Chef MD Way

CHAPTER 6

The Eight-Week Program for Optimal Health:

EAT, DRINK, AND BE HEALTHIER

One cannot think well, love well, sleep well, if one has not dined well.

—VIRGINIA WOOLF

Okay, you're now an expert on culinary medicine, bioavailability, anti-nutrients, and satiety.

You know how to build a kitchen medicine chest (your pantry!) stocked with the healthiest foods in the world and you know how to make some truly scrumptious and healthy meals. You've taken stock of your doctor inside and absorbed a lot of information, along with some very healthy nutrients.

Now you're ready to put it into everyday action. What follows is an easy, step-by-step plan for optimal health that builds on itself. You start slowly and then keep adding on to what you know. Each week you'll practice what you did the week before, plus add a new color-coded food, a new recipe, and a new exercise skill. New habits can give you a new future.

Every other week, I'll suggest wines that complement the recipes in the plan. I'll bet this is sounding better already.

By the time you complete the plan, you'll have more energy, be sleeping better, have less joint pain, and feel less anxiety. Your skin will be clearer and your sleep will be sounder. You'll be at less risk for developing cancer, diabetes, and heart disease. Although this is not a diet plan, you'll also probably have lost weight. When you're finished, you'll look better and feel better.

Ask yourself:

1. Can I sincerely commit to trying the plan for the whole eight weeks?
2. Am I and my family worth the hard work it takes to achieve optimal health?
3. Do I want to prevent and control common chronic conditions?
4. Do I love myself enough to try?

If you answer yes to these four questions, you're ready for the ChefMD plan! If you answer no to any of them, decide to develop better habits—they make your life easier. Work on ways to "get to yes," and then try the plan.

Before We Start . . . Where Are You Now?

When you're trying to get somewhere, you need to know your starting point. To help you figure out where you are, health-wise, I've put together a list of sixteen essential questions for you to answer.

Write down the answers! On paper! So you can see them! You're creating a road map for success. For example, if you want to lower your blood pressure, take your own blood pressure after first sitting for five minutes, write it down, and in eight weeks, take it again, in exactly the same way, at the same time. Be clear about your goal and be consistent. You can create a lifestyle of great health. Knowing where you started will make it easier to know how far you've come.

It can be painful to look at the scale and see that you're thirty pounds overweight (since when can't I see my feet?). It can be scary to learn that your blood pressure is in the danger zone. Once you know where you are, you can do something about it, and you'll feel better than ever. Believe in yourself!

YOUR OPTIMAL HEALTH

What is my LDL level?

(Most desirable is 100 milligrams per deciliter or less; 160 milligrams per deciliter or above is danger zone.)

Where I am now   _____

Where I want to be   _____

Where I am after the ChefMD program   _____

What is my HDL level?

(For men, above 50 milligrams per deciliter is ideal; 40 milligrams per deciliter or less is danger zone.)

(For women, above 60 milligrams per deciliter is ideal; 45 milligrams per deciliter or less is danger zone.)

Where I am now   _____

Where I want to be   _____

Where I am after the ChefMD program   _____

What is the level of my triglycerides?

(Below 150 milligrams per deciliter is normal; above 150 milligrams per deciliter is danger zone.)

Where I am now   _____

Where I want to be   _____

Where I am after the ChefMD program   _____

What is my resting blood pressure?

(The ideal is 115/76 millimeters of mercury; 130/85 millimeters of mercury and above is danger zone.)

Where I am now   _____

Where I want to be   _____

Where I am after the ChefMD program   _____

What is my resting heart rate?

(Average is 60 to 76 beats per minute; 80 beats per minute or over is danger zone.)

Where I am now   _____

Where I want to be   _____

Where I am after the ChefMD program   _____

What is my fasting blood sugar level?

(Up to 110 milligrams per deciliter is considered normal; levels between 110 and 125 milligrams per deciliter are risk factors for type 2 diabetes.)

Where I am now _____

Where I want to be _____

Where I am after the ChefMD program _____

What is my body mass index (BMI)?

(Figure out your BMI by multiplying your weight in pounds by 703 and dividing that number by your height in inches squared. Or calculate it for free on www.ChefMD.com. Ideally your BMI should be less than 25 kilograms per square meter; over 30 kilograms per square meter is obese; 40 kilograms per square meter and over is severely obese.)

Where I am now _____

Where I want to be _____

Where I am after the ChefMD program _____

What is my waist-to-hip ratio (WHR)?

(Figure out your WHR by dividing your waist by your hips. Or calculate it for free on www.ChefMD.com. You want it to be less than 0.8 if you are a woman, and less than 1.0 if you are a man, to prevent heart disease: it is more important than waist size alone or weight.)

Where I am now _____

Where I want to be _____

Where I am after the ChefMD program _____

How much do I sleep per night?

(You should get, on average, 6.5 to 8.5 uninterrupted hours per night.)

Where I am now _____

Where I want to be _____

Where I am after the ChefMD program _____

How much tobacco do I smoke, including cigars?
(You should not smoke at all.)
Where I am now   _____
Where I want to be   _____
Where I am after the ChefMD program   _____

How much alcohol do I drink?
(You should have fewer than 3 drinks per day if you are a man, and
    fewer than 2 drinks if you a woman.)
Where I am now   _____
Where I want to be   _____
Where I am after the ChefMD program   _____

How often and for how long do I exercise per week?
(You should be active at least 6 days a week, for 30 minutes, bare
    minimum.)
Where I am now   _____
Where I want to be   _____
Where I am after the ChefMD program   _____

**Rate the following on a scale of 1 to 10, where 1 is virtually none
at all and 10 is the highest possible for you:**

What is my stress level?
(Stress is a killer. Yoga, meditation, exercise, time spent with friends,
    and laughter all reduce it.)
Where I am now   _____
Where I want to be   _____
Where I am after the ChefMD program   _____

What is my anxiety level?
(This can decrease with exercise and good nutrition.)
Where I am now   _____
Where I want to be   _____
Where I am after the ChefMD program   _____

What is my level of fatigue?
(This can also decrease with exercise and good nutrition.)
Where I am now   _____
Where I want to be   _____
Where I am after the ChefMD program   _____

The most powerful part of the ChefMD program is simply that you are doing it: to read this far and to begin to listen to the doctor inside is to begin to put your knowledge into action.

Again, knowing where you are starting is essential in knowing whether what you are doing is working. Here's where you get to witness the real healing power of quality food, and prepare for success, great health, and a long life. Set concrete goals so it will be easier to reach them. Let's get started!

Week 1

WHAT TO EAT, WHAT NOT TO EAT

This week, avoid as much as you can of breaded, creamed, and deep-fried foods. Instead of these, have foods that are steamed, baked, sautéed, or grilled.

Also, switch out white processed foods, such as white bread, white rice, sugary cereals, and white pasta, for less-processed whole-grain versions, including whole-grain bread, brown or wild rice, steel-cut oats, and whole-wheat pasta. You can mix regular and wheat pasta the first few times you eat it to help your taste buds make the transition.

Avoid iron supplements, as they increase oxidation and risk for heart disease, unless you are a premenopausal woman, and avoid more than twenty-five hundred international units of beta-carotene in your multivitamin, if you take one, as beta-carotene may increase lung cancer in smokers and precancerous colon polyps in some people.

Choose leaf lettuce (the darker varieties are by far the best) from the front of store shelves rather than the heads in back: those in front have more flavonoids. The outer leaves have ten times the concentration as the inner leaves.

At least twice this week have breakfast, whether or not you're hungry, first thing when you get up, and include a chewy low-sugar carb such as whole-grain cereal, whole-grain bread, apple, or berries and a lean protein, such as egg whites, chicken, veggie burger, or tofu. Protein stays in your stomach longest and the carbs give your brain and body great start-up energy.

SPECIAL TO WEEK ONE

Take an hour this week to go through your kitchen and pantry and do the following:

- Check the labels on your foods. If they have trans fats (the ingredients say "partially hydrogenated" or the label says "trans fats") or high-fructose corn syrup, which is in many breads, cereals, and crackers, toss them in the trash, and start a shopping list to replace them with healthier versions.
- Throw out all cooking fats and oils except olive oil, nut and seed oils, avocado, and canola. Toss any bottles that have lost their caps: the oil will have oxidized.
- Check all canned and packaged food for high-sodium and high-sugar levels. Throw away those with more than eight hundred milligrams of sodium and twelve grams of added sugar per serving—even the cans of soup and boxes of Froot Loops you were saving in case of nuclear disaster. Put low-sodium and low-sugar versions on your shopping list, and read the label once you find them: they are often full of tricks.
- Pick up a filtration system for your tap water. Some are inexpensive and efficient, like pitchers with filters.

Once you have done this, you will have given your kitchen a great ChefMD face-lift to launch you on your way.

To reward yourself, treat yourself to a good eight-inch chef's knife from a department store or specialty store with a high carbon-steel alloy blade and a plastic handle. I like the simple Forschners with an eight-inch blade, and matching steel (the tapered rod to hone the blade), but there are many other good ones. Learn how to hold and use your new knife. Grip the handle as if you were shaking hands with it, or if you play tennis, like a forehand grip. Resist the impulse to put your index finger down the back of the blade: it is too easy to lose control. The knife should feel balanced in your hand.

THIS WEEK'S COLOR: YELLOW-ORANGE

Pick a yellow-orange food you've never had before or haven't had in years and try it: butternut squash, apricot, tangerines, crookneck squash, yellow peppers, honeydew melon, pumpkin, persimmons, oranges, papaya, or peaches. That yellow shouts the presence of the antioxidant beta-cryptoxanthin, which appears to reduce colon and lung cancer risk and the risk for rheumatoid arthritis. Keep lemons on hand to brighten whole grains and salads—nothing could be quicker or simpler for a no-fat, no-sodium, almost no-calorie flavor boost. And a quarter cup of juice gives you almost half your reference daily intake (RDI) of vitamin C. Here are two recipes to help you eat yellow-orange.

RECIPES TO TRY
Cinnamon Orange Dreamsicle (page 141)
        or
Papaya Filled with Gingered Blueberries (page 142)

MOVE IT TO LOSE IT

Comfortable clothes, good shoes, fun music, and a positive attitude will get you started. Walk for thirty minutes six times this week (everyone needs a day off), with no excuses, at any pace that is comfortable for you. Even if you already have an exercise routine, also do this walk. If it is snowy or raining, go to the mall, or go to your office before anyone arrives in the morning and walk up and down the hall. If you are really stuck, you can walk circles around your house or living room. Just get those legs moving!

If thirty minutes of walking is over your limit and you feel you cannot do more, but you're committed to doing less—say fifteen minutes—six times a week, that's great. Work up to thirty. Be consistent. Being a moderate exerciser is almost as good for your health as being a serious athlete—it's doing nothing at all that's the killer.

Week 2

WHAT TO EAT, WHAT NOT TO EAT

This week, eat breakfast at least four times. Try to avoid sweet, drinkable foods with added refined sugar, such as soda, punch, and energy drinks. Instead, drink water, tea, coffee, and vegetable and diluted fruit juices. If this is too hard, alternate them with the higher sugar drinks, or dilute them by half, or just pour a little in the bottom of a glass and fill it with sparkling water.

Start to minimize—meaning eat no more than two servings total each day, and less if you can—foods high in solid, saturated and trans fats (such as butter, cream, full-fat cheese, and dairy; most processed and other red meat; and store-bought baked goods). These fats coat your palate so you can't taste other foods as clearly, and so you overeat. Start to use oils that are rich in omega-3 fatty acids (such as sesame, walnut, cold-pressed canola and flax, plus extra-virgin olive oil), and choose low-fat dairy, fish, chicken, and turkey.

Starting this week (and continuing for the rest of the plan), always sit down when you eat—even if you are only having a snack. Don't eat over the sink or while standing in front of the refrigerator. You taste more when you are sitting, the flavors become more pronounced, your mind is more on your food and meal, and you will achieve satiety faster. Don't make an exception because you are too busy. Treat yourself to a seat.

THIS WEEK'S COLOR: RED

Pick a red food you've never had before or haven't had in years and have it: rhubarb, cherries, radicchio, watermelon, pink grapefruit, red bell peppers, red cabbage, or radishes. The red in these foods—some red-purple, others red-pinks—tell you they contain colorful anthocyanins, the pigments that help protect you from oxidative stress. Have some red onion—its isothiocyanates will help reduce the inflammation that can cause arthritis pain. Also, have a tomato, tomato sauce, or tomato paste every day if you can, as you already know the value of tomatoes. Here are two recipes to help you eat red.

RECIPES TO TRY

Pasta e Fagioli (Pasta and Bean) Soup (page 102)
     or
Cherry Tomato and Mozzarella Morsel Salad (page 134)

WINES THAT COMPLEMENT

With that Cherry Tomato and Mozzarella Morsel Salad, try a glass of good Pinot Grigio or Pinot Gris. Their light, slightly spicy flavors will balance the delicate mozzarella. With the soup, try a juicy, smooth Chianti or a simple Sangiovese, the principal grape in Chianti.

If this sounds like a bunch of wine mumbo jumbo, ask your local wine merchant or the department head at your local grocery to help you find a great wine.

MOVE IT TO LOSE IT

Continue walking six of seven days for thirty minutes. This week, learn how to walk with purpose—at least three miles per hour. Stroll for a few minutes, which will begin to warm up your muscles. Pick up the pace slightly so that you can feel your pulse go up a little. Bend your arms at the elbows so that they are parallel to the ground or floor and make a loose fist as you walk. The difference between an easy walk and a walk with purpose is burning 25 percent more calories. Move your arms slightly, like pistons. Walk this way, purposefully, for thirty minutes.

Week 3

WHAT TO EAT, WHAT NOT TO EAT

Starting to get the hang of this? You should be, and I hope you are even starting to enjoy yourself. This week, eat breakfast every day. Eat all your nuts, fruits, and vegetables with the skin on, when feasible: most antioxidants are in the skin or just beneath it, and so is much of the fiber. Antioxidants in food lessen free radical damage, reduce inflammation, and protect your DNA.

Begin buying organic foods whenever you can, especially fruits and vegetables. Some organic vegetables have from 30 percent to 1,000 percent higher levels of powerful flavonoids than conventional vegetables. That's as much as ten times the antioxidant power, without the artificial synthetic chemical pesticides and herbicides. And I think most organics taste better.

If you want to eat out this week, make deliberate, good ChefMD choices that will keep you on the plan. Eat out with authority: plan what you are going to order before you open the menu. Avoid using no-fat dressing in a salad, as you'll absorb only 13 percent of the lutein and 6 percent of the beta-carotene in the vegetables, but don't drown the salad in good dressing—just dress it. Also, order whole-grain pasta al dente (literally, "to the tooth" in Italian). It means ever so slightly undercooked. This lowers the pasta's glycemic index and makes it more filling. Enjoy marinara sauce with a little extra-virgin olive oil so you'll absorb extra carotenoids.

This week, try getting into the habit of eating a water-dense, volume-rich food at the start of the meal. Remember, you determine your future with your habits. Eat a bowl of soup or a large green, red, and yellow salad with a lower calorie but not nonfat dressing at the start of at least two dinners this week: a large first course of a low-calorie salad or vegetable soup helps you eat more slowly, absorb more nutrients, and lowers the rate at which you digest the rest of the meal. I hope you will come to love soups as much as I do—they are a great way to get your nutrients when you don't feel like eating vegetables by themselves.

THIS WEEK'S COLOR: PURPLE-RED

Purple-red foods include purple cabbage, purple onions, red apples, prunes, plums, figs, purple grapes, raisins, and of course berries of every kind—straw, rasp, black, blue, cran, and mixed. This week, try some eggplant, best during their high season, August to October. The antioxidant that gives eggplant's skin its rich purple color is called nasunin, and it helps fight cancer. Also, eat some berries every day if you can—with your breakfast, or as an afternoon snack: buy frozen ones, so they'll last. Blueberries and blackberries contain some of the highest levels of anthocyanins and phenolics, which are some of the most powerful fighters against those nasty free radicals that damage DNA and accelerate aging. Here are two recipes to help you eat purple-red.

RECIPES TO TRY
Chocolate Blackberry Breakfast Smoothie (page 95)
        or
Maple Syrup Triple Berry Parfait (page 141)

MOVE IT TO LOSE IT
Continue your routine of a few minutes of warm-up strolling followed by purposeful walking. Try to exercise in clean air or sunshine or both. This week, stretch after walking to keep your muscles limber; stretching before walking is overrated. Focus on your legs. Step forward with one foot and then bend that knee slowly until you feel a gentle stretching sensation across the back of the calf of the unbent

leg. Do not bounce. Switch and do the other leg. Stretch your quads by standing on one leg and holding the foot of the other leg behind you, pulling it gently toward your butt. You can stretch your Achilles tendon by standing on a stair on the balls of your feet and letting your heels gently lower below the stair. Again, do not bounce. Hold on to something to steady yourself while stretching, and remember to be *gentle*—forcing a stretch could tear a muscle or tendon.

Week 4

WHAT TO EAT, WHAT NOT TO EAT

Check your grains—they should be all whole. Try a grain you've never tried before, like spelt, which is fabulous and chewy simmered in chicken stock and dressed with a little olive oil and some real Parmigiano-Reggiano. Begin three dinners this week with a salad or vegetable soup.

Continue to make your kitchen into a ChefMD kitchen. Toss out your scratched, weary Teflon pans (all produce toxic gas when you leave an empty pan on a hot burner too long). While you're at it, toss your copper-lined pans, too. They put copper into food, and people who eat a lot of saturated fat (such as butter, red meat, or full-fat dairy) who also have a high copper intake develop Alzheimer's disease 143 percent more often than people who do not. Use cast-iron, stainless steel, or ceramic pans instead.

This week, cook your vegetables. Try a cooking technique you haven't used in a while that will maximize bioavailability (body readiness)—steam, simmer, marinate, dry rub, roast, or grill.

Try eating more slowly to taste and enjoy more of your food. It takes at least twenty minutes for your brain to register satiety. So take at least twenty minutes to eat each meal, with whatever trick works for you: put down your fork between bites, chew each mouthful ten times, count to twenty aloud between bites, or watch the clock. Make yourself do it. At first, twenty minutes may seem like forever, but by the end of eight weeks it will seem ordinary, and to eat faster would feel like you are gulping your food, which you might be.

THIS WEEK'S COLOR: ORANGE

Pick an orange food you've never had before or haven't had in years and try it: apricots, sweet potatoes, chili peppers, carrots, peaches, mangoes, persimmons, kumquats, or winter squash. That bright orange is a sign of beta-carotene and its anti-rusting potential: have one of these foods every day if you can. This week, try some pumpkin—and don't forget the seeds, which may prevent testosterone from being transformed into dihydrotestosterone, which is associated with an enlarged prostate. Also, have some cantaloupe—sweet, succulent, and at only fifty-six calories a cup, it's no surprise it's America's favorite melon. Here are two recipes to help you eat orange.

RECIPES TO TRY
Warm Beef Tenderloin Salad with Mango and Avocado (page 133)

or

Portuguese Caldo Verde (page 104)

WINES THAT COMPLEMENT
The sweetness of the mango layers over the lean tenderloin, so a wine with real zing will cut through it: look for a young California Zinfandel or even a fresh, hardly-at-all-tannic Beaujolais. And for the Caldo Verde, a clean dry crisp Sauvignon Blanc from Chile or New Zealand would be delicious.

MOVE IT TO LOSE IT
Continue your routine of warm-up, walking with purpose for thirty minutes, and gentle stretching. Now, add intervals twice a week to build your stamina. Intervals help you burn fat, even after you walk. After your warm-up and five minutes of walking with purpose, try two minutes of faster, speed walking, so that you can really feel your heartbeat and perhaps even start to sweat a little. After two minutes, pull back to purposeful walking and cool down. Then, after another five minutes, pick up the pace again. Do three sets of picking up and cooling down during your thirty-minute walk.

By now you should be noticing that you have more stamina, better energy, and better sleep—this is just some of what your daily walk does for you.

You're halfway through the plan—celebrate! Buy yourself a treat like a new pair of walking shoes, a terra-cotta planter for growing herbs, or tickets to see your favorite sports team or theater group.

Week 5

WHAT TO EAT, WHAT NOT TO EAT

Now, bump the number of days you are having a soup or salad as a first course for dinner to five. You're eating a daily breakfast, and your whole-grain efforts are daily. These things should start to feel normal—like you'd miss them if you stopped. You are creating good habits.

This week, be more aware of how the meats you eat are cooked. Charred meats can contain carcinogens. Marinate meats (red meat, poultry, and fish) in a low-sugar marinade before grilling or roasting them, to avoid charring and minimize carcinogen formation: cook to medium or medium-rare and cut off any accidental char and discard.

Also, every day this week, take a moment to relax and drink a cup of tea. Tea drinking has been linked to a reduced risk of heart attacks. But don't drink it with milk—new research has found that adding milk undoes the heart-healthy effect. The culprits are proteins in milk called caseins that interact with tea, decreasing the concentration of catechin—the flavonoids in tea that are likely responsible for its protective effects against heart disease. Try tea with honey and lemon instead—the honey has antioxidants and the lemon has vitamin C, and the flavor combination is very refreshing.

Make "small is beautiful" your new mantra, and put quality before quantity. Start buying foods in smaller packages, even if it means losing out on the "bulk" discount. Studies show that when people pour liquid (for example, olive oil or corn syrup) from a small bottle they pour anywhere from 15 percent to 48 percent less when than when they pour from a big one. Researchers think that perhaps the smaller bottle makes the liquid seem more valuable, or that just by being small itself, the sight of the bottle prompts you to use less. Also, most people will eat more from a big bag of food than a small one, since having to open another bag makes you realize that maybe you've had enough.

THIS WEEK'S COLOR: WHITE

Pick a naturally white or white-brown food that you've never had before or haven't had in years and try it: garlic, onions, shallots, or sunchokes. They are all rich in vitamin-like flavonoids—especially quercetin and kaempferol—to protect your arteries, heart, and brain. Have one of these white foods every day if you can. Have cauliflower, too, which when cooked with turmeric is a powerfully synergistic way to fight prostate cancer. Cut the cauliflower into bite-size florets and let sit for five to ten minutes; this gives it time to produce phenethyl isothiocyanates, which form when cruciferous vegetables are cut and which fight human cancer cells. Then steam it briefly to keep those anticarcinogens. You might also eat a pear once this week—this juicy and elegant fruit ripens faster when next to a banana, because of the natural hormone ethylene that it gives off. Here are two recipes to help you eat white.

RECIPES TO TRY
Roasted Winter Vegetables with Cranberry-Studded Quinoa (page 126)
> or
Sauerkraut with Onion, Apple, and Toasted Caraway (page 136)

MOVE IT TO LOSE IT
On one of the days when you are not doing intervals, incorporate stair-climbing into your walking. If you need more time, give yourself more. Warm up, walk for ten minutes, climb stairs slowly both up and down for five minutes, walk for another ten minutes, cool down, and stretch. You could climb your own stairs, the stairs in front of a public building, or the stairs inside a tall office building. Don't worry about looking silly—everyone else will be taking the elevator.

Week 6

WHAT TO EAT, WHAT NOT TO EAT
By this time you should be having breakfast every day, and only rarely eating processed white foods. Your taste buds and digestive system should have started becoming used to having more vegetables. Chances are you have started feeling more alert, and no longer get the crash and burn that happens after you eat foods that are high in sugar and fat. You may no longer need the four o'clock pick-me-up of a sugary soda.

This week and from now on, drink no more than one serving of alcohol daily for women, two for men. Make it really good wine, beer, or spirits: it's quality and consistency, not quantity, that matters. If you're not sleeping well or can't get up in the morning, cut out the coffee, tea, and alcohol altogether for one month and then see how you feel. If overused, caffeine and alcohol can dehydrate you, interfere with sleep, and increase fatigue. If you want to get the health benefits of your daily tea without the caffeine, pour off the water after thirty seconds—you pour off the caffeine as well. Have half a banana within an hour of bedtime: the banana's melatonin helps reorient your circadian rhythm, and the banana's magnesium is a muscle relaxant.

This week, try a food combination that is synergistic. The combination of broccoli and tomatoes, for example, is more effective at slowing tumor growth than either tomato or broccoli alone and more effective than purified lycopene, an antioxidant in tomatoes, alone. Add broccoli and tomatoes to a traditionally heavy dish you might need to prepare—for example, lasagna, casseroles, or seven-layer salad. You'll eat less meat and trans fat, and more vegetables.

Eat a smooth food, like yogurt, cottage cheese, or pudding, with another differently textured food such as a few sunflower seeds, a few mini–chocolate chips, diced berries, salsa, or a little cereal. You will take smaller bites as the food is now thicker and not so smooth. The variability in a food's texture helps you eat more slowly and be satisfied with less.

THIS WEEK'S COLOR: GREEN

Pick a green food you've never had before or haven't had in years and try it: kale, broccoli rabe, collard greens, brussels sprouts, or cabbage. Also seek out young broccoli, and try it at least once. Green means go! These foods are powerful messages to your immune system: their sulforaphane tells your genes to help break down cancer-causing chemicals. Try some turnip greens at least once—one cup has 662 percent of your RDI of vitamin K, which is necessary for healthy blood clotting. Try some bok choy at least once. The Chinese started eating it in the fifth century, and even back then, they believed it had medicinal qualities. Stir-fry the stems with dark sesame oil for five minutes and the leaves for two.

RECIPES TO TRY

Cedar-Planked Roast Salmon with Candied Ginger and Berry Salsa (page 112)

or

Broccoli, Cheese, and Kalamata Olive Pizza (page 101)

WINES THAT COMPLEMENT

Pinot Noir, a sleek, smooth wine, complements dark, oily fish like wild salmon. Try chilling the Pinot—from Oregon, Washington, or California—for just thirty minutes in the fridge. It will be just as soft and easy to drink as most California Chardonnays. With pizza, food-friendly soft reds like a well-made Chilean Merlot or Spanish Grenache are a slam dunk.

MOVE IT TO LOSE IT

Add a few minutes of strength training (i.e., weight lifting) to your routine three days a week. Don't worry that you might look like Arnold. Even lifting moderate weights for just a few minutes a few times a week has a great ChefMD benefit—it especially helps you burn fat and keeps your bones strong. Free weights are inexpensive and can be used in the privacy of your home.

Focus on your arms, shoulders, chest, and back to balance the strength you are now gaining in your legs. Ideally, you should first have a session with a trainer so that you learn good technique that can safeguard you from injury. If you can't afford to hire a trainer, have a friend show you the ropes or pick up a basic book or DVD on strength training. It may seem a challenge at first, but do a little at a time—you won't regret the results!

Week 7

WHAT TO EAT, WHAT NOT TO EAT

From now until the end of the plan, avoid artificial sweeteners: they daze your taste buds into thinking "sweet" means "no calories" and you overeat. Try stevia, buckwheat, or another dark honey, or use mint instead to sweeten food. See if you still miss artificial sweeteners by the end of the eight weeks—I bet you won't.

Roasting, steaming, and frying do not affect flavonoids as much as boiling. When you boil food you lose about 30 percent of your flavonoids and minerals like potassium. Starting this week, don't boil your vegetables unless you're making soup. You don't lose flavonoids in soup since you also eat the broth.

Know some basic numbers, and recall them before you eat: if you have been walking for thirty minutes at least four days weekly, your daily caloric needs are your weight times 15; if you haven't, it's your weight times 13. One ounce of tortilla chips, about fourteen chips, has 140 calories; one cup of cooked white pasta has 160 calories; one twenty-ounce soda has 250 calories. And few of those calories are filling, aromatic, or aesthetically appealing. Skip the bread on the restaurant table and hand back the basket to the server: it's not why you are out to eat.

THIS WEEK'S COLOR: BROWN

This week, eat foods that are brown, such as grains, nuts, and seeds. Try small portions of whole-wheat bread, brown rice, kasha (which are roasted buckwheat groats), quinoa, millet, walnuts, pecans, peanuts, macadamia nuts, hazelnuts, or sesame seeds. Have some sunflower seeds—they are crunchy and tasty, and just a quarter cup will give you almost your full reference daily intake of vitamin E. Or try some cashews—not only do they have less fat than most nuts, but more than half of that fat is oleic acid, the same heart-healthy monounsaturated fat in olive oil.

RECIPES TO TRY

Sardine and Arugula Salad with Ratatouille (page 129)
     or
Roasted Turkey Tenderloin Stuffed with Cranberries and Pecans
    (page 125)

MOVE IT TO LOSE IT

This week, add two twenty-minute sessions of aerobics to your schedule. Jogging, in-line skating, running, using the elliptical trainer, swimming, spinning, or kickboxing—choose something you enjoy, and do it. This will give your arteries and immune system a big boost.

Week 8

WHAT TO EAT, WHAT NOT TO EAT

By now, you're eating breakfast every morning; eating plenty of vegetables, salads, and soups; and are no longer eating any processed white foods. The healthy diet you are following by now should taste good to you, and you might find yourself choosing fruit when before you would have reached for a cookie.

Release, absorb, and experience the hundreds of flavor compounds in chocolate. Hold a small piece of dark chocolate in your mouth for one minute and let it melt. Is it any wonder we love chocolate? Remember, only dark chocolate has positive health benefits, and white chocolate too often is made with shortening, not chocolate.

You are now doing your best to sit when you eat and are eating more deliberately. You are doing your best to avoid exceptions. Now, add another satiety trick to your meals—when you prepare food, cut it smaller and into strips. Smaller pieces create the illusion of a greater amount or volume. Strips are more successful at creating this illusion than small cubes or blocks. Peel cheese sticks into shreds so it looks like more atop a salad or main dish. The appearance of more food helps to fill you up, even before you start to eat. You can sometimes fool your brain (and your stomach) even when it knows it's being fooled.

THIS WEEK'S COLOR: NEW GREENS

Try new greens—collard greens, mustard greens, or watercress. Look for green peas, avocado, and nopales (cactus paddles, an effective food for lowering blood sugar), and green melons: they are all rich in lutein and zeaxanthin, which will help keep your eyesight sharp. You've never seen a rabbit with glasses, have you? Try some spinach—it is rich in a flavonoid called kaempferol, which guards against ovarian cancer. Eat cooked spinach—spinach reduces in volume so much when it's cooked, you'll get up to six times the nutrients per cup than when it's raw. Have some romaine lettuce in a salad at least once, for a one-two ChefMD punch—you'll be getting your folate and helping yourself reach satiety faster at the same time.

RECIPES TO TRY

Red Pozole with Shredded Chicken and Avocado (page 124)
   or
Skillet Chilaquiles with Cactus Paddles, Eggs, and Kale (page 98)

WINES THAT COMPLEMENT

Mexico is not known for its wine, but there are some surprisingly good Cabernets and Tempranillos coming out of Baja. Or explore an Italian Barbera for bright, clear flavors that will cut against the richness of the warming pozole. And for the chilaquiles (traditionally for breakfast, but hey, who doesn't like to have breakfast for dinner?), the chipotle salsa would work with a good Argentinean Malbec (it has its own smoky finish), or even a lovely Australian Shiraz (which has less alcohol than most California Syrahs). Talk to your local wine merchant for help with picking a brand for you and your pocketbook.

MOVE IT TO LOSE IT

This week, try a physical activity that masquerades as pure fun. Get your family or friends together and do something other than going out for dinner as a group—go ice skating, play tennis, play a game of hockey or Frisbee or basketball, or go dancing. There is no set time requirement—the only requirement is that you have fun.

You Did It!

That's it! You did it! Celebrate with a massage, a session with a personal trainer, or a funny movie with a loved one, and then look at the numbers you wrote down at the start and see where you stand. What progress did you make? Chances are good you may have lost a few pounds, are feeling less joint pain, and are sleeping better. You've just scratched the surface with what you can do to find and train the doctor inside—there's even more and better success and health ahead.

I would love to hear how you live the ChefMD plan: how you change it, adapt it, improve on it; what you're able to follow and what you're not, and how it makes a difference in your life and your health. Follow it for eight weeks or more, and then write me with your story at drjohn@ChefMD.com.

Now that you're on track for a long, healthy life, let's look at what else you can do to optimize your health. Read on to find out what to eat for common conditions.

CHAPTER 7

What Do You Eat for That?

He that takes medicine and neglects diet wastes the skills of the physician.

—Chinese proverb

Male pattern baldness and a love of practical jokes are not the only things that run in families. So does a risk for diseases. And if you know that a certain disease runs in your family, or you're otherwise at risk, you probably want to know how to prevent it. Or maybe you've already had a diagnosis of a disease, and you want to know what good nutrition can do.

In the past, we thought that having extra nutrients, especially antioxidants, helped people function at their peak level and prevented heart disease and cancer. However, so far this has not been shown to be true. For example, vitamin C–rich food may prevent oral precancer, but vitamin C supplements do not. Nuts and seeds rich in vitamin E fight prostate cancer, but vitamin E supplements do not, and actually increase the risk of heart failure in people with diabetes. Beta-carotene-rich carrots protect against lung cancer, but beta-carotene supplements have been shown to increase the rate of lung cancer in smokers and precancerous colon polyps in people at high risk.

Too much supplementation is a safety concern, because too

many supplements of the wrong kinds can do harm—especially iron, zinc, vitamin A, E, beta-carotene, niacin, and calcium. People who take multivitamins are more likely to have too much iron, zinc, vitamin A, and niacin. Many foods now are fortified with multivitamins, so what you take in pill form often doubles your dose. And supplements can interact with prescription medication and sometimes do not contain what they say they do. For these reasons, if you choose to take a multivitamin or supplements, please follow the ChefMD guidelines to make sure you are not taking too much, and speak with your doctor.

How Do You Know If You Need a Multivitamin?

You need to take a multivitamin or supplements if you are or may become pregnant, are seriously undernourished or underweight, taking a diet pill that causes nutrient loss (for example, weight-loss drugs Alli or Xenical), or have a poor diet (for example, you are hospitalized, you are malnourished because of difficulty eating or an eating disorder, you eat only junk food, or you are in a long-term care facility). If any of these are the case for you, here is a suggested maximal intake for vitamins and minerals in a multivitamin: lower amounts will also be safe. Only vitamin B12 and vitamin D are difficult to get from food in these amounts. If you can get a multivitamin that has them, it is probably worth taking.

VITAMINS
- Vitamin A: No more than twenty-five hundred international units (1.6 milligrams) daily
- Vitamin B6: No more than two milligrams daily
- Vitamin B12: No more than twenty-five micrograms daily. (It is not toxic, and B12 malabsorption is common in adults over age fifty.)
- Vitamin C: No more than approximately two hundred milligrams up to twice daily
- Vitamin D: Eight hundred to one thousand international units daily, vitamin D3 preferred (unless you have kidney stones and then less than two hundred international units daily; if you

have dark-pigmented skin, you may need two thousand international units.)

- Vitamin E: No more than thirty international units (about fifteen milligrams) up to twice daily, mixed tocopherols preferred. (Again, vitamin E is best gotten from food, as you get all eight forms of the vitamin.)
- Folate (vitamin B9): Four hundred micrograms daily

MINERALS

- Iron (premenopausal women only): Eighteen milligrams. Ferrous gluconate is easiest on the stomach.
- Magnesium: 320–400 milligrams daily (although this is better obtained from food, especially whole grains, and this dosage of magnesium is too bulky to fit in most multivitamins)
- Selenium: No more than fifty-five micrograms daily (but none if you have had invasive squamous cell skin cancer or are at risk for diabetes)
- Zinc: No more than fifteen milligrams daily

In addition, you may want to supplement with nutrients that do not fit in a multivitamin, especially calcium and essential fatty acids.

- Calcium: Up to one thousand milligrams daily; men do not need it, as it may increase the risk of prostate cancer. Calcium citrate is well absorbed.
- Omega-3s from fish: Up to two grams total daily. This should be molecularly distilled and tested for heavy metals, such as mercury and lead, and contaminants, such as PCBs. If you take anticoagulants such as Coumadin, or if you take flax, fish, black currant, borage, or evening primrose oil, you should have your coagulation status monitored by a physician.

WHAT SHOULD NOT BE IN YOUR MULTIVITAMIN

- Iron (for men and postmenopausal women). Iron is an oxidant and increases damage to your blood vessels. In men, it increases the risk of gallstones.
- Too much vitamin A: Men who ingest an average of more than forty-three hundred international units daily have a dramati-

cally increased risk of hip fracture over those who ingest the least.

- Too much beta-carotene (more than twenty-five hundred international units per day).
- More than one hundred milligrams vitamin B6 daily (it can cause peripheral neuropathy).
- Excessive intakes of iron, zinc, and niacin—make sure your multivitamin has 100 percent or less of the reference daily intake (RDI) of these.
- Too much synthetic vitamin E.

GOOD FOOD SOURCES OF VITAMINS AND MINERALS

Vitamin B6	• General Mills Total Raisin Bran • Chickpeas • Yellowfin tuna • Beef liver	• Turkey giblets • Rice • Chestnuts • Buckwheat flour
Vitamin B12	• Clams • Beef liver • Turkey giblets • Oysters • Chicken giblets • New England clam chowder	• Alaska king crab • Sockeye salmon • Sardines • General Mills Whole-grain Total
Vitamin C	• Orange juice • Red peppers • Grapefruit juice • Peaches • Papayas	• Grape juice • Green peppers • Hot chili peppers • Strawberries • Broccoli
Vitamin D	• Cod liver oil • Herring • Salmon • Mackerel • Tuna fish	• Sardines • Nonfat milk • Eggs • Liver • Swiss cheese

GOOD FOOD SOURCES OF VITAMINS AND MINERALS

Vitamin E	• General Mills Whole-grain Total	• Spinach
	• Canned tomato paste	• Sunflower oil
	• Sunflower seeds	• Turnip greens
	• Almonds	• Hazelnuts

Folate	• General Mills Whole-grain Total	• Lentils
	• Cornmeal	• Orange juice
	• Turkey giblets	• Pinto beans
	• General Mills Wheat Chex	• Okra

Calcium	• General Mills Whole-grain Total	• Collards
	• Canned milk	• Rhubarb
	• Ricotta cheese	• Sardines
	• Cornmeal	• Spinach
	• Yogurt	• Soybeans

Iron	• Clams	• Soybeans
	• Swiss chard	• Baked beans
	• Cream of Wheat	• Canned tomato paste
	• Bison	• Beef
	• Spinach	

Magnesium	• Buckwheat flour	• Spinach
	• Bulgur	• Barley
	• Oat bran	• Cornmeal
	• Halibut	• Pumpkin seeds
	• Whole-grain flour	• Soybeans

Selenium	• Brazil nuts	• Orange roughy
	• Whole-grain flour	• Halibut
	• Tuna	• Flounder
	• Turkey giblets	• Rockfish
	• Barley	

GOOD FOOD SOURCES OF VITAMINS AND MINERALS

Zinc	• Oysters	• Alaska king crab
	• General Mills Total cornflakes	• Lean lamb shoulder meat
	• Baked beans	• Lean beef ribs
	• Turkey neck meat	• Duck
	• Lean beef chuck	
Essential fatty acids	• Salmon	• Shellfish
	• Sardines	• Flaxseed
	• Trout	• Walnuts
	• Herring	• Canola oil
	• Mackerel	• Purslane

For each of the forty conditions cited in this chapter are lists of foods to consume and foods to avoid. (Of course, if you are allergic to a food, avoid it!) Only major recommendations are listed, as there simply isn't space for all there is to say. Some common folklore—avoid nuts and popcorn if you have diverticular disease, for example—turns out not to be true at all.

Some conditions benefit from a certain eating pattern (for example, diets that are low fat, high fiber, low sugar, low glycemic load, rich in a mineral, Mediterranean, and vegetarian)*. Only a little is known about eating patterns, but they combine the effect of foods, adding up the small bits of good each ingredient does to work together.

The Western eating pattern, for example, is high in dairy, red and processed meats, refined grains, and sweets. Men with West-

*Because foods are not simply a sum of nutrients, these suggestions are based, whenever possible, on studies of actual foods.

Quickie definitions: Recipes that are low fat contain less than 30 percent calories from fat; low saturated fat means less than 7 percent calories from saturated fat. Recipes that are high in fiber have at least fourteen grams of fiber per thousand calories. Recipes that are low in sugar and low glycemic have less than sixteen grams of sugar per serving. Recipes that are low glycemic load are those in which the amount of carbohydrate in the recipe is digested slowly.

Recipes rich in a mineral, such as magnesium or calcium, contain at least 33 percent of the RDI for that mineral.

Recipes that adhere to the Mediterranean diet pattern contain ingredients central to this region, such as olive oil, wine, fish, whole grains, dark leafy greens, garlic, and tomatoes.

Vegetarian recipes do not contain meat, poultry, or fish but may contain eggs and dairy.

ern eating patterns and who are sedentary are twice as likely as other men to develop diabetes. An inflammatory eating pattern—high in sugar-sweetened soda and in diet soda, refined grains, and processed meat but low in wine, coffee, cruciferous vegetables, and yellow vegetables—raises the risk of diabetes in women; an anti-inflammatory pattern (just switch high and low) should lower the risk.

I also recommend three recipes for each condition, using the ChefMD-Approved System. ChefMD Approved is simple in concept and complex in math. The ChefMD scientific team analyzed over one thousand peer-reviewed, published scientific studies done in people to determine which eating patterns and which individual foods had the greatest effect on forty common conditions.* The team assigned point values to the eating patterns and the foods and then analyzed fifty of our best, easiest, and tastiest recipes to identify which ones were best for which conditions. All the recipes are in this book.

Each recipe earned ChefMD-Approved points when it fit a condition's best eating pattern(s), and points when it contained foods that can help that condition. Recipes were disqualified as ChefMD Approved for a particular condition if they contained an eating pattern or food to be avoided for that condition.

Enjoy!

ACNE

WHAT IT IS: Acne is a skin condition in which skin pores or hair follicles become clogged and infected.

YOU ARE AT INCREASED RISK IF YOU
- are between the ages of twelve and seventeen
- are under stress or are taking a prescription drug for depression or stress
- have a family history of acne
- use toiletries, hair products, or cosmetics that are oil- or talc-based

*Many thanks to Elizabeth Ko, now a University of Miami medical student, for her keen insights and analyses.

CULINARY MEDICINE

FOODS TO INCREASE

- Foods with low glycemic indexes. These include nonstarchy, minimally processed fruits and vegetables, whole-grain products, beans, nuts, chicken, eggs, meat, and fish. Forty-three men who ate a low glycemic load diet for twelve weeks reduced their number of acne lesions by more than 20 percent, possibly by avoiding the high insulin levels and increased androgen bioavailability brought on by high glycemic load foods.
- Green tea. Epigallocatechin-3-gallate, the catechin in green tea, affects the hormones that cause acne.

FOODS TO AVOID

- Nonfat and low-fat milk. They *may* contribute to acne, although the data have been hotly argued on both sides. It is suspected that hormone-rich dairy fat is not the cause—but rather the imbalance of hormones, specifically excess insulin growth factor 1.

TOP CHEFMD-APPROVED RECIPES FOR ACNE

- Healthy Real Hamburgers (page 119)
- Roasted Turkey Tenderloin Stuffed with Cranberries and Pecans (page 125)
- Toasted Walnut and Creamy White Bean Pitas (page 109)

WATER-COOLER FACT: As adolescents, boys are more likely to suffer acne scarring than are girls. But as adults, women are more likely to get acne than men. Acne can persist past age sixty-five.

ALLERGY

WHAT IT IS: An allergy is a reaction by your immune system in response to a foreign substance such as mold or pet dander.

YOU ARE AT INCREASED RISK IF YOU

- have a family history of allergies
- were not exposed to allergens in childhood (because being exposed as a child can prevent some allergies later in life)

CULINARY MEDICINE

FOODS TO INCREASE

- Yogurt and kefir. Lactic acid bacteria have been shown to lower the risk of allergies in junior high school students who habitually eat foods rich in these healthy bacteria. The probiotics in yogurt stimulate the gut immune system.

- Food rich in eicosapentaenoic acid (EPA), an omega-3 fatty acid. People who eat omega-3-rich foods such as wild salmon, herring, mackerel, anchovies, and sardines often are less than half as likely to get allergies as those who do not. Also, when pregnant women eat fish two or three times a week, their children are less likely by one-third to have food allergies and eczema than children of women who eat little or no fish during pregnancy. The anti-inflammatory effects of fish's omega-3s may make the baby's developing immune system less prone to allergic reaction.

- Hempseed oil. In a twenty-week trial it helped alleviate the symptoms of eczema, probably because of its omega-3s.

- Fruits and vegetables. People with high blood levels of carotenoids from food, in a German study, had less than half the risk of those who had the lowest.

- Seaweed. A study done on over one thousand pregnant women showed that eating it decreases the risk of allergic rhinitis, possibly because of the anti-inflammatory effects of its flavonoids.

- Foods rich in calcium, phosphorous, and magnesium. They reduce the risk of allergies.

- Unripe apples. A small Japanese study showed that an apple drink rich in polyphenols taken daily for a month reduced sneezing attacks in people with persistent allergic rhinitis.

FOODS TO AVOID

- Cheese, hard-cured sausage, pickled cabbage, wine, beer, and other foods high in histamine, which is an inflammatory chemical. When one hundred people with allergies avoided such foods for four weeks, more than half had considerable improvement, and fifteen had complete remission. Once they started eating histamine-rich food again, 50 percent had a recurrence of atopic eczema.

- Red meat. People who eat a meat-rich diet have almost three times the risk of having hay fever as those who eat little or no meat (probably because of its inflammatory effects).
- Foods high in saturated fat for women who are breast-feeding. When infants were tested at three months old, those whose mothers ate a diet high in saturated fat had a 16 percent increased chance of atopic disease compared with those whose mothers ate little or no saturated fat.

TOP CHEFMD-APPROVED RECIPES FOR ALLERGY
- Cedar-Planked Roast Salmon with Candied Ginger and Berry Salsa (page 112)
- Grilled Citrus Trout over Crunchy Mediterranean Slaw (page 118)
- Saffron Scallop, Shrimp, and Chickpea Paella (page 128)

WATER-COOLER FACT: Almost one in five Americans suffer from allergies.

ALZHEIMER'S

WHAT IT IS: Alzheimer's disease is a slowly progressive, irreversible brain disease that results in memory loss, impaired thinking ability, and ultimately changes in behavior or personality.

YOU ARE AT INCREASED RISK IF YOU
- are sedentary
- are depressed or lonely
- have heart disease or diabetes

WHAT ARE MY DOGS' NAMES?

Ellen is a fifty-eight-year-old information technology specialist in Colorado whose seventy-eight-year-old mother has Alzheimer's disease. Ellen became worried that she might be getting it, too, when she couldn't remember her border collies' names while driving home from work.

She went to see her family physician, who sent her for neuropsychological testing. She had no medical problems, and her weight, blood sugar, and blood pressure were all normal. Although her judgment and orientation tests were normal, the neurologist said she was developing mild cognitive impairment, which can be the start of Alzheimer's disease.

When Ellen came to see me, I told her that Alzheimer's is not an inevitable stage of aging, and with some changes in her diet, she could slow the progress of the disease. Ellen agreed to avoid eating saturated and trans-fat foods together with high copper foods, such as cashews, soy, and barley, to reduce her risk. She changed her favorite snack (soft pretzels from a street cart, which are full of trans fats) to still-convenient store-bought bags of presliced apples. At my urging, she promised to replace aluminum- and copper-lined cookware and to drink filtered water.

Ellen started eating omega-3-rich fish three times a week, because people with Alzheimer's have less omega-3 docosahexaenoic acid (DHA) in their brain-cell membranes than people without Alzheimer's. She began drinking fresh brewed green tea, which lowers the risk of cognitive impairment—and brewed tea has ten times the antioxidants of bottled tea. She began eating more green leafy vegetables, since three servings a day means a 40 percent slower rate of cognitive decline than just one serving. She started drinking red wine, as it contains resveratrol, which reduces the amyloid beta peptides that form senile plaques in the brain. She agreed to become more active, because even just half an hour daily of brisk walking helps maintain memory. She signed up for training sessions in memorizing, reasoning, and processing, which help improve skills in people over age sixty-five—and may work for people like her who are younger, too. And when I asked her to consider following the Mediterranean diet, she said she'd start eating more nuts and olive oil as well as continuing to eat fish.

A year later, Ellen feels great. She has not experienced any further mental decline, and her changes in diet and lifestyle have increased her overall health. She has the peace of mind of knowing she is doing everything she can to minimize her risk of developing Alzheimer's and feels she is making a difference in others' lives by volunteering at her local Alzheimer's association.

CULINARY MEDICINE
FOODS TO INCREASE

- Water. Drink at least sixty-four ounces every day.

- Green tea. People who drink two or more cups of it a day are 54 percent less likely to have cognitive impairment than people who drink it only three times a week. An antioxidant named epigallocatechin-3-gallate may reduce plaque buildup in the brain.

- Apple juice. It contains S-adenosylmethionine for neuroprotection, as well as antioxidants. Unfiltered apple juice contains one and a half times the antioxidant effectiveness as filtered.

- Red wine. In a French study, people who drank three or four five-ounce glasses a day were at less risk of dementia than teetotalers, possibly because wine's polyphenols may protect the brain.

- The Mediterranean diet of fish, fresh vegetables, fruits, legumes, whole-grain bread, grain cereals, and nuts and seeds. More than two thousand New Yorkers were tracked over four years; those who ate a diet rich with foods from the Mediterranean diet were found to be at 40 percent lesser risk of Alzheimer's than those who ate few or none of those foods. Those people most adherent lived 3.9 years longer than those least adherent.

- Asparagus, spinach, kale, and other dark green vegetables. Their folate has been associated with a slower rate of cognitive decline. Spinach is rich in zeaxanthin, a carotenoid linked to better mental performance in healthy older people. Those who ate three servings a day of leafy vegetables had a 40 percent decrease in mental decline.

- Vegetables in general. Those who ate four servings a day of vegetables had a 40 percent decrease in mental decline compared to those who ate less than one.

- Oily fish. Salmon and tuna are high in omega-3s. People who eat fish at least weekly have 40 percent less risk of developing Alzheimer's than those who rarely or never eat fish.

- Fortified whole-grain cereals. They are rich in folic acid and of almost one thousand people over the age of sixty-five, those whose diets were the richest in folate were found to be at only half the risk of developing Alzheimer's compared with those eating diets with the least folate.

- Foods rich in niacin. In a nine-year study of more than six thousand Chicago residents age sixty-five or older, those who ate foods rich in niacin such as chicken breast, yellowfin tuna, and Chinook salmon had up to a 70 percent decreased risk of Alzheimer's and mental decline, although the exact mechanism is not known.
- Sunflower seeds, almonds, and other foods rich in vitamin E. A study of people over the age of sixty-five showed that an increase of five milligrams of dietary vitamin E per day lowered their risk of Alzheimer's by 26 percent, perhaps because of vitamin E's antioxidant properties.

FOODS TO AVOID

- Foods rich in copper. These include calves' liver, turnip greens, molasses, and crimini mushrooms. A Chicago study of thirty-seven hundred people over age sixty-five showed that those with the highest levels of copper (2.75 milligrams per day) added the equivalent of nineteen years' worth of mental decline if they also ate a high saturated and trans-fat diet compared with those who ate the least copper. An imbalance of iron, zinc, and copper is thought to be important in the formation of Alzheimer's plaques.
- Foods high in saturated fats and trans fats. Avoiding them cuts your risk of Alzheimer's by almost 50 percent.

TOP CHEFMD-APPROVED RECIPES FOR ALZHEIMER'S
- Cioppino (page 114)
- Portuguese Caldo Verde (page 104)
- Roasted Red Pepper, Wine, and Red Lentil Soup (page 105)

WATER-COOLER FACT: Using nonsteroidal anti-inflammatory drugs and getting regular physical exercise both reduce the risk of Alzheimer's, as may coffee . . . Stay tuned.

ANEMIA

WHAT IT IS: Anemia is a lower than normal number of red blood cells. There are different types of anemia, including but not limited to anemia from iron deficiency, folic acid deficiency, and vitamin B12 deficiency.

YOU ARE AT INCREASED RISK IF YOU
- are a premenopausal woman (because of menstrual bleeding)
- are an alcoholic
- have gastrointestinal bleeding
- have a chronic disease that causes bleeding, such as kidney or liver disease
- have a hereditary defect, such as sickle-cell anemia, or thalassemia (a blood disease)
- were not breast-fed or were under-breast-fed as an infant
- drink water contaminated with lead, which lowers the level of iron in your blood

CULINARY MEDICINE
FOODS TO INCREASE
For iron deficiency

- Foods with readily absorbable heme iron. These include beef liver, lean sirloin, and fortified (with iron) breakfast cereal.
- Foods with non-heme iron. These include pumpkin seeds, bran, blackstrap molasses, soybeans, and spinach.
- Foods rich in vitamin C, especially together with foods with non-heme iron. Kiwi, citrus fruits, and red bell peppers all improve the absorption of non-heme iron.
- Alcohol, in moderation. People who drink two drinks a day have a 40 percent decreased risk of iron-deficiency anemia than those who do not drink. More than two drinks a day increases the risk of iron overload.

For folic acid deficiency

- Foods rich in folate. They include chicken and beef livers, vitamin B12–fortified breakfast cereal, soy flour, chickpeas, pinto beans, lima beans, and spinach.

For vitamin B12 deficiency
- Clams, oysters, snails, trout, salmon, beef liver, and fortified breakfast cereal. They are all rich in vitamin B12.

FOODS TO AVOID
- Cakes, candy, and other sweet foods. A Chinese study found that people who ate a diet high in these foods had more than twice the risk of anemia as those who ate few or none.
- Coffee and tea. They both inhibit the ability of the body to absorb non-heme iron if drunk at the same time that iron-rich food is eaten.

TOP CHEFMD-APPROVED RECIPES FOR ANEMIA
- Bison Steak and Broccoli Salad (page 110)
- Parmigiano Caesar Salad with Shrimp (page 121)
- Sardine and Arugula Salad with Ratatouille (page 129)

WATER-COOLER FACT: People over age fifty often need extra vitamin B12, because it is less well absorbed as we age.

ASTHMA

WHAT IT IS: Asthma is a chronic inflammatory respiratory disease that causes wheezing and difficulty breathing. It is potentially life-threatening.

YOU ARE AT INCREASED RISK IF YOU
- are sensitive to food additives and preservatives
- are obese
- are underweight
- have alcohol, food, or environmental allergies
- are insecure, fearful, anxious, or stressed
- have overused antibiotics, particularly in early childhood
- have a family history of asthma or eczema
- have a mother who did not get enough vitamin D while pregnant with you

FOODS TO INCREASE

- Water. Drink 1.5 to 2 liters (a little more than 1.5 to 2 quarts) of water daily.

- Whole grains, Brazil nuts, walnuts, and beef. They are all rich in the mineral selenium, which activates an antioxidant enzyme to reduce inflammation. Participants in a study with the highest intakes of selenium—54 to 90 micrograms a day—were only about half as likely to have asthma as those who consumed the least selenium, about 23 to 30 micrograms daily. The U.S. RDI for selenium is 55 micrograms.

- Oily fish. Mackerel, tuna, salmon, and trout are all rich in anti-inflammatory omega-3s and vitamin E, magnesium, and selenium.

- Flaxseed oil. It is rich in some omega 3-fatty acids and not omega-6 fatty acids; children who have a low ratio of omega-6s to omega-3s in their diet have a lowered risk of asthma.

- Garlic, rosemary, turmeric, red pepper, cloves, ginger, cumin, anise, fennel, and basil. They all prevent inflammation.

- Soy foods. In a study of over one thousand adults with asthma, the greater the level of soy phytoestrogen genistein in the bloodstream, the better the lung volume.

- Organic fruits and vegetables. They do not have synthetic artificial chemical additives and are less likely to provoke asthma than conventionally grown produce.

- Tomatoes, eggplant, cucumber, green beans, and summer squash. Kids who ate just one and a half ounces of these five vegetables were least likely to have childhood asthma or wheeze. The vegetables' flavonoids protect cells lining the airway from inflammation.

- Apples. They seem particularly effective at protecting against asthma, perhaps because of a bronchodilator flavonoid called khellin. People who eat apples twice weekly are at an 11 percent reduced risk of asthma compared with those who eat few or none.

- Citrus fruits. They are high in vitamin C and have an anti-inflammatory effect. People who ate 46.3 grams a day of citrus fruits (about an ounce and a half daily) had a 41 percent reduced risk of asthma compared with those who ate none.

- Orange juice. In a twelve-month study of Italian children ages six and seven, those who ate foods rich in vitamin C five to seven times a week had a 36 percent reduced rate of wheezing than those who ate vitamin C–rich foods less than once a week.
- Milk. Pregnant women who ate a diet richest in vitamin D—about 724 international units per day—had about half the risk of having a child who would have a wheezing illness at age three, and less than half the risk of having a child at high risk for asthma than women who ate very little vitamin D–rich food. Every daily increase of one hundred international units of vitamin D reduced the asthma risk for the child by 20 percent.

FOODS TO AVOID
- Alcohol (especially white wine, if it triggers an allergic response).
- Margarine. In a Greek study, consumption of it more than doubled the risk of wheezing and rhinitis.
- Processed carbohydrates and sweets. They are likely to contain colorings, preservatives, and other additives that can cause allergic-response-related asthma.
- Red meats. They very often contain saturated fats, which stimulate your genes to make inflammatory proteins.
- Soft drinks. They are likely to contain artificial food additives, such as yellow dye #5 (tartrazine), sodium benzoate, alluva red, monosodium glutamate, and sulfites.

TOP CHEFMD-APPROVED RECIPES FOR ASTHMA
- Cedar-Planked Roast Salmon with Candied Ginger and Berry Salsa (page 112)
- Cheese Ravioli with Tofu and Baby Peas (page 113)
- Sicilian Pasta with Swiss Chard, Goat Cheese, and Basil (page 130)

WATER-COOLER FACT: Ounce for ounce, the Himalayan goji (pronounced "Go-Gee") berry contains more vitamin C than oranges.

Vitamin C has been shown to reduce medication dependence in adults with mild asthma.

ATTENTION DEFICIT HYPERACTIVITY DISORDER

WHAT IT IS: Attention deficit hyperactivity disorder (ADHD) is a mental disorder that causes people to be impulsive, hyperactive, and to have difficulty concentrating. The disorder starts in childhood but remains throughout life.

YOU ARE AT INCREASED RISK IF YOU
- are male
- are a smoker
- drink alcohol
- have a family history of ADHD
- have had a head injury
- have had lead poisoning
- have a mother who smoked while pregnant
- have a mother who was under great stress while pregnant
- were breast-fed for less than three months
- were born prematurely

CULINARY MEDICINE
FOODS TO INCREASE
- Organic fruits
- Organic vegetables
- Flaxseed oil
- Fish oil. People with ADHD usually have low levels of omega-3s. Girls ages nine to twelve with ADHD who ate fish oil–fortified foods (bread, sausage, and spaghetti) for a total weekly intake of 3,600 milligrams of docosahexaenoic acid (DHA) and 840 milligrams of EPA showed significantly decreased impulsive behavior after three months.
- Foods rich in iron. A French study showed that 84 percent of the fifty-three children between ages four and fourteen with ADHD had abnormally low levels of iron in the blood compared with 19 percent in the control, non-ADHD group.

- Any food to which you are sensitive or allergic or that seems to provoke hyperactive behavior.

- Foods with artificial food coloring or additives. They may cause neurobehavioral toxicity, and taking them out of the diet has been shown to decrease impulsive behavior in children with ADHD. Sodium benzoate, tartrazine, sunset yellow, and allura red have prompted hyperactive behavior in three-year-olds and eight- to nine-year-olds without ADHD.

- Chemicals in food, such as leads, dyes, and pesticides.

- Food preservatives, such as bread preservative #282. It causes irritability, restlessness, inattention, and sleep disturbance in children with ADHD. Children eating bread with this preservative every day had 52 percent "worsened" behavior compared with 19 percent in a control group that did not eat the bread.

- Foods with trans fats and highly refined sugars: both affect cognitive development.

TOP CHEFMD-APPROVED RECIPES FOR ADHD
- Cedar-Planked Roast Salmon with Candied Ginger and Berry Salsa (page 112)
- Cinnamon Orange Dreamsicle (page 141)
- Cioppino (page 114)

WATER-COOLER FACT: Yoga has been found to help the symptoms of boys with ADHD, particularly in the evening.

BENIGN BREAST DISEASE

WHAT IT IS: Benign breast disease (BBD) is a noncancerous condition in which a woman's breasts become lumpy and tender, especially before menstruation. It was formerly known as fibrocystic breast disease.

YOU ARE AT INCREASED RISK IF YOU
- are a woman between the ages of thirty and fifty
- are premenopausal
- do not take birth control pills

CULINARY MEDICINE

FOODS TO INCREASE

- Flaxseed. Women who eat ground flax have half the risk of BBD compared with those who do not eat flax.
- Vegetables with fat. The more vegetable fat that women ate, the less risk they had of BBD.
- Fruits, both citrus and noncitrus. A Mexican study following women for two years showed that a high consumption of fruit reduces the risk of benign breast disease by more than half.
- Breakfast cereal. Women who ate cereal daily had less BBD than those who ate cereal weekly.

FOODS TO AVOID

- Alcohol, especially when you are young. Drinking more than 2.5 glasses of wine a day when women are between the ages of eighteen and twenty-two increases their risk of BBD by up to 46 percent.
- Caffeinated foods such as coffee or tea. Women who drank the most caffeinated beverages were almost 2.5 times more likely to have BBD than those who drank the least, although these data are controversial.

TOP CHEFMD-APPROVED RECIPES FOR BENIGN BREAST DISEASE

- Maple Syrup Triple Berry Parfait (page 141)
- Strawberry Pomegranate Blender Blaster (page 144)
- Fresh Tomatillo Guacamole (page 138)

WATER-COOLER FACT: Women who have fewer than three bowel movements per week have a four to five times greater risk of BBD than women having at least one movement daily. It is thought that food that sits in the colon is more likely to pass waste products into the bloodstream, which creates a toxic environment that can result in the disease.

BENIGN PROSTATIC HYPERPLASIA

WHAT IT IS: Benign prostatic hyperplasia (BPH) is a noncancerous enlargement of the prostate gland in men.

YOU ARE AT INCREASED RISK IF YOU
- are a man *and*
- are black or Hispanic
- are obese, especially with a waist over forty inches or a waist-to-hip ratio of one or greater
- have a family history of BPH
- live in a city

CULINARY MEDICINE
FOODS TO INCREASE

- Foods rich in beta-carotene. Eating more foods like carrots, spinach, lettuce, tomatoes, sweet potatoes, broccoli, cantaloupe, oranges, winter squash, and bell peppers was inversely related to BPH occurrence.
- Foods rich in lutein. They include spinach, kale, and turnip greens. Cooked vegetables have the top effect on reducing risk; soups are next.
- Foods rich in vitamin C. The more vitamin C–rich food men ate in a large study, the less they were at risk for BPH.
- Foods rich in vitamin E.
- Foods rich in vitamin A, such as carrots, spinach, kale, cantaloupe, apricots, papaya, mangoes, oatmeal, and peas. All of the fruits and vegetables in this short list shorten the healing process after BPH surgery is performed.
- Vegetables. An Italian study showed that men who eat vegetables every day have a 32 percent reduced risk of lower urinary tract symptoms compared with those who eat few or no vegetables.

FOODS TO AVOID

- Alcohol and caffeinated drinks, especially in the evening, because of their disturbing diuretic effect.
- Eggs and poultry. Men who eat them the most often have the greatest risk of BPH.
- Red meat. Men who eat it every day are at 2.5 times greater risk of lower urinary tract symptoms than those who eat it infrequently or never.

- Starchy foods. Men who eat the most starchy foods such as white bread, cereal, pasta, and rice have a 69 percent greater risk of BPH than those who eat very little.

TOP CHEFMD-APPROVED RECIPES FOR BENIGN PROSTATIC HYPERPLASIA
- Garlicky Potato Salad with Spinach and Lemon (page 135)
- Sardine and Arugula Salad with Ratatouille (page 129)
- Portuguese Caldo Verde (page 104)

WATER-COOLER FACT: BPH affects 80 percent of men over the age of seventy.

BREAST CANCER

WHAT IT IS: The most common cancer in women.

YOU ARE AT INCREASED RISK IF YOU
- are a woman (less than 1 percent of breast cancer occurs in men)
- are postmenopausal
- are tall
- are overweight or obese
- are taking hormone replacement therapy
- are from the upper-middle or upper class
- have a mother or sister who has had breast cancer
- have over 75 percent dense breast tissue (ask your doctor for your ultrasound results)
- have never given birth, or gave birth after age thirty
- have had a primary cancer of the endometrium or ovary
- have been exposed to environmental toxins (including excess estrogen)
- were born in a North American or a northern European country
- work the graveyard shift

CULINARY MEDICINE
FOODS TO INCREASE
- Green tea. Women who drink one cup of tea daily have an almost 40 percent reduced risk of breast cancer.

- Cruciferous vegetables. Premenopausal women who eat the most broccoli have a 40 percent reduced risk of breast cancer compared with those who eat little or none. Broccoli contains an antioxidant called sulforaphane that helps the liver disable cancer cells. Chinese women with the highest levels of isothiocyanates—which also kill leukemia and melanoma cells—in their urine cut their risk of breast cancer in half as compared with those with the lowest levels.

- Olive oil. Women who ate two teaspoons of olive oil a day had a 74 percent reduced risk of breast cancer compared with those who ate little or none. The healthy monounsaturated fat found in olive oil—called oleic acid—may deactivate a gene that makes breast cancer cells grow and divide.

- Fruits with high levels of the carotenoids vitamin A and C. Women who ate five servings a day had a reduced risk of breast cancer, especially premenopausal women with a family history of breast cancer. Also, in a New York study, women who ate the most foods with vitamin C had almost half the incidence of breast cancer versus those who ate few or none, but this was not true of vitamin C supplements.

- Pomegranates. Pomegranate extract has been shown to inhibit the growth of human cancer cells, perhaps because of its many antioxidants and high polyphenol content.

- Pumpkins and carrots. Both are rich in beta-carotene, and women who ate the most foods with beta-carotene had a 54 percent lower breast cancer rate than those who ate few or none.

- Chicken liver (simmered), fortified breakfast cereal, chickpeas, and pinto beans. They all have high levels of folate, which may reduce the risk of breast cancer, especially in women who drink half an ounce or more of alcohol per day. When those women consumed three hundred micrograms a day of folate, their breast cancer risk was only 5 percent higher than nondrinkers. Among nondrinkers, those who ate the most foods rich in folate had their breast cancer risk reduced by 29 percent. Folate is involved in DNA synthesis and repair.

- Flax and foods containing flax meal. Ground flaxseed has shown the potential to reduce tumor growth in breast cancer in postmenopausal women. In one study, women ate a muffin with 0.88 ounces of flax meal a day for thirty-two days. An increase in mutated cell death of 30.7 percent was observed in the flaxseed group but not in the placebo group.

• Milk, kefir, yogurt, and cheese. Cheese contains conjugated linoleic acid, which may be anticarcinogenic. In a three-year Finnish study, women who ate the most cheese had their risk decrease by as much as 60 percent compared with those who ate little or no cheese. Premenopausal women with the highest intake of dairy products had a 65 percent reduction in breast cancer risk over those who ate the least.

FOODS TO AVOID

• Alcohol. Women who drink the equivalent of 2.5 glasses of wine daily have an increased risk of 37 percent, although a high consumption of vegetables may reduce this risk somewhat. Alcohol raises estrogen levels, which when prolonged can increase cell mutations.

• Grapefruit. Just one quarter of one daily in postmenopausal women increased risk by up to 30 percent, perhaps because grapefruit increases estrogen levels by interfering with liver metabolism.

• Red meat (especially processed red meat) and saturated animal fats. Saturated fats more than double the risk of breast cancer. Also, a British study showed that women who ate the most nonprocessed red meat had a 20 percent greater risk of breast cancer than women who ate little or none, and women who ate the most processed red meats had a 64 percent higher risk than those who ate few or none.

• Soy foods, if you are at increased risk and are perimenopausal or postmenopausal. They contain phytoestrogens that may further increase your risk, although the data on soy are mixed.

TOP CHEFMD-APPROVED RECIPES FOR BREAST CANCER
• Broccoli, Cheese, and Kalamata Olive Pizza (page 101)
• Maple Syrup Triple Berry Parfait (page 141)
• Strawberry Pomegranate Blender Blaster (page 144)

WATER-COOLER FACTS: High vitamin D levels give premenopausal women half the breast cancer risk of those with low levels, perhaps because vitamin D helps your "proofreader" genes to work and kicks out bad cells. Women can make about two thousand units of active vitamin D with about twelve minutes of sunshine on arms, legs, and face—and no sunscreen. Overweight women do not convert vitamin D to its active form as well as normal weight women. Gaining twenty-one to forty pounds after age eighteen increases metastatic breast cancer risk by 68 percent.

BRONCHITIS, CHRONIC

WHAT IT IS: Chronic bronchitis, with a recurrent, phlegm-producing cough, is often part of chronic obstructive pulmonary disease (COPD), the number-four cause of death worldwide. Ninety percent of people who get COPD are smokers.

YOU ARE AT INCREASED RISK IF YOU OR YOUR CHILD (SOME OF THESE RISK FACTORS ARE SPECIFICALLY FOR CHILDREN)
- are under six months old
- are exposed to other children who have bronchitis
- are a smoker or have been exposed to cigarette smoke or other toxins
- have a heart and lung condition
- were never breast-fed
- were born prematurely

CULINARY MEDICINE
FOODS TO INCREASE

- Foods rich in beta-carotene but not beta-carotene supplements. People who eat the most of these foods are at a 22 percent reduced risk of bronchitis compared with people who eat few or none of these foods—this is true even for people who smoke twenty or more cigarettes a day. Being a heavy smoker and having a low level of beta-carotene or vitamin E means the most FEV1 (forced expiratory volume in one second) lost: 52.5 cubic centimeters per year. FEV1 measures respiratory health.

- Mediterranean diet. People who eat this type of diet have 50 percent of the risk for COPD when compared with those eating in the Western pattern.
- Foods rich in vitamin A. A lack of vitamin A has been shown to contribute to airway blockage, particularly in smokers.
- Foods rich in vitamin C. In a nine-year British study, it was found that FEV1 was improved by 50.8 cubic centimeters per hundred milligrams of vitamin C.
- Foods rich in vitamin E. People who eat foods rich in vitamin E have lower rates of bronchitis by 22 percent.
- A diet rich in vegetables. It has been shown to protect against the development of COPD by 50 percent, possibly because of the diet's antioxidant and polyphenol content. Antioxidants protect against oxidative stress, which contributes to airway obstruction.

FOODS TO AVOID
- Alcohol in excess. People who drink more than three drinks a day have an 80 percent greater risk of chronic bronchitis than those who drink less.
- Meats preserved with nitrites, such as bacon, salami, and cured ham. People who eat such foods every other day or more are more likely to get COPD, because nitrites damage the elastin and collagen in the lung.
- The Western eating pattern. It is high in refined grains, red meats, simple sugars, and unhealthy fats and may increase the risk of developing COPD, possibly because the diet promotes chronic inflammation.

TOP CHEFMD-APPROVED RECIPES FOR BRONCHITIS
- Grilled Citrus Trout over Crunchy Mediterranean Slaw (page 118)
- Portuguese Caldo Verde (page 104)
- Spicy Gazpacho with Crab (page 137)

WATER-COOLER FACT: Men who smoke can help protect themselves from chronic bronchitis by frequently drinking black tea: at least three eight-ounce cups daily.

CATARACTS

WHAT IT IS: A cataract is a cloudy or opaque protein deposit area on the lens of the eye, obscuring vision, and exposing the eye to free radical damage: early cataract starts at around age forty-five.

YOU ARE AT INCREASED RISK IF YOU

- have been exposed to lots of sunlight without eye protection
- have been exposed to radiation
- have had an eye injury or eye disease
- have taken corticosteroids

CULINARY MEDICINE

FOODS TO INCREASE

- Fish and seafood that are high in omega-3s (EPA and DHA). They reduce the risk of nuclear cataract. Women who eat omega-3 rich fish three or more times a week have a 12 percent reduced risk of cataracts compared with those who eat fish less than once a month.
- Foods rich in niacin, such as beef, chicken liver, turkey, and fish, which helps protect against posterior subcapsular cataracts.
- Foods rich in vitamin C. A five-year Japanese study found that men and women who ate the most of these foods were at a 35 percent to 41 percent reduced risk of getting cataracts compared with those who ate few or none of these foods.
- Foods rich in thiamin. People who eat foods rich in thiamin are at a 40 percent reduced risk of cataracts compared with those who eat few or none.
- Foods rich in riboflavin. People who eat the most foods rich in riboflavin have half the risk of people who eat few or none.
- Spinach and broccoli for men, and spinach and kale for women. These foods are also rich in the carotenoids lutein and zeaxanthin. Women who eat such foods have a 22 percent reduced risk of cataracts, and men have a 19 percent lower risk than women and men who rarely or never eat these foods. (Lutein and zeaxanthin are stored in the macula of the retina, act as blue light filters, and help protect the eye.)

- Cheese. It is high in vitamin A, which protects you against cataracts. People who eat a diet rich in vitamin A have half the risk of cataracts of those who eat few or no foods rich in it.
- Cruciferous vegetables, tomatoes, citrus fruit, and melon. Over ten years, thirty-five thousand women studied who ate the most of these foods had a reduced cataract risk of 50 percent for each food compared with those people who did not eat those foods. A high consumption of peppers showed a reduced risk of cataracts by 30 percent; a similar consumption of spinach showed a reduced risk of 40 percent.

FOODS TO AVOID

- Butter and any fats and oils (except olive oil and oils rich in omega-3s). Other fats have been found to significantly (by up to 80 percent) increase the risk of having a cataract that requires extraction. People with the highest butter intake had an almost three times greater risk of cataract than those who eat little or none.
- Salt. Those who eat the most salt are at twice the risk of getting a cataract than those who eat little or none. Eighty percent of salt intake comes from processed food, not from that used at the table or in your cooking.

TOP CHEFMD-APPROVED RECIPES FOR CATARACTS
- Creamy Goat Cheese Pesto Omelet (page 96)
- Parmigiano Caesar Salad with Shrimp (page 121)
- Rosemary Grilled Chicken and Summer Vegetables (page 127)

WATER-COOLER FACT: Many cataracts are age related, but the term *age related* is misleading. You don't have to be a senior citizen to get an age-related cataract. You can get one even if you are in your forties or fifties.

CELIAC DISEASE

I DON'T SLEEP, I'M TIRED, AND I HAVE AN UPSET STOMACH . . . BUT I EAT A HEALTHY DIET. WHAT'S WRONG?

Terri is a fifty-eight-year-old who traced her gastrointestinal problems back to high school. She had periodic insomnia, fatigue, abdominal cramping, gas, bloating, and mood swings. She had strong reactions to high-fiber foods, including the protein supplements she had recently purchased, had periods of "shakiness" if she went four hours without eating, and was at her wit's end about what and how to eat. Her physician referred her as a "diagnostic dilemma."

She had taken many medications, had psychotherapy, tried different diets of many kinds, and weighed more or less the same for years, give or take ten pounds: she was a size 12.

Her lab tests showed mild anemia of uncertain origin, and a borderline elevated blood sugar. Her exam was otherwise normal.

I explained that the best way to discover the cause of her problems was to eliminate all the major allergens in her diet and then add them back, one by one, over a period of several months. She did this first with dairy; then fish, seafood, and eggs; then nuts and peanuts; then soy; and then foods that contained gluten (such as wheat, barley, rye, and by contamination, oats). She could eat everything except gluten—after two months without it, she had fatigue, upset stomach, and irritability all within a day of eating it. We went through the hidden gluten gamut: spelt and triticale have gluten, millet does not, and neither does chestnut. Blue cheese is off limits unless you know how it is made—its pungent mold sometimes starts with bread.

Terri switched to a gluten-free soy sauce and found she loved the ancient grain quinoa for its nutty flavor. She learned to cook brown rice and amaranth, and she gave up tabouli and oatmeal. She read the GlutenFreeGirl blog and traveled to Seattle to eat at Impromptu Wine Bar Café, for its gourmet yet reasonably priced gluten-free menu. She swapped out her regular beer for New Grist, a delicious gluten-free beer from Milwaukee, brewed from sorghum and rice instead of malted barley, with yeast grown on molasses.

Although her blood tests suggested that she had celiac disease, her results were not conclusive, but Terri was convinced she had it: off gluten, she felt better than she had in forty years. On her new, gluten-free diet, she gained muscle and stamina, while dropping to a size 8.

Terri did so well that she inspired me to create the Gluten Free Quiz (www.glutenfreequiz.com), a free self-assessment of your risk for celiac disease, and a Gluten Free Recipe Search (www.gluten-free-recipes-swicki-eurekster.com), a specialized search engine for gluten-free recipes. Over one hundred thousand people have used the quiz and search since 2007.

WHAT IT IS: Celiac disease is an inherited condition in which gluten inflames the small intestine and causes an autoimmune reaction and malabsorption.

YOU ARE AT INCREASED RISK IF YOU
- have a family history of celiac disease
- have type 1 diabetes
- have osteoarthritis
- have Down's syndrome

CULINARY MEDICINE
FOODS TO INCREASE
- Fresh vegetables. They can provide the fiber that a person with celiac disease needs and may miss.
- Quinoa, amaranth, sorghum, brown and wild rice, buckwheat, oats, and millet. They are high in B vitamins and antioxidants. (Although all these grains are gluten-free, they are often subject to cross-contamination from processing or field rotation, so make sure they are certified gluten-free.) Thirty-seven percent of patients with celiac disease who were tested had low levels of folate, and 20 percent had low levels of B6.
- Foods certified as "gluten-free."

FOODS TO AVOID
- Foods with added gluten, like some soy sauces, candy bars, malt vinegar, and vitamins.
- Wheat, rye, barley, triticale, spelt, and kamut. They are high in

gluten, and a person with celiac disease should eat less than fifty milligrams of these foods a day (and preferably none).

TOP CHEFMD-APPROVED RECIPES FOR CELIAC DISEASE
- Roasted Winter Vegetables with Cranberry-Studded Quinoa (page 126)
- Saffron Scallop, Shrimp, and Chickpea Paella (page 128)
- Warm and Nutty Cinnamon Quinoa Cereal (page 100)

WATER-COOLER FACT: A person with celiac disease may have no symptoms but still have celiac disease and be at risk of malnutrition. Ninety-seven percent of people with celiac disease in the United States are undiagnosed, and nearly 1 percent have it.

COMMON COLD

WHAT IT IS: The common cold is a short-term viral infection of the nose and throat.

YOU ARE AT INCREASED RISK IF
- it is spring or fall
- you work and/or socialize with a lot of people
- you do not wash your hands frequently

CULINARY MEDICINE
FOODS TO INCREASE
- Kefir and yogurt. Their probiotic bacteria stimulate the immune system. They also reduce potentially pathogenic bacteria in the nose. A study in which people were given just over two ounces of kefir daily for three weeks showed that kefir's probiotics can reduce potentially pathogenic bacteria in the upper respiratory tract by 19 percent and decrease the incidence and duration of upper-respiratory infection.
- Chicken soup. It helps clear nasal passages and thus ease the symptoms of a cold. Chicken soup may also have an anti-inflammatory effect that alleviates upper respiratory tract infections. Chicken soup and foods with vitamin C are the traditional cures for the cold, but foods with vitamin C have not yet been proven to help.

- Red wine. People who drink two glasses a day have a 40 percent reduced risk of getting a cold compared with people who do not drink at all. Beer and hard liquor do not have the same effect. Women should weigh the potential health benefits against the fact that drinking more than one glass per day increases the risk of other diseases.

FOODS TO AVOID

- Any foods to which you are allergic. An allergy can weaken the immune system, making you more susceptible to catching a cold.

TOP CHEFMD-APPROVED RECIPES FOR COMMON COLD

- Açai Berry and Banana Dessert Soup (page 139)
- Papaya Filled with Gingered Blueberries (page 142)
- Roasted Red Pepper, Wine, and Red Lentil Soup (page 105)

WATER-COOLER FACT: Thirty studies of vitamin C and colds have found that those people who are physically stressed (skiers, marathon runners, and soldiers) had colds that lasted 8 percent shorter than average when they were given vitamin C—and then just two hundred milligrams did it. No difference for everyone else.

CONSTIPATION

WHAT IT IS: Constipation means having a bowel movement three times a week or less and passing hard, dry stool.

YOU ARE AT INCREASED RISK IF YOU

- are over sixty-five
- are a woman
- don't use the bathroom when you should
- have a metabolic disorder, such as an underactive thyroid
- have an endocrine problem such as diabetes
- have a neurological illness, such as Parkinson's disease
- take one of over seven hundred medications known to cause constipation

CULINARY MEDICINE

FOODS TO INCREASE

- Foods that are high in fiber. These include:
  - Whole-wheat breads, brown rice, barley, oats, rye, spelt, and quinoa.
  - All-bran, or any cereals that contain bran.
  - Nearly all vegetables, especially tomatoes, bean sprouts, brussels sprouts, celery, broccoli, carrots, parsnip, spinach, zucchini, asparagus, and eggplant.
  - Soybeans, lentils, peas, nuts, and seeds.
  - Apples, pears (skins on), oranges, raisins, raspberries, strawberries, bananas, avocados, kiwis, and mangoes.
  - Dried fruits, such as dried apricots, dates, and prunes.
- Any fermented dairy product that contains *Lactobacillus casei*—a good-for-you probiotic. Women in a four-week study who took about a quarter cup of such a dairy food along with fiber (in the form of rye bread) had softer stools and more frequent defecation than those who did not eat a fermented dairy food.
- Water, especially along with high-fiber foods. During a two-month trial, people with chronic constipation who ate a little less than an ounce of fiber and drank a little over two quarts a day of water had significantly improved bowel movements compared with those who drank just over four cups of water a day. Carbonated water may be more effective than noncarbonated water.

FOODS TO AVOID

- High glycemic load foods, especially potatoes, bread, soft drinks, and sweets, when combined with eating few whole grains.
- Low-fiber foods. They include soft drinks, concentrated fruit juice, white rice, white bread, white pasta, refined sugar, potatoes, and many processed foods.

TOP CHEFMD-APPROVED RECIPES FOR CONSTIPATION

- Cheese Ravioli with Tofu and Baby Peas (page 113)
- Quick Steel-Cut Oats with Apples, Ginger, and Walnuts (page 97)
- Teriyaki Tofu, Vegetables, and Buckwheat Noodles (page 108)

WATER-COOLER FACT: Wood ear mushroom, a fungus that grows on a tree and is used in Chinese cooking, has 50 percent more fiber than other mushrooms and has been shown to help constipated people get relief with less straining and more frequent bowel movements.

DEPRESSION

PASSED OVER IN PORTLAND

Barbara is a fifty-two-year-old married woman from Portland, Oregon. She teaches college biology. Several years ago, she began to feel hopeless and sad much of the time. She had counted on getting tenure and had worked her whole career for it, but the committee had passed her by again. It didn't seem worth further struggle. She felt stressed and demoralized, as though life would never get better. She had also gained forty-two pounds over the previous year. Her physician referred her to me for a weight-loss program.

When I saw her, Barbara told me she had no appetite, couldn't sleep, and was tired all the time. She drank diet Red Bull and coffee every day, smoked, and had almost a bottle of cheap wine every night. The only vegetables she ate were french fries. I told her that these habits were responsible for both her mood swings and her weight gain. I referred her to a psychiatrist for an evaluation of her suicide risk and for medication and follow-up.

She began taking antidepressants and started to feel better. I asked her to drink juice instead of the diet Red Bull, because aspartame may worsen depression in some people. I tested her vitamin D level, which was low, and so I asked her to take two thousand international units of vitamin D3 a day. I also asked her to go for a daily walk with a friend or colleague. I asked her not to drink wine. She did most of the things I asked, and within a few weeks started to feel a little better.

At my request, she started to eat mood-stabilizing food—those rich in omega-3s, such as wild salmon, anchovies, sardines, flax meal, walnuts, and even omega-3-enriched eggs. She increased her vitamin B—rich foods, especially those rich in folate. She learned to love New Zealand Marmite, a vitamin-enriched dark yeast spread that she put on toast and which she once told me was almost as good as french fries. Once a week, she cooked what she called her "depression dish": saffron lentils with garlic and three chilies. (The dish is rich in B vitamins, and small studies suggest saffron has antidepressant effects.)

Slowly, Barbara started to feel better. She gained new energy, lost weight, and her depression lifted. When it did, she adopted two dogs, who love her. Life is now once again looking good for her.

WHAT IT IS: Depression is a medical condition that causes people to feel overwhelmingly sad, worthless, apathetic, fatigued, and hopeless.

YOU ARE AT INCREASED RISK IF YOU
- abuse alcohol or drugs
- are a woman (especially one who has just had a baby)
- have a family history of depression
- have been depressed in the past
- have recently been diagnosed with a serious illness such as cancer

CULINARY MEDICINE
FOODS TO INCREASE
- Foods high in DHA and EPA, the omega-3 fatty acids in fish and seafood. Depressed patients given 0.23 grams of omega-3s a day for eight weeks experienced significant recovery from their depression. A meta-analysis of ten studies of at least four weeks duration found that the omega-3s significantly improved depression in patients, and that dosage didn't matter. DHA affects cell membranes in the brain; EPA appears to have a role in improving blood flow.
- Dark chocolate. It has been found to elevate mood and decrease a feeling of loneliness in clinical studies, including one in Finnish elderly men.
- Saffron. Depressed men who ate thirty milligrams a day of saffron extract had as beneficial an effect as experienced by those taking Prozac.

- Foods rich in folate such as potatoes, bananas, lentils, chili peppers, tempeh, liver, turkey, tuna, and molasses. Folate is sometimes deficient in people with depression.
- Foods rich in vitamin D. Of eighty people tested (forty with mild Alzheimer's and forty without), those with vitamin D deficiencies were almost twelve times more likely to have a mood disorder than those who were not deficient.

FOODS TO AVOID

- Alcohol. It can cause mood swings and, as a sedative, can worsen depression. It does not help people cope.
- Foods with the artificial sweetener aspartame. Depressed patients given thirty milligrams per kilogram per day for seven days had their symptoms worsen so severely that the study was halted.
- Caffeine. A study of thirty-six hundred adult twins showed a link between lifetime caffeine consumption and major depression.
- Foods with simple sugars. They increase hypoglycemia, which is linked to mood swings and depression.

TOP CHEFMD-APPROVED RECIPES FOR DEPRESSION
- Saffron Scallop, Shrimp, and Chickpea Paella (page 128)
- Sardine and Arugula Salad with Ratatouille (page 129)
- Chocolate Blackberry Breakfast Smoothie (page 95)

WATER-COOLER FACT: It has been shown that people with elevated homocysteine in their blood are more prone to depression. Just drinking juice fortified with B vitamins can lower your homocysteine level.

DIABETES (TYPE 2)

GARAGE EATER BY NIGHT, DIABETIC 24/7

Carol is a forty-eight-year-old mother of two and a successful litigator. She is now obese, though she was once a competitive swimmer in college. Her father died suddenly three months ago of heart disease, which has made her worried about her own health. She is in my office because she has diabetes, does not know what to eat, and has to go to a reception and dinner tonight.

She eats out ten times weekly, usually orders chicken Caesar salad, and snacks on cheese, chocolate, and energy bars. She eats cornflakes and drinks orange juice in the morning and often eats at night, out of sight of her family, consuming the last of her Taco Bell take-out meal in the front seat of her car in her garage. She drinks four bottles of green tea daily but no alcohol, and she trains on her home treadmill for forty-five minutes every day. She says she is stressed.

On exam, she is five feet ten inches tall, 254 pounds, with a body fat of 42.4 percent. Her waist is forty-two inches. She takes aspirin and Byetta (a newer drug for diabetes). Her blood sugar is 299; her glycohemoglobin is 8.2. She has a swelling, tender rash on her right shin where she has a sore from bumping her leg.

I explain that she may have a cellulitis, a bacterial disease of the skin that can be life-threatening, and which she needs antibiotics to treat, immediately, so I prescribe Bactrim and Clindamycin to treat it aggressively. I tell her that she must treat eating like her best client: regular appointments, genuine curiosity, careful record keeping, and innovative thought. The high-calorie foods she is eating are low in fiber and not filling, and her eating late at night is worsening her insulin resistance.

I asked her to start eating a standard breakfast: a bran-containing cereal with at least ten grams of fiber per serving, every day, with a half-cup of frozen or fresh berries, sprinkled with cinnamon to improve her insulin sensitivity; coffee and a part-skim cheese stick, twelve almonds or a hard-boiled egg (their protein improves satiety). I asked her to avoid red and processed meat for twelve weeks: the heme iron increases diabetes risk. If she encountered food with the words *hydrogenated, high-fructose corn syrup, enriched flour, sugar, rice,* or *corn syrup* on the package I asked that she put it back on the shelf. I asked her to try several new foods. For that evening's reception, I said she should have two dinner salads with a good vinaigrette over twenty minutes and bring her own prepackaged one-ounce almonds to eat with dinner. After her salads and almonds, she should order a half portion of grilled fish with a double portion of vegetables instead of starches.

Twelve weeks later, Carol's blood sugar was 121, and her glyco-hemoglobin was 7.1—a decrease of cardiac risk of over 30 percent. She no longer ate secretly in the garage, had lost sixteen pounds, and had started taking yoga to reduce her stress. Her cellulitis had long since healed, she had started swimming again, and now has a much improved diet. She now practices law, teaches water aerobics, has her diabetes under control, and feels better than she has in years.

WHAT IT IS: Type 2 diabetes is a chronic metabolic disease in which the body cannot properly regulate its glucose level.

YOU ARE AT INCREASED RISK IF YOU
- are an African American, Asian American, Pacific Islander, Latino or Latina, or Native American
- are over age forty
- are obese, especially with a waist of thirty-five inches or more for a woman and forty for a man
- have an HDL cholesterol of thirty-five milligrams per deciliter or lower and/or triglyceride level of 250 or higher
- have blood pressure of 140/90 millimeters of mercury or higher
- have a parent or sibling with diabetes

CULINARY MEDICINE

FOODS TO INCREASE
- High-fiber foods. They can lower blood sugar after meals, help your body to combat obesity and diabetes, and can reduce your risk by 35 percent. High-fiber foods include:
  - Low-sugar cereals (bran). Fiber from cereal has been shown to be the most effective and accessible food that helps prevent and control diabetes. Cereal that contains psyllium can lower blood sugar.
  - Whole-grain products. These include rye, whole wheat, brown rice, barley, oats, millet, spelt, and quinoa.

- High-fiber vegetables. These include cauliflower, kale, bean sprouts, brussels sprouts, celery, broccoli, carrots, parsnips, spinach, asparagus, eggplant, and cabbage.
- Foods with plant sterols. People with diabetes who ate a fortified margarine containing 1.8 grams of plant sterols a day reduced their levels of cholesterol, which is important because diabetes is a risk factor for heart disease and stroke. Soybeans, lentils, peas, nuts, and seeds are all good sources.
- Foods high in magnesium. For every hundred-milligram increase in magnesium intake, type 2 diabetes risk drops 15 percent. Barley, buckwheat flour, and almonds have magnesium.
- Nopal (the "meat" of the prickly pear cactus paddle, used in Mexican cuisine). A 30 percent reduction in blood sugar was observed in type 2 diabetics fed chilaquiles with nopales, and 20 percent in those fed scrambled egg and tomato burritos, both with about three ounces of cooked nopales, probably because they slowed carbohydrate absorption.
- Cinnamon. Although the data are controversial, less than a teaspoon of cinnamon daily turns on insulin receptors, increases insulin sensitivity, keeps food in the stomach longer, and lowers blood sugar; it does not appear to help people with type 1 diabetes.
- Vinegar. Subjects given 0.71 ounce of apple cider vinegar raised their whole-body insulin sensitivity by 34 percent when tested one hour later.
- A Mediterranean diet, rich in whole grains, nuts, fish, and vegetables. It prevents insulin resistance.
- A vegetarian diet. Vegetarians, who consume more legumes, fruits, and nuts and do not eat meat, have a lowered risk of diabetes.
- Coffee. Caffeinated or decaffeinated, instant or drip, as little as two and as many as four cups per day lowers the risk of diabetes in young and middle-aged women over the course of ten years.

FOODS TO AVOID
- Potatoes. People who eat potatoes in place of a whole grain once a day have a 30 percent increased risk of developing diabetes compared with those who do not eat potatoes.

- Heme iron, which is found primarily in red meat. It increases the risk of type 2 diabetes. More than eighty-five thousand women were followed for twenty years, and those who ate foods that contained more than 2.25 milligrams of heme iron a day were 52 percent more likely to develop diabetes than those who ate less than 0.75 milligrams a day. A high level of iron in the body has been tied to insulin resistance.
- Low-fiber cereals. These include Cheerios, Special K, cornflakes, and Rice Krispies.
- Starchy foods. These include white rice, white bread, doughy bagels, Italian bread, and white pasta.
- Sugary foods. Soft drinks and candy spike sugar levels in the blood and lead to the obesity and inflammation that put you at risk for diabetes.
- Foods with trans-fatty acids. Replacing trans-fatty acids with polyunsaturated fat lowers your risk of diabetes by 40 percent.
- Alcohol. Women should have no more than one drink a day; no more than two drinks a day for men.

TOP CHEFMD-APPROVED RECIPES FOR DIABETES
- Grilled Citrus Trout over Crunchy Mediterranean Slaw (page 118)
- Skillet Chilaquiles with Cactus Paddles, Eggs, and Kale (page 98)
- Teriyaki Tofu, Vegetables, and Buckwheat Noodles (page 108)

WATER-COOLER FACT: Low vitamin D levels worsen insulin resistance found in many people with type 2 diabetes.

DIARRHEA

WHAT IT IS: A condition marked by watery stools and a frequent need to defecate.

YOU ARE AT INCREASED RISK IF YOU
- are Latino or Latina, Asian American, Native American, or African American, and therefore more likely to suffer from lactose intolerance, which can cause diarrhea

- are traveling internationally, where you may be subjected to bacteria such as *E. coli*
- are taking a medication new to you
- have been hospitalized recently
- have recently been on antibiotics

CULINARY MEDICINE
FOODS TO INCREASE

- Yogurt. Its probiotics—beneficial bacteria—stimulate the immune system and can prevent antibiotic-related diarrhea in children. In one study, babies with diarrhea from viral gastroenteritis given about half an ounce per 2.2 pounds of body weight along with their regular pharmacological treatment for diarrhea got better faster than babies not given yogurt. They were out of the hospital on average in 2.7 days rather than the 3.1 days for the babies not given yogurt. Hospitalized older adults taking antibiotics who drank 3.3 ounces of liquid probiotic-rich yogurt twice daily developed diarrhea 65 percent less often than those who did not drink the probiotic-rich yogurt.
- Oat bran. Soluble fiber absorbs the water in stool. Eighty-four percent of patients getting treatment for HIV who ate oat bran either a half hour before meals or right before taking their medication for two weeks had less diarrhea—some dramatically so.
- Green bananas, because of their resistant starch. Children with diarrhea who were given green banana daily were 82 percent recovered after four days compared with 23 percent recovered for those given a placebo.
- Foods rich in pectin. Boys with diarrhea were given one teaspoon of pectin a day for every 2.2 pounds of body weight for seven days along with rice; another group was just given rice. After four days, 82 percent of those given pectin had recovered, compared with 23 percent of those just given rice. Pectin has an antimicrobial effect and is especially found in oranges, lemons, berries, grapefruit, apples, and pineapple.
- Salty foods. They replace the electrolytes that are lost when you have diarrhea.

- Alcohol. Especially when drunk in excess, it injures the lining of the small intestine, which pours out fluid that is poorly absorbed.
- Caffeinated foods, such as coffee or chocolate. Their effect on secretions of the small intestine may play a role in causing diarrhea.
- Candy with the sweetener sorbitol. Individuals given 1.4 ounces of candy with sorbitol per day had diarrhea within one to three hours after eating the candy. This happened even when subjects were given only 80 percent of the amount that might have a "laxative effect," according to the label.
- Chilies. The capsaicin in chilies can irritate the intestine and worsen diarrhea.
- Foods with high-fructose corn syrup. Some people have difficulty absorbing fructose, and fructose not absorbed can draw water from the intestine, leading to diarrhea, cramping, and discomfort.

TOP CHEFMD-APPROVED RECIPES FOR DIARRHEA
- Pasta e Fagioli (Pasta and Bean) Soup (page 102)
- Rosemary Grilled Chicken and Summer Vegetables (page 127)
- Strawberry Pomegranate Blender Blaster (page 144)

WATER-COOLER FACT: It is easy to get dehydrated when you have diarrhea. Drink plenty of fluids.

DIVERTICULITIS

WHAT IT IS: Inflammation and often infection of small "pouches" or sacs in the intestine's inner lining.

YOU ARE AT INCREASED RISK IF YOU
- are middle aged or elderly
- have excess belly fat

CULINARY MEDICINE
FOODS TO INCREASE
- Foods that are rich in soluble and insoluble fiber. These include apples, berries, grapefruits, mangoes, nectarines, or-

anges, peaches, pears, dried fruits, asparagus, bean sprouts, broccoli, brussels sprouts, cabbage, carrots, cauliflower, and celery. Eating a diet rich in dietary fiber reduces your risk of diverticulitis by 40 percent compared with eating little or no dietary fiber.

- Foods rich in insoluble fiber. Popcorn is a good source: eating popcorn twice weekly reduces the risk of diverticulitis by 28 percent, probably because it keeps your gut moving.

- Nuts. They have been associated with a 20 percent reduced rate of the complications of diverticulitis.

FOODS TO AVOID

- Foods that are high fat. A low-fat diet has been shown to decrease the risk of diverticular disease.

- Red meat. Avoiding red meat has been shown to decrease the risk of diverticulitis.

TOP CHEFMD-APPROVED RECIPES FOR DIVERTICULITIS

- Blackberry, Kiwi, and Mango Fruit Salad (page 140)
- Curried Turkey Tenderloin with Penne and Roasted Asparagus (page 116)
- Red Pozole with Shredded Chicken and Avocado (page 124)

WATER-COOLER FACT: Diverticulitis is rare in Africa and India, where people eat much more fiber than people in the United States do. In contrast, half of all Americans over the age of sixty have the disease. The common advice to avoid nuts and seeds is not supported by most studies.

GALLBLADDER DISEASE

WHAT IT IS: Gallbladder disease is often related to obstruction of the flow of bile from the gallbladder to the intestine, caused by inflammation, stones, polyps, or cancer.

YOU ARE AT INCREASED RISK IF YOU

- are a man and you yo-yo diet (lose and gain weight in cycles)
- are a woman (because estrogen increases cholesterol in bile, which in turn causes stones)

- are obese, especially in the abdomen
- have diabetes
- have metabolic syndrome
- have a history of gallbladder disease in your family

CULINARY MEDICINE
FOODS TO INCREASE

- Foods rich in insoluble fiber. Women who ate the most foods with fiber were 13 percent less likely to get gallbladder disease compared with those who ate the least. Bran and flax are good sources.
- Leafy green vegetables, vegetables and fruits that are rich in vitamin C, and cruciferous vegetables. A fifteen-year study showed that women who eat the most of these groups of foods have 21 percent less risk of needing surgery to remove gallstones than those who eat the least.
- Alcohol. A twelve-year study showed that men who drink alcohol every day or almost every day have fewer gallstones than men who only drink once or twice a week. Regularity, and not quantity or type of alcohol, seemed to be the important factor. A twenty-year study in women showed similar beneficial effects.
- Caffeinated foods, such as coffee. Four generous cups (on average, eight ounces of brewed coffee has ninety-five milligrams per cup) of coffee daily reduces the risk of gallbladder disease by 45 percent; eight hundred milligrams safeguards you even more, but buckle your seat belt. "Bold" and "mild" in coffee describes flavor, not caffeine level.
- A vegetarian diet. Vegetarians have only half as many problems with gallbladder disease. Only 12 percent have gallstones (as compared with 25 percent of nonvegetarians).
- Olive oil, avocados, and nuts. During a fourteen-year study it was found that men who ate foods with the most monounsaturated fats had a 17 percent reduced risk of gallstone disease compared with those who ate few or none.
- Tea. A Chinese study showed that women who drank at least one cup per day were at a 27 percent reduced risk of getting gallstones, and at almost half the risk of getting gallbladder cancer, compared with women who did not drink tea, perhaps

because of the antiproliferative and anti-inflammatory properties of tea polyphenols, in particular epigallocatechin-3-gallate.

FOODS TO AVOID

- Foods with high glycemic loads. In a study with a sixteen-year follow-up, women who ate foods with the most carbohydrates had a 35 percent increased risk of surgery for gallbladder disease compared with those who ate the least. In a twelve-year study of men, the highest compared with the lowest consumption of carbohydrate more than doubled the risk of gallstones.
- Foods high in heme iron. Eating too much iron-rich food such as red meat can cause biliary cholesterol crystal formation. A high intake of heme iron increases the risk of gallstones in men by about 20 percent.
- Foods high in trans-fatty acids. These include those made with shortening, margarine, and hydrogenated fats and oils. More than forty-five thousand men reported on their diets; after a fourteen-year follow-up, it was found that those who ate foods with the most trans fats had a 23 percent increased risk of gallstones compared with those who ate the least.

TOP CHEFMD-APPROVED RECIPES FOR GALLBLADDER DISEASE
- Cinnamon Orange Dreamsicle (page 141)
- Fresh Tomatillo Guacamole (page 138)
- Toasted Walnut and Creamy White Bean Pitas (page 109)

WATER-COOLER FACT: Ninety percent of gallbladder disease is accompanied by gallstones.

GOUT

WHAT IT IS: Gout is a painful type of arthritis associated with a buildup of urate crystals, which deposit in and around joints and are then "swallowed" by white blood cells, which release inflammatory, painful chemicals.

YOU ARE AT INCREASED RISK IF YOU
- are obese
- are sedentary

- are an African American man or a postmenopausal woman
- drink a lot of alcohol
- have been exposed to lead
- have hyperlipidemia, kidney disease, diabetes, leukemia, arteriosclerosis, or enzyme defects
- have a disease that interferes with uric acid excretion, including untreated high blood pressure
- have had a sudden or serious illness or injury
- take cyclosporine, diuretics, or aspirin

CULINARY MEDICINE
FOODS TO INCREASE

- Oranges and other citrus fruits. They have a high vitamin C content and are rich in dietary fiber, both of which have been shown to aid in the prevention and management of gout.

- Water. It dilutes increased urates.

- Coffee. Women who drink ten cups of coffee a week, and men who drink even one per day, caffeinated or decaf, have a decrease in serum uric acid level and a significantly lower risk of developing gout.

- Nuts, eggs, cheese, highly refined pastas, breads and grains, chocolate, and ice cream. These foods are low in a compound called purine, which raises uric acid in the blood.

- Low-fat dairy products. They are associated with a decreased risk of gout and have been shown to decrease the level of uric acid in the blood by 0.21 milligrams per deciliter, which can make a difference. In a twelve-year study, men who ate the most dairy were at a 44 percent reduced risk of gout compared with those who ate little or none. Even just one serving of milk a day or one serving of yogurt every other day reduces the serum uric acid level.

- Wine. One daily glass of wine seems to protect against gout, possibly because of its polyphenols.

FOODS TO AVOID

- Beer and hard liquor. A twelve-ounce glass of beer a day raises your risk of gout by half; a shot of hard alcohol daily raises it by 15 percent.

- Iron-rich foods. Many meats and seafood, and some fortified cereals, are rich in iron. When patients with gouty arthritis were brought to near-anemic levels of iron deficiency, the frequency of their attacks lessened, and the attacks were also less severe when they did occur.
- Meat and seafood. Over a twelve-year study, it was found that men who ate the most meat were at a 41 percent increased risk of gout compared with those who ate the least, and those who ate the most seafood were at a 51 percent increased risk compared with those who ate the least. Limit meat, fish, seafood, poultry, and tofu to eight ounces a day. Tofu has been found to be the safest protein source, since it doesn't raise uric acid levels as high as the other sources.
- Purine-rich foods. These include poultry, fish, shellfish, anchovies, gravies, sweetbreads, bouillon, cauliflower, kidney beans, lentils, lima beans, mushrooms, navy beans, steel-cut oats, bran, peas, spinach, asparagus, and tripe. They all raise levels of uric acid in the blood.

TOP CHEFMD-APPROVED RECIPES FOR GOUT
- Butternut Barley Risotto with Goat Cheese and Toasted Almonds (page 111)
- Walnut-Scented Dessert Pancakes with Bananas and Agave Nectar (page 145)

WATER-COOLER FACT: Bing cherries may help protect you from gout by reducing the levels of urate in the blood.

HAIR, SKIN, AND NAIL PROBLEMS

WHAT IT IS: Nails may be deformed, discolored, brittle, weak, or flaking. Skin may be dry, wrinkled, or sunburned. Hair may be dull, oily, dry, or thinning.

YOU ARE AT INCREASED RISK IF YOU
- are taking medication that affects your hair, skin, or nails
- are a smoker
- have a family history of hair, skin, or nail problems

- have an autosomal recessive disease (such as trichothiodystrophy) that makes hair brittle
- have yellow nail syndrome
- have onychomycosis (a fungal infection of the nails)
- have an eating disorder, are malnourished, or have nutritional deficiencies
- have food allergies that cause skin inflammation

CULINARY MEDICINE
FOODS TO INCREASE

- Eggs, wheat germ, and oatmeal. They are rich in biotin, which thickened nails in one study by 25 percent over six months.
- Chocolate. The skin of women who consumed a high flavonol (326 milligrams) cocoa powder dissolved in about 3.5 ounces of water every day for twelve weeks became 12 percent thicker and retained more moisture. Cocoa also acts as a UV blocker.
- Omega-3 rich foods. They act as a sunscreen and decrease the risk of squamous cell skin cancer by more than 20 percent.
- Tomato juice and tomato paste. Men given about 1.5 ounces of tomato paste with two teaspoons of olive oil for ten weeks were found to have 40 percent less sunburn than those who ate just olive oil, probably because of increased skin carotenoids and decreased free radical absorption generated by UV light.
- Foods rich in vitamin C. The babies of nursing mothers who ate more vitamin C–rich foods had a 70 percent reduced risk of eczema. Men who ate the most foods rich in vitamin C had their risk of oral premalignant lesions cut almost in half compared to those who ate few or none. This was not true of men who took vitamin C supplements.
- Vegetables, olive oil, fish, and legumes. An international study of Greek and Swedish people living both in their native countries and abroad showed that those who ate the most of these foods had less skin wrinkling than those who ate the least.
- Tea, and black tea with citrus peel. A study showed that the risk of skin cancer was reduced by as much as one-half by regularly drinking tea, especially in those who had been drinking it for a long time (forty-seven years or more) and those who drank two or more cups a day. The polyphenols in tea may protect

against the carcinogenic effect of UV radiation. The anticancer results were even more marked when citrus peel was combined with the tea: in an Arizona study, those who reported consuming both hot black tea and citrus peel had an 88 percent reduced risk of squamous cell carcinoma of the skin.

FOODS TO AVOID

- Alcohol (especially in binges). Of almost thirty thousand people polled, those who reported binge drinking also reported the highest incidence of sunburn. Sunburn can lead to melanoma or basal cell carcinoma.

TOP CHEFMD-APPROVED RECIPES FOR HAIR, SKIN, AND NAIL PROBLEMS

- Broccoli, Cheese, and Kalamata Olive Pizza (page 101)
- Creamy Goat Cheese Pesto Omelet (page 96)
- Pasta e Fagioli (Pasta and Bean) Soup (page 102)

WATER-COOLER FACT: Women who are very stressed are eleven times more likely to experience hair loss than those who are not. Squamous cell skin cancers appear more often on the left side of the face because of sun exposure while driving.

HEART DISEASE

A PICKY EATER WHO IS NEVER HUNGRY HAS A HEART ATTACK IN THE BRAIN

Susan was just sixty when her cousin Nick became disabled with vascular dementia. Always significantly overweight, she nevertheless felt healthy. She was energetic, took no medicines, and ran a small scrap-booking business. However, she was also mildly hypertensive, had smoked like a chimney for twenty years, and was sedentary.

Nick's disability affected her deeply, and at sixty-one, she had a transient ischemic attack, which is like a small heart attack in the brain. When she came to see me, I saw that she was mildly hypertensive, a borderline diabetic, had high triglycerides, and was at risk for a major stroke. She needed to make some changes.

Susan was a very picky eater: she had been raised on corn casserole, peanut brittle, and beef, and she kept to those foods. I recommended the Mediterranean diet, with its higher healthy fats and fewer starches.

Susan had trouble changing her pattern of eating, because she did not feel hunger (although she ate a lot, to deal with stress). So I asked her to stop eating when her plate was 80 percent empty. I explained that it took eight weeks to change how new foods would taste to her and that I'd like her to try a rule of ten: try a food ten times over a year before she decided she didn't like it. I asked her to avoid butter, shortening, cheese, and sugary foods and to commit to eating up to six servings per day of fruits and vegetables, especially high-folate ones: one citrus (she chose oranges), one vitamin C–rich (red peppers), one leafy green (spinach), and three cruciferous (brussels sprouts, watercress, and broccoli). Just by making these changes in her diet, she reduced her risk of stroke by 55 percent.

She switched from beef to halibut (which has more folate), first twice a week and then every day. She upped her potassium level with baked sweet potatoes. She started a walking program, at first just around the block, then increasing her distance each week. And then she quit smoking cold turkey, munching on crisp jicama until the cravings passed.

After four years, Susan is like a new person. She has lost seventy-two pounds, decreased her triglycerides, increased her HDLs, and is smoke-free. She has drastically reduced her risk of stroke, and every morning enjoys walking twenty blocks to her new job as a textile buyer for a major department store in Seattle.

WHAT IT IS: Heart disease means coronary artery disease. Its main cause is atherosclerosis, in which plaque builds up in the arteries and prevents the heart and vessels from getting enough blood.

YOU ARE AT INCREASED RISK IF YOU
- smoke
- are sixty-five or older
- are male
- are a postmenopausal woman

- are African American
- are physically inactive
- are overweight or obese
- are under chronic stress
- have diabetes mellitus
- have a family history of heart disease
- have high blood cholesterol
- have high blood pressure

CULINARY MEDICINE
FOODS TO INCREASE

- Tea, onions, and apples. They contain flavonoids, and a five-year study found men who ate the most flavonoids were at less than half the risk of coronary heart disease compared with those who ate the least. The flavonoids rutin and quercetin stabilize small blood vessels, and increase artery-dilating nitric oxide levels. And the risk of heart attack decreases by 11 percent with tea consumption of three cups or more per day.

- Alcohol. A Finnish study found that when alcohol-containing beverages are drunk in moderation and with consistency, they reduce the risk of heart disease as they raise HDL cholesterol levels.

- Oily fish. It reduces platelet aggregation, thereby lowering the risk of cardiovascular disease. (And does so more effectively as part of a low-fat rather than a high-fat diet.) A Chinese study showed that people who ate almost 2.5 pounds of fish a week had a 93 percent reduced risk of coronary atherosclerosis compared with those who ate little or none.

- Extra-virgin olive oil. A Greek study showed that extra-virgin olive oil reduces the risk of acute coronary syndrome by 47 percent in people who cook with no other fats.

- Nuts, especially walnuts and almonds. A seventeen-year study that followed more than twenty-one thousand men showed that those who eat nuts twice a week or more cut their risk of sudden cardiac death almost in half, although we don't know exactly why.

- Whole grains, which contain antioxidants as well as fiber and B vitamins. People who eat the most whole grains have a 25 percent reduced risk of coronary heart disease compared with those who eat the least.

- Legumes. A nineteen-year study found that people who eat foods such as beans, peas, and lentils four times or more a week have a 22 percent lower risk of coronary heart disease than those who only eat them once a week.

- Citrus fruit. Their flavonoids reduce inflammation.

- Dark chocolate (eaten in moderation—about an ounce a day). Its flavonoids reduce LDL and increase HDL cholesterol, dilate the arteries, and inhibit platelet activity, which fights heart disease. Cocoa also reduces blood pressure, which reduces the risk of heart disease.

- Vegetables. An Italian study showed that those who ate the most vegetables had a 21 percent reduced risk of heart attack and an 11 percent reduced risk of angina pectoris. Even increasing your intake by just an ounce and a half a day can make a difference in your risk of death from heart disease.

- The Mediterranean diet. People who have already had a heart attack halve their risk of having a second by adhering to this eating pattern.

FOODS TO AVOID

- Alcohol in excess. Men who binge drink raise their risk of cardiovascular disease by half.

- High-trans-fat foods. Women who eat foods with the most trans fats have levels of the inflammatory marker called C-reactive protein in their blood that are 73 percent higher than women who eat foods with little or no trans fats. C-reactive protein is a risk factor for cardiovascular disease.

- Red meat. A twenty-year study showed that its heme iron increases the risk of heart disease among women with type 2 diabetes by up to 50 percent.

- Salty foods, especially for men who are overweight. In one study, participants who lowered their sodium intake reduced their risk of a cardiovascular event by 25 percent.

- Sugary foods. Especially for those with diabetes or prediabetes.
- Potatoes, bread, soft drinks, and sweets, if you are an overweight woman. These foods contribute most to glycemic load (a measure of how fast a carb-rich food raises your blood sugar and how much carbohydrate you eat) and probably to inflammation, part of the heart disease cascade. A study of more than seventy-five thousand women over ten years found that those who ate the most foods with a high glycemic load almost doubled their risk of cardiovascular disease compared with those who ate few or no such foods.

TOP CHEFMD-APPROVED RECIPES FOR HEART DISEASE
- Cioppino (page 114)
- Sardine and Arugula Salad with Ratatouille (page 129)
- Toasted Walnut and Creamy White Bean Pitas (page 109)

WATER-COOLER FACT: Cocoa is rich in phenols, compounds that fight heart disease and aging.

HEARTBURN

WHAT IT IS: Heartburn, or gastroesophageal reflux disease (GERD), is a burning irritation or inflammation of the esophagus and throat caused by stomach contents backing up.

YOU ARE AT INCREASED RISK IF YOU
- are a smoker
- are obese
- drink alcohol or coffee
- eat food very rapidly

CULINARY MEDICINE
FOODS TO INCREASE
- Foods that are low in calories. People who eat a low-calorie diet have a higher pH (translation: lower acid) in the throat than those who eat a high-calorie diet.
- Low-carbohydrate foods. A low-carbohydrate diet has been shown to reduce acid in the throat and the symptoms of heartburn, especially in people who are obese.

- Sugar-free gum. Chewing it for half an hour after a meal can reduce heartburn as it raises pH levels in the throat.

FOODS TO AVOID
- Carbonated beverages. They reduce your throat's ability to keep out stomach acid.
- Coffee. It causes heartburn; decaffeinated coffee causes less heartburn, but caffeine is not thought to be the culprit.
- High-calorie processed foods, fatty meats, and fried foods. They lead to weight gain, and reflux is more common in obese people.
- Peppermint and spearmint. They loosen the esophageal sphincter, allow you to burp, and make your throat burn.
- White wine and beer. People with GERD and without GERD who drank one and a quarter cups of white wine or a pint of beer with their meals reported increased heartburn.

TOP CHEFMD-APPROVED RECIPES FOR HEARTBURN
- Chocolate Blackberry Breakfast Smoothie (page 95)
- Ginger Peanut Grilled Chicken with Sweet Potatoes and Sugar Snap Peas (page 117)
- Shrimp and Egg Burritos with White Beans and Corn (page 106)

WATER-COOLER FACT: According to surveys, almost half (44 percent) of Americans have heartburn at least once a month.

HIGH CHOLESTEROL

WHAT IT IS: Hypercholesterolemia means that you have a high level of cholesterol in your blood. It can lead to inflammation and hardening of the arteries, which can cause impotence, premature wrinkling, memory loss, a heart attack, or stroke.

YOU ARE AT INCREASED RISK IF YOU
- are a man over the age of forty-five
- are a woman over the age of fifty-five (especially if you have gone through menopause)
- are overweight

- are sedentary
- are a smoker
- have low thyroid gland activity, diabetes, or a kidney or liver disorder
- have a family history of high cholesterol
- take certain drugs such as drugs for high blood pressure, endocrine drugs, female hormones, steroids, or dermatologic drugs

CULINARY MEDICINE
FOODS TO INCREASE

- Black tea. In one study, five cups a day for three weeks reduced LDL cholesterol by 7.5 percent.
- Dark chocolate. In a Finnish study, 2.5 ounces a day for three weeks increased HDL cholesterol by between 11.4 percent and 13.7 percent.
- Yogurt. In a study, people who ate just under seven ounces of yogurt a day for four weeks reduced blood cholesterol by 2.9 percent, perhaps because of yogurt's probiotics.
- Cinnamon. Barely a teaspoon daily for four weeks lowered LDL (bad) cholesterol between 7 percent and 27 percent in sixty people with type 2 diabetes. Cinnamon improves insulin sensitivity.
- Ground flaxseed. About 1.8 ounces a day over four weeks reduced LDL in people with normal cholesterol by 8 percent and significantly decreased both total cholesterol and LDL levels, probably because of its phytosterol content and lignan content. Two tablespoons twice daily is a maximal dose.
- Rice bran and oat bran. In a six-week study, people ate three ounces of either rice bran or oat bran. LDL levels decreased 14 percent in the rice bran group and 17 percent in the oat bran group.
- Barley. Men fed a diet that included barley (providing six grams of soluble fiber a day) for five weeks saw their total cholesterol lowered by 20 percent and their LDL cholesterol lowered by 24 percent.
- Avocado. In people with high cholesterol, a diet of two thousand calories and forty-nine grams of monounsaturated fatty

acids enriched with avocado decreased bad cholesterol by 22 percent, and increased good cholesterol by 11 percent.

- Macadamia nuts. They are 75 percent fat by weight, 80 percent of which is monounsaturated. Men with high cholesterol who were given 1.5 to 3 ounces a day for four weeks decreased their LDL cholesterol by 5.3 percent, and increased HDL by 7.9 percent.
- Hazelnuts. In an eight-week study, men who ate 1.5 ounces a day for four weeks increased their HDL cholesterol by 12.6 percent. (Hazelnuts are high in soluble fiber, which lowers bad cholesterol. So do their phytosterols.)
- Sunflower oil and canola oil. They both reduce LDL—even more than olive oil.
- Alcohol. One to two alcoholic drinks per day increases HDL cholesterol by about 12 percent, and decreases LDL cholesterol by 5 percent to 17 percent: the type of alcohol is not relevant.
- Egg whites. A Japanese study that gave female subjects cheese, tofu, or egg whites as 30 percent of their daily protein found that those given egg whites had lowered total cholesterol levels in the blood and increased "healthy" HDL cholesterol.
- The Mediterranean diet. A study of people aged sixty-five to one hundred in Cyprus showed that adherence to this dietary pattern, as opposed to the Western pattern, reduces total cholesterol.

FOODS TO AVOID

- Saturated fats. In an Australian study, people who ate forty grams of high-fat dairy a day for four weeks had significantly raised LDL levels. Oxidized LDL injures arteries.
- Foods with trans fats. They both lower HDL and raise LDL.
- Unfiltered coffee. Five cups of French press raises LDL and total cholesterol by 6 percent to 8 percent over four weeks because of a chemical called cafestol.

TOP CHEFMD-APPROVED RECIPES FOR HIGH CHOLESTEROL

- Cinnamon Orange Dreamsicle (page 141)
- Papaya Filled with Gingered Blueberries (page 142)
- Roasted Red Pepper, Wine, and Red Lentil Soup (page 105)

WATER-COOLER FACT: Say *adios* to bad cholesterol with Fresh Tomatillo Guacamole (page 138), which will lower your LDL and raise your HDL.

A REPORTER EATS HIS WAY TO LOWER CHOLESTEROL

Tom Burton is a Pulitzer Prize–winning health reporter for the *Wall Street Journal.* He knew about cholesterol—both because of his work, and because he was health conscious. A daily runner and not a bit overweight, he'd given up most cheese and red meat because of their saturated fat. He ate fish, whole grains, and chicken. But his (lousy) LDL was 169 milligrams per deciliter, far above the optimal 100.

I knew he could do better. He was skeptical but agreed to try.

He regularly filled out daily logs of what he ate and when, although as the single father of two hungry teens, he already had a lot on his plate. His logs showed that he sometimes snacked on cheese and often skipped vegetables except for rosemary potatoes caressed in Cajun slow-roasted chicken fat. And, of course, there was the chicken skin.

Tom gradually eliminated the weekly chicken and potatoes and, on his own, cut out shrimp and squid, which are high in cholesterol, despite my advice: these are minor contributors to LDL. The real bonus came, however, when he added meals that actively lower cholesterol to the weekly cycle at home. He loved Mediterranean foods, so he added an eggplant skillet recipe and a white bean soup with escarole and tomato to his repertoire. He found a steel-cut oatmeal, rich in soluble fiber, and learned to cook unrefined (not pearled) barley. He started using recently ground flaxseed (in his coffee grinder) and tried roasted soybeans for a snack. He traded white pasta for whole wheat and got his kids to try brussels sprouts. He used a cholesterol-lowering butter substitute instead of margarine. And he was happy to hear that alcohol can raise HDL cholesterol by up to 12 percent in just three weeks, and that his liver worked normally.

It wasn't all easy. He took the two tablespoons of flaxseed like it was cod liver oil—just down the hatch. He had to drink more water: a high-fiber diet can cause constipation. His kids had to go along. And progress was slow: after three months, his LDL was down only 10 points. But he kept at it, and he actually accelerated his program by running six days out of seven, at least sixty minutes.

After nine months, he got a third blood test. His internist was shocked: his LDL was 114 milligrams per deciliter and his HDL was 75 milligrams per deciliter. His C-reactive protein and homocysteine levels, markers of inflammation linked to heart disease, had also dropped to optimal levels. A repeat blood test a week later showed a higher LDL—142 milligrams per deciliter—but far better than he'd expected. His HDL remained protectively high, and his internist judged he did not need medicine.

The best part? His kids love the food. His daughter has become a steel-cut-oatmeal-for-breakfast fan and loves the split pea and carrot soup with tarragon, nutmeg, and barley Tom has mastered. And that slow-roasted chicken? Now, grilled salmon with honey-mustard marinade, his son's favorite Sunday dinner. Hard to find that in a pill.

Source: Adapted from T. Burton, "A Reporter Eats His Way to Lower Cholesterol," *Wall Street Journal,* July 22, 2003.

HIGH TRIGLYCERIDES (HYPERTRIGLYCERIDEMIA)

WHAT IT IS: Hypertriglyceridemia is a condition in which the level of triglycerides—a fat in the blood—is too high. It is one of the diagnostic criteria for metabolic syndrome, which itself is caused by toxic belly fat.

YOU ARE AT INCREASED RISK IF YOU
- are obese
- are on antiretroviral therapy
- drink alcohol to excess
- eat carbohydrates to excess
- eat more calories than you burn
- have diabetes
- have a family history of high triglycerides
- have nonalcoholic fatty-liver disorder

- take steroids, beta-blockers, diuretics, estrogen, birth control pills, antipsychotic medications, or tamoxifen

CULINARY MEDICINE
FOODS TO INCREASE

- Avocado. People who ate a diet of two thousand calories enriched with avocado for seven days had a 22 percent decrease in triglycerides.
- Cod liver oil. In a six-week trial, healthy men taking four teaspoons of cod liver oil a day reduced levels of triglycerides in their blood. The omega-3 fatty acids stop the liver from making triglycerides and accelerate their metabolism there.
- Fish, cereals, legumes, fruits, and vegetables. Each has been separately shown to lower triglycerides.
- Foods that are rich in calcium. A Danish study found that people eating a test meal high in calcium reduced their triglycerides by 19 percent. Calcium supplements did not provide the same benefit.
- Eggs laid by hens that have been fed foods with omega-3s, such as walnut, flax, and algae. In one study, people who ate five such eggs a week had a 16 percent to 18 percent decrease in their triglycerides and could not taste the difference in the eggs.
- Red grapefruit. An Israeli study showed that coronary bypass patients who ate red grapefruit every day for thirty days had their triglyceride levels decrease from 206 milligrams per deciliter to 150 milligrams per deciliter, or 27 percent.

FOODS TO AVOID

- Alcohol.
- Foods that have a high glycemic index. They cause weight gain, which raises triglycerides.
- Foods high in saturated and trans fats.
- Sugary and starchy foods. They cause the synthesis of fatty acids, which in turn elevates triglycerides.

TOP CHEFMD-APPROVED RECIPES FOR HIGH TRIGLYCERIDES

- Ginger Peanut Grilled Chicken with Sweet Potatoes and Sugar Snap Peas (page 117)

- Shrimp and Egg Burritos with White Beans and Corn (page 106)
- Spicy and Rich Sausage and Kidney Bean Chili (page 107)

WATER-COOLER FACT: Triglycerides are the marbling you see in corn-fed steaks.

HYPERTENSION (HIGH BLOOD PRESSURE)

WHAT IT IS: Hypertension means that you have high blood pressure.

YOU ARE AT INCREASED RISK IF YOU
- are a man over age thirty-five or a woman over age fifty-five
- are an African American
- are a smoker
- are obese
- have a family history of hypertension
- have obstructive sleep apnea
- have type 2 diabetes

CULINARY MEDICINE
FOODS TO INCREASE

- Sesame oil. People who substituted sesame oil for their regular cooking oil for forty-five days had reduced sodium levels in the blood and increased potassium levels, and both help fight hypertension.

- Mineral water. People with borderline hypertension who drank it for four weeks had a significant decrease in blood pressure. It contains magnesium and calcium, both of which decrease blood pressure.

- Omega-3 rich foods, especially fish. An international 4,680 person study in men and women showed slightly lower blood pressures among those with the highest omega-3 intake, even in people without high blood pressure—about one millimeter of mercury, both systolic and diastolic.

- Foods that are rich in vitamin C. People who increased foods rich in vitamin C such as citrus fruits, strawberries, sweet red peppers, and broccoli, and foods that are rich in carotenoids, such as carrots, sweet potatoes, spinach, kale, collard greens, and tomatoes in their diets for one year saw their blood pressure go down by an average of 2.7 millimeters of mercury.

• Foods that are rich in folic acid. These include spinach, turnip greens, dried beans, dried peas, romaine lettuce, broccoli, cauliflower, lentils, collard greens, mustard greens, brussels sprouts, celery, red bell peppers, summer squash, cabbage, fennel, and liver.

• Olive oil. It regulates blood pressure and is so effective that some participants in a six-month study on average cut their need for hypertensive drugs in half after eating a diet rich in extra-virgin olive oil, and 35 percent did not need to take any drugs at all. Its polyphenols raise the levels of nitric oxide in the blood, which regulates blood pressure.

• Soy nuts. Substituting soy nuts for nonsoy protein in a lower-fat, higher-fiber diet reduces blood pressure by up to 10 percent systolic and 7 percent diastolic in postmenopausal women.

• The Mediterranean diet. Adherence to a Mediterranean food pattern reduces the risk of hypertension among healthy adults.

• The DASH (Dietary Approaches to Stop Hypertension) diet. Low in fat, red meat, and sweets and high in fruits, vegetables, and low-fat dairy, it has reduced blood pressure on average 11 points (systolic) and 5.5 points (diastolic), possibly because it is rich in the minerals calcium, magnesium, and potassium.

FOODS TO AVOID

• Caffeine supplements. The systolic and diastolic blood pressures of men given three hundred milligrams (in, on average, just over three cups of brewed coffee) of caffeine increased by as much as by six points. Drinking coffee increases the risk of being treated with drugs for high blood pressure, except for those people drinking less than four or more than twenty-six ounces of coffee, showed a study of twenty-four thousand adults over thirteen years.

• Energy drinks. Two drinks daily with eighty milligrams caffeine and one thousand milligrams taurine raised blood pressure on average of ten points (systolic) and six points (diastolic) within two hours.

- Foods high in salt and sodium, if you are sodium-sensitive (only about half of people with hypertension are: people at greatest risk are those who are elderly, obese, or African American).

TOP CHEFMD-APPROVED RECIPES FOR HYPERTENSION
- Grilled Citrus Trout over Crunchy Mediterranean Slaw (page 118)
- Rosemary Grilled Chicken and Summer Vegetables (page 127)
- Spicy Gazpacho with Crab (page 137)

WATER-COOLER FACT: Weight loss is an effective way to lower high blood pressure.

INSOMNIA

WHAT IT IS: Insomnia is the inability to get to sleep or to stay asleep for the night.

YOU ARE AT INCREASED RISK IF YOU
- are a smoker
- are stressed, anxious, or depressed
- have a loud or light sleeping environment
- have a condition such as sleep apnea

CULINARY MEDICINE

FOODS TO INCREASE

- Foods that contain tryptophan. Good choices are turkey, chicken, fish, cottage cheese, bananas, eggs, nuts, avocados, milk, cheese, beans, and peas, especially for children and especially at breakfast. Tryptophan metabolizes into melatonin, a hormone that regulates our sleep cycles.
- Carbohydrates with a high glycemic index—rapidly absorbed carbs—eaten four hours before bedtime to get to sleep faster. Men who ate the high glycemic index meal four hours before bedtime got to sleep in an average of 9 minutes in contrast to men who ate the low glycemic index meal, who took 17.5 min-

utes to get to sleep. The same foods eaten one hour before bedtime did not have the same effect.

FOODS TO AVOID

- Alcohol. A study of people living in northwest Russia showed that those who abuse alcohol are more likely to have sleeping disorders. Alcohol can relax the upper airway and worsen sleep apnea, which can cause insomnia.
- Any liquids prior to two hours before bedtime, as the need to urinate may wake you during the night.
- Foods to which you are allergic. In one study, seventeen toddlers (average age 13.5 months) who had unexplained sleeping problems and suspected undiagnosed milk intolerance had cow's milk excluded from their diet. Within six weeks, fifteen of the seventeen children had normalized sleep patterns, falling to sleep faster (in ten minutes instead of fifteen) and sleeping longer (for 13 hours instead of 5.5).
- Spicy foods, especially those that may cause heartburn and especially at dinner.
- Tea and coffee. People who did not lower their overall tea and coffee consumption had more sleep problems than people who did lower it.

TOP CHEFMD-APPROVED RECIPES FOR INSOMNIA
- Creamy Goat Cheese Pesto Omelet (page 96)
- Pasta e Fagioli (Pasta and Bean) Soup (page 102)
- Shrimp and Egg Burritos with White Beans and Corn (page 106)

WATER-COOLER FACT: Eating breakfast every day can help you get a good night's sleep. A Japanese study found that those who skipped breakfast were more likely to experience insomnia.

IRRITABLE BOWEL SYNDROME

WHAT IT IS: Irritable bowel syndrome is a condition in which spasms of the colon disrupt regular digestion, leading to constipation, diarrhea, or both.

YOU ARE AT INCREASED RISK IF YOU

- are a woman
- are under stress
- have a family history of irritable bowel syndrome
- have food allergies and sensitivities

CULINARY MEDICINE
FOODS TO INCREASE

- High-fiber foods. Patients who ate an ounce of wheat bran a day for twelve weeks experienced reduced symptoms of irritable bowel syndrome. Fiber is a bulking agent and has lubricating properties.
- Guar gum, a soluble fiber. People with irritable bowel syndrome who took a heaping teaspoon daily for twelve weeks had less abdominal pain and more regular bowel movements. Their symptoms were better than those patients taking wheat bran, and they seemed to tolerate the guar gum better than the wheat bran.

FOODS TO AVOID

- Alcohol. It aggravates the symptoms of irritable bowel syndrome, and is named by many women with irritable bowel syndrome as a "trigger food."
- Any food to which you may be allergic. These may include the major allergens, which are wheat, fish, shellfish, eggs, dairy products, nuts, peanuts, and soy. (People with irritable bowel syndrome are more prone to food allergies than people who do not have the condition and may also be hypersensitive to beef, pork, and lamb.)
- Coffee and tea. They also aggravate the symptoms of irritable bowel syndrome, probably because of their caffeine content.

TOP CHEFMD-APPROVED RECIPES FOR IRRITABLE BOWEL SYNDROME

- Blackberry, Kiwi, and Mango Fruit Salad (page 140)
- Papaya Filled with Gingered Blueberries (page 142)
- Sauerkraut with Onion, Apple, and Toasted Caraway (page 136)

WATER-COOLER FACT: Women who have irritable bowel syndrome seem to have more symptoms during their menstrual periods.

KIDNEY STONES

WHAT IT IS: Kidney stones are hard mineral deposits that form inside your kidneys. Different types of stones include calcium oxalate and uric acid, and the diet recommendations are the same, except for oxalates.

YOU ARE AT INCREASED RISK IF YOU
- are a man
- are Caucasian
- have a medical condition such as cystic kidney disease, hyperparathyroidism, chronic urinary tract infections, or gout
- have had bariatric surgery
- have a family history of kidney stones

CULINARY MEDICINE
FOODS TO INCREASE
- Fluids. Men and women drinking the most fluids—an average of over 2.5 liters per day—had significantly fewer stones those drinking just 1.2 liters per day.
- Cranberry juice. Men who drank about seventeen ounces of juice diluted with tap water for two weeks significantly reduced their risk of kidney stones. Women who drank cranberry juice regularly over twelve months decreased their symptomatic urinary tract infections, reducing the risk for stones. Cranberry juice causes a decrease in oxalate and phosphate and an increase in citrate excretion—all of which lower your risk of developing kidney stones. It also decreases the supersaturation of calcium oxalate—another risk reducing factor.
- Tea and coffee, either caffeinated or decaffeinated. Tea reduces the risk of kidney stones in women by 8 percent, coffee reduces it by 10 percent, and decaf coffee reduces it by 9 percent when an eight-ounce cup is drunk daily. (The mechanism is not known, although it may be the diuretic effect of these beverages.)
- Lemonade. It is rich in citric acid, which may reduce the risk of kidney stone formation in people with recurrent calcium stones. People who ingested four ounces a day for six days decreased their urinary calcium by thirty-nine milligrams, and

were less likely to form stones. The citric acid is credited—lemon juice has five times the citric acid as orange juice.

- Red wine. It has been shown to reduce kidney stones by 59 percent in women who drank eight ounces a day.
- Beer. The risk of stones was reduced by 40 percent by drinking a twelve-ounce bottle of beer daily.
- Foods high in magnesium. Such foods, like lentils and nuts, bind oxalate in the intestine, preventing its excretion in the urine. Men eating the most magnesium-rich foods had the fewest kidney stones, when compared with those eating the least magnesium-rich foods.

FOODS TO AVOID
- Apple juice. A prospective study in men showed that apple juice increased the risk of stone events.
- Grapefruit juice. People who drink one eight-ounce glass have a 44 percent increased risk compared with those who drink none.
- High-fat foods.
- Meat, fish, and poultry. Restricting animal protein intake has been shown to reduce the risk of kidney stones in people who get recurrent calcium oxalate stones.
- Spinach, rhubarb, beets, chocolate, wheat bran, and strawberries. These foods are high in oxalate and promote stone formation in people who form stones.

TOP CHEFMD-APPROVED RECIPES FOR KIDNEY STONES
- Blackberry, Kiwi, and Mango Fruit Salad (page 140)
- Broccoli, Cheese, and Kalamata Olive Pizza (page 101)
- Cinnamon Orange Dreamsicle (page 141)

WATER-COOLER FACT: One in ten Americans will pass a kidney stone in his or her lifetime. Low-calcium diets actually create a higher overall risk for kidney stones.

MACULAR DEGENERATION

WHAT IT IS: The macula is the part of the eye responsible for central vision. Macular degeneration is the leading cause of blindness in people over age sixty-five in the United States.

YOU ARE AT INCREASED RISK IF YOU

- are obese
- are a smoker
- have high blood pressure
- have high cholesterol
- have a family history of macular degeneration (this increases your risk by four times)

CULINARY MEDICINE

FOODS TO INCREASE

- Spinach and collard greens. Eat them cooked—cooked vegetables have more lutein and zeaxanthin than raw vegetables, and lutein and zeaxanthin absorb short wavelength light in the retina to protect the eyes. Those who eat the most of these foods—just two or more servings daily—have a 47 percent reduced risk of macular degeneration compared with those who eat the least of them. Kale, romaine, eggs, and brussels sprouts are also rich in lutein and zeaxanthin.
- Wine, in moderation. A study of more than three thousand people showed that those who drink wine moderately and regularly have a 34 percent reduced risk of macular degeneration.
- Fatty fish, such as salmon or tuna. A study of elderly twins found that those who ate the most omega-3s had a 45 percent reduced risk of macular degeneration compared with those who ate the least. A study of people with acute macular degeneration (AMD) showed that for some, eating fatty fish once monthly reduced risk for age-related maculopathy by 60 percent.
- Nuts. They have been shown to slow the progression of AMD.
- Foods rich in beta-carotene, vitamin C, vitamin E, and zinc. A study in the Netherlands showed that elderly people who ate more than average quantities of these foods had a 35 percent reduced risk of macular degeneration compared with those who ate less of these foods.

FOODS TO AVOID

- Beer. It has been shown to increase the risk of retinal pigment degeneration in people with macular degeneration by 13 percent—although we don't know why.

- Foods rich in fat. Even "healthy" fats like monounsaturated fats fall under this category—all except omega-3s. People who have AMD and who eat the most fatty foods have more than twice the risk of progression of the disease than those who eat little or no fat.
- Foods with a high glycemic index. A ten-year study of 526 people from Boston showed that such foods—sugars and highly processed starches—make you more than 2.5 times more likely to suffer macular degeneration. The increased oxidative stress of such rapidly absorbed high-carb foods may increase inflammation.
- Processed (commercial) baked goods. They doubled the rate of AMD progression over 4.6 years.

TOP CHEFMD-APPROVED RECIPES FOR MACULAR DEGENERATION
- Toasted Walnut and Creamy White Bean Pitas (page 109)
- Cedar-Planked Roast Salmon with Candied Ginger and Berry Salsa (page 112)
- Cioppino (page 114)

WATER-COOLER FACT: Macular degeneration is more common in whites than in African Americans and is one of the few conditions in which a specific vitamin-mineral combination (zinc, copper, beta-carotene, vitamin E, vitamin C available as Ocuvite Preservision, iCaps AREDS Formula, and VisiVite Original Formula) has been shown to prevent progression of the disease.

MALE INFERTILITY

WHAT IT IS: Male infertility is any condition that interferes with a man's ability to get a woman pregnant.

YOU ARE AT INCREASED RISK IF YOU
- are overweight
- have an endocrine problem (such as diabetes mellitus, or a thyroid disorder or have a hypothalamic disorder)
- have had cancer, cryptorchidism, varicocele, physical groin injury, hydrocele, or the mumps

- have testicular factors, such as genetic defects on the Y chromosome and chromosomal abnormalities
- have posttesticular causes such as infection (for example, prostatitis), obstruction, retrograde ejaculation, or a hypospadia
- have oligospermia (you produce few sperm) or azoospermia (you produce no sperm)
- have asthenozoospermia (you produce a normal number of sperm but they have poor motility)
- have taken anabolic steroids, cimetidine, spironolactone, sulfasalazine, or nitrofurantoin as your medications
- have celiac disease
- experience impotence

CULINARY MEDICINE
FOODS TO INCREASE
- Lean beef, wheat germ, oysters, and dark-meat turkey. These foods all have zinc, and a zinc deficiency can cause a decreased sperm count. Men put on a zinc-restricted diet of less than five milligrams daily for up to forty weeks had a decreased sperm count, but this normalized within twelve months when they ate zinc-rich foods.
- Tomatoes and tomato-based foods, because of their lycopene content, in theory only. Thirty men were given two thousand micrograms of lycopene supplements twice a day for three months. Two-thirds had increased sperm counts by the end of the study. Free oxygen radicals are a major cause of male infertility, and lycopene squelches free radicals.
- Foods high in vitamin C, in theory only. They increase sperm count and motility, perhaps by reducing oxidative stress. Infertile men given one thousand milligrams of vitamin C twice a day had their sperm counts increase by an average of over 125 percent.
- The Mediterranean diet. It improves impotence and erectile function in men with metabolic syndrome.
- Organic foods, so that you are not exposed to some synthetic chemical pesticides. Men who are exposed show damaged sperm and a prolonged time to first pregnancy.

FOODS TO AVOID

• Alcohol. It decreases sperm count and motility, and the more you drink, the more the count and motility decrease.

• Coffee. An Italian study showed that the more coffee men drank, the greater their risk of sperm that do not work. Even having just one cup a day has a negative effect.

• Mercury-containing fish (such as shark, swordfish, marlin, king mackerel, tilefish, or albacore tuna). In one study, mercury concentrations were found to be significantly higher (40 percent) in the hair of subfertile males, who had 4.5 parts per million, than fertile males, who had 3.9 parts per million. Vegans who had not eaten fish for the previous five years had only 0.38 parts per million.

TOP CHEFMD-APPROVED RECIPES FOR MALE INFERTILITY
• Cherry Tomato and Mozzarella Morsel Salad (page 134)
• Sardine and Arugula Salad with Ratatouille (page 129)
• Toasted Walnut and Creamy White Bean Pitas (page 109)

WATER-COOLER FACT: Stress has been shown to decrease the quantity and motility of sperm—so meditate, do yoga, or relax with friends.

METABOLIC SYNDROME

WHY IS MY HDL LOW? WHY IS MY BLOOD PRESSURE HIGH? MY HIP HURTS.

Dan was a middle-aged Wall Street executive who was working even more now that he had "retired." A serious limo accident had left him with chronic hip pain, and that, coupled with pressure from two new ventures, made it all too easy for him to gain weight. His annual physical showed he had high triglycerides, a low HDL cholesterol, mildly high blood sugar, high blood pressure (his systolic had always been more than 140 millimeters of mercury, but now his diastolic was 95 millimeters of mercury), and a waist of forty-four inches. He never skipped his twice weekly handball game, but his hip pain was getting worse, and he drank to relieve the pain. He weighed 251 pounds.

"Dr. John, I'll level with you. I'm scared," he said, handing me a six-page summary of his medical records over eighteen years, including current prescriptions for pain meds and Viagra, and recent lab values and test results.

Dan had metabolic syndrome. His low HDL, high blood pressure, and large waist size greatly raised his heart attack risk. So did taking Viagra, which I advised him to stop. He ate like many people: a morning muffin, a sandwich at his desk at noon, chips around 4:00 p.m., and whatever he could manage for dinner (which was often take-out or a restaurant meal).

Dan started the Mediterranean diet to reduce the inflammatory effects of metabolic syndrome and to help with his impotence. He had no wine (alcohol is metabolized first: its seven calories per gram go straight to the liver to be stored) or ice cream in the first twelve weeks. No steaks or full-fat cheese, either, except on four special occasions per year. I told him that high-fiber, whole-grain cereals lowered diabetes risk and insulin resistance, unlike most muffins, so he switched to cereal in the morning. And I said that learning to cook—even a little—would help. I showed him how to use a chef's knife and how to sauté: he had never cooked before, but he quickly got the hang of it. I suggested he switch from espresso to herbal tea, as caffeine raises blood pressure, and unfiltered coffee raises LDL cholesterol.

I persuaded him to play handball three days a week, and he eventually added two more sessions. He began a simple treadmill walking regimen, which he made easier by watching *Hawaii Five-0* reruns. Executives like to compete, so he found 5Ks to walk with a buddy. After twelve weeks he had lost sixteen pounds, his systolic had dropped ten millimeters of mercury and diastolic five millimeters of mercury, his glucose fourteen milligrams per deciliter and triglycerides seventy-four milligrams per deciliter. I told Dan that these were all typical measurements for someone with metabolic syndrome who had lost about 6 percent of his weight, but Dan wanted to do better. And he did.

After nine months, Dan's waist was thirty-nine inches, his blood pressure was normal, and he had raised his HDL to forty-five. He had walked a 10K and lost forty-one pounds. His pain was reduced and quality of life had greatly improved—both in the kitchen and in the bedroom. "Dr. John, I just want to thank you. I didn't believe you when you said the lentils, olive oil, and nuts would help my sex life. But they did, even without the Viagra!"

WHAT IT IS: Metabolic syndrome means having three out of five risk factors—large waist size, low HDL, elevated blood sugar, blood pressure, and triglyceride level—for heart disease. Together they pose a greater risk than each one alone. The cause of metabolic syndrome is visceral (on the inside) belly fat and increased insulin resistance.

YOU ARE AT INCREASED RISK IF YOU
- are overweight, especially around the waist
- are obese
- are sedentary
- have elevated triglycerides
- have low HDL cholesterol
- have high blood pressure
- have a hormone imbalance
- have a family history of metabolic syndrome

CULINARY MEDICINE
FOODS TO INCREASE

- Milk, yogurt, cheese, and other dairy products. A study of more than ten thousand women over the age of forty-five showed that those who eat the most calcium-rich foods have a 36 percent reduced risk of metabolic syndrome compared with those who eat the least. A study of twenty-four hundred middle-aged men showed that those who drank two cups of milk daily were 62 percent less likely to have metabolic syndrome than those who rarely drank milk.

- The Mediterranean diet. Eating a diet rich in whole-grain cereals, fish, legumes, fruits, and vegetables has been shown to reduce the risk of metabolic syndrome by 13 percent, and over two years it has improved sexual function in women with metabolic syndrome.

- Fruits and vegetables in general. An Iranian study found that people who ate the most fruit had a 34 percent reduced risk of metabolic syndrome, and people who ate the most vegetables had a 30 percent reduced risk of metabolic syndrome, compared with those who ate the fewest of these foods.
- High-fiber cereals and grains. People who eat the most cereal fiber have a 38 percent reduced risk of metabolic syndrome and people who eat the most whole grains have a 33 percent reduced risk of metabolic syndrome compared with people who eat few or none of these foods.
- Foods rich in magnesium such as halibut, almonds, cashews, soybeans, spinach, nuts, oatmeal, and peanuts. The current RDI for magnesium is 310–420 milligrams. People who get half or less are at a 75 percent increased risk of metabolic syndrome compared with those who get the full RDI. Magnesium may act as an anti-inflammatory.
- Soy nuts. When substituted for red meat for eight weeks among women with metabolic syndrome, soy nuts reduced blood sugar and LDL cholesterol; other soy foods did not.

FOODS TO AVOID

- Alcohol. It has been shown to increase the risk of metabolic syndrome by 26 percent.
- Red meat. In a seven-year study, men who ate the most meat had a 4.7 times greater chance of developing metabolic syndrome than men who ate the least, though this was attributed to the saturated fat content of the meat.
- Foods high in saturated fat. A Greek study showed that 35 percent of those who ate a diet high in saturated fat had metabolic syndrome compared with only 9 percent of those who ate a Mediterranean diet that was low in saturated fat.
- The Western diet. Women who eat a diet low in whole grains and high in saturated fat have up to a 68 percent increased risk of developing metabolic syndrome.
- High-fructose corn syrup (HFCS) for men. HFCS raises uric acid levels, which lowers nitric oxide levels, and increases insulin resistance. HFCS does not raise uric acid levels in women.

- Parmigiano Caesar Salad with Shrimp (page 121)
- Curried Turkey Tenderloin with Penne and Roasted Asparagus (page 116)
- Tangy and Cool Buttermilk and Avocado Breakfast Smoothie (page 99)

WATER-COOLER FACT: It is estimated that one in four or five adults in the United States—up to 25 percent—has metabolic syndrome.

MIGRAINE

FLASHING LIGHTS AND BRIE ON ENGLISH MUFFINS

Mary C. is a twenty-nine-year-old Houston attorney and mediator. She plays softball after work and can pound beers with the boys. She works long hours. One night, she noticed flashing lights and colors in her vision. She had a blind spot and a terrific headache on her left side. She became nauseated. Worried, her boyfriend brought her to the emergency room.

A CAT scan of her brain showed no bleeding. Her blood tests were normal except for mild anemia. She was given Imitrex, and her headache stopped.

She came to see me to find out how to prevent future migraines, and I learned that she loved the frozen pizzas and Pop-Tarts she grew up with as much as she loved Houston's famous Café Annie. She was a poster child for high-tyramine foods, especially sauerkraut, pickles, olives, nuts, pepperoni, and liverwurst. She liked having brie on English muffins for breakfast, and downed a six-pack of diet soda every week. She was weight conscious and regularly went a whole day without eating.

There were several factors that could have been triggering her migraines—stress, birth control, artificial sweeteners, beer, nitrates, and the tyramine in her food. The best way to find out which was the trigger would be to stop all of these, and add them back one at a time. She didn't want to do that, or to be tested for food allergies, and she thought giving up the soda would be very hard.

So we worked around the edges of the problem. Skipped meals are the most common migraine trigger, which she solved with energy bars in her desk, handbag, and car. Instead of snacking on high tyramine foods, I recommended that she try several high-iron cereals (such as Total and Product 19). Instead of cheeses, I recommended she have avocado (which was fine with her, because of its spreadability) to replace the brie. I asked her to drink water instead of beer or soda, since alcohol, sucralose, and aspartame have all been reported to trigger migraines.

She worked at it for over two months. She lost a little weight and decided she did not need to fast anymore. She found she liked toasted pumpkin seeds, which are high in magnesium and therefore help reduce the frequency of headaches. She learned to make a weekly dish of toasted chickpeas and lentils, with wilted spinach, which is high in riboflavin, which also reduces the frequency of headaches. She doused the dish in olive oil, which further reduces the frequency, severity, and duration of headaches. As a result of her change in diet, her migraines have become much less frequent and much less severe.

WHAT IT IS: A migraine is an intensely painful headache on one or both sides of your head, accompanied by nausea, vomiting, and sensitivity to light.

YOU ARE AT INCREASED RISK IF YOU
- are under stress
- are a woman, especially between the ages of thirty-five and forty-five
- don't get enough sleep
- have a family history of migraines
- have celiac disease

CULINARY MEDICINE
FOODS TO INCREASE

- Water. Drinking at least eight eight-ounce glasses of water a day can guard you against migraines, and can lessen their length and severity. Patients who drank this much water had twenty-one hours less headache over a two-week period than they typically did. (Dehydration may be one cause of headache.)

- Fish oil. Of participants who took fish oil as a dietary supplement in a five-month study, 87 percent reported a reduction in headache frequency, 74 percent reported a reduction in the duration of headaches, and 83 percent reported a reduction in headache severity.

- Olive oil. Of participants who took olive oil as a supplementary placebo in the same study as the fish oil, 78 percent reported a reduction in headache frequency, 70 percent reported a reduction in the length of headaches, and 65 percent reported a reduction in headache severity.

- Regular meals. Skipping meals is one of the most common triggers for migraine attacks.

FOODS TO AVOID

Note: because food migraine triggers vary so much from person to person, you might eliminate all of these foods if you want, and then add them back slowly, checking for effect.

- Artificial sweeteners. These include sucralose and aspartame.

- Beer. In a British study, 28 percent of migraine patients reported that drinking beer gave them headaches.

- Chocolate and red wine. These are the classic triggers of migraine. Thirty-one percent of headache patients reported they got headaches from wine. It is probably the phenols that cause migraines. Conversely, before a migraine, sufferers may crave chocolate.

- Citrus fruit and cheese. They can reportedly trigger migraines, although less so than red wine or chocolate. Eighteen percent of patients said they got migraines from cheese, and 11 percent from citrus fruits.

- Monosodium glutamate. Thirty-six percent of people given five grams of MSG experienced headaches or other reactions.

- Foods rich in tyramine (such as any aged, dried, fermented, salted, smoked, or pickled foods). These include pepperoni, salami, liverwurst, pickled herring, aged cheese, sauerkraut, and pickles.

- Cumin-Crusted Salmon over Silky Sweet Potatoes (page 115)
- Saffron Scallop, Shrimp, and Chickpea Paella (page 128)
- Spicy Gazpacho with Crab (page 137)

WATER-COOLER FACT: Women are three times more likely to suffer from migraines than men, possibly because the waves of brain activity thought to excite migraines are activated more quickly in women than in men.

MULTIPLE SCLEROSIS

WHAT IT IS: Multiple sclerosis (MS) is a relatively rare disease in which the immune system attacks the myelin sheath, which covers nerves, causing increased difficulty moving and progressive physical weakness.

YOU ARE AT INCREASED RISK IF YOU
- are a woman
- are of European ancestry
- are a smoker
- are underweight, with a low body mass index
- are sedentary

CULINARY MEDICINE
FOODS TO INCREASE

- Low-fat foods. People with MS who eat a very low-fat diet (less than twenty grams of fat a day) have significantly less physical deterioration in at least one study. Of 144 people with multiple sclerosis who ate a low-fat diet over thirty-four years, 95 percent survived and remained physically active.
- Fish oil and fish, especially fatty fish such as salmon and tuna. They contain omega-3 fatty acids, which were shown in a one-year trial to decrease the relapse rates in people with MS but not affect disease progression.
- Foods high in vitamin D3. Milk, soy milk, cod liver oil, mackerel, and sardines all have vitamin D. Deficiency of vitamin D is common in people with multiple sclerosis, and lower levels

of vitamin D are associated with greater disability. Vitamin D3 helps to confirm the signals sent between nerves and the immune system.

FOODS TO AVOID

- Coffee. When people with MS were compared with healthy individuals, they were 70 percent more likely to be coffee drinkers.
- Hard liquor. People who drink it are more than six times more likely to be diagnosed with MS than people who do not.
- Foods rich in saturated fats, especially milk and cream. People with MS who ate a high-fat diet had higher rates of deterioration and death.

TOP CHEFMD-APPROVED RECIPES FOR MULTIPLE SCLEROSIS

- Blackberry, Kiwi, and Mango Fruit Salad (page 140)
- Cedar-Planked Roast Salmon with Candied Ginger and Berry Salsa (page 112)
- Chocolate Blackberry Breakfast Smoothie (page 95)

WATER-COOLER FACT: Being in the sun reduces your risk of MS, especially when you're a child, probably because your skin normally makes the vitamin D it needs with just ten minutes on your arms and legs twice weekly. A study on twins (so that a genetic tendency toward MS could be ruled out) showed that the longer the twins had spent time in the sun as children, the less likely they were to get MS—by up to more than 40 percent.

OBESITY

TELL ME WHAT TO DO TO LOSE WEIGHT AND I WILL DO IT

Kathi is wildly successful. She writes, produces, and directs movies seen all over the country. She owns homes in Vancouver, Chicago, and Hollywood. She has a personal chef and a personal assistant. She also has been seriously overweight since she was in second grade. A patient of mine dragged her to a public lecture I gave.

Kathi had to use seat-belt extenders on airplanes, and airplane trays rode up on her stomach. Her seat in her car was back as far as it could go. Sometimes she stopped breathing when she slept, waking every few minutes at night, with dark circles under her puffy eyes to show for it in the morning. Her sister died of diabetic ketoacidosis last year.

Kathi's body mass index was forty-eight, and her diagnosis was class III obesity. Like 3 percent of American adults five-feet six-inches tall, she weighed nearly 100 percent more than she should: in her case, 297. (A normal weight is 155 pounds or less.)

She hated the idea of stomach surgery. And she had already been through psychotherapy, Jenny Craig, Weight Watchers, LA Weight Loss, e-diets, and Overeaters Anonymous. She had taken every diet pill ("except Orlistat—no oily leakage for this girl!") and intimidated every dietitian she had met. She rejected theories of genetic fatalism. She hoped that I could help her.

I agreed to try. I drew a plate. Three-quarters vegetables and one-quarter other foods—foods she chose. She was to eat her vegetables first at lunch and dinner. She would see her physician regularly, and her chef and I would collaborate. She was to call me twice a week, no matter where she was, and fax her records of what, where, when, how, and how long she ate. (She dismissed this latter idea: she had spent her entire career being free of a time-card punch; she had no time to write down what she ate.)

But we continued to work at it until it did just that: worked. As Oprah has said, "I've been through lots of diet programs, and there's nothing like getting up and going for a walk in the morning." And that's what Kathi learned to do—put one foot in front of the other, literally. She began with a two-minute walk: that was all she could do. She learned to use a perceived exertion scale, and aim for seven out of ten. And she slowly increased her walking time, intensity, and frequency.

Over three years Kathi lost 120 pounds. And she has kept off sixty, after five years. Not perfect—but much better than where she was before.

WHAT IT IS: Obesity is defined by a body mass index of more than 30 kilograms per square meter. For a five-foot six-inch person, that's about thirty pounds overweight. Wanting food is a biologic drive, not greed, but eating more calories than you burn off causes obesity.

YOU ARE AT INCREASED RISK IF YOU
- are under stress at work or home
- have parents or close friends who are overweight or obese
- live in a Western or Westernizing country
- regularly use food as a reward, companion, stress-reliever, or emotional balm
- vary your eating schedule significantly

CULINARY MEDICINE

FOODS TO INCREASE
- Whole fruits and vegetables, which are high in fiber, moisture, and volume.
- Small amounts of solid, higher-protein foods. These include poultry, tofu, eggs, beans, and lower-fat cheese.
- Small amounts of foods with healthy flavorful fats. These include olives and olive oil; salmon, trout, eel, herring, sardines; and nuts and seeds of all kinds.
- Foods with resistant starch. These include firm bananas, most legumes (lentils, chickpeas, edamame), and whole grains.
- Any effective reduced-calorie diet plan. Recipes from Atkins (very low carb), Ornish (very low fat), Zone (lower carb, higher protein) and LEARN (balanced) all are lower in calories than average, and all help people reduce weight very modestly over a year.

FOODS TO AVOID
- Alcoholic beverages. They contain seven calories per gram unlike protein and carbs, and these calories are both metabolized and stored—in the liver—first.
- Crackers, breads, chips, and other starchy foods. They are high calorie, low satiety, and low nutrient.
- Foods with artificial sweeteners. They do not facilitate weight loss and may actually increase overweight and obesity, perhaps because people tend to overeat them.

- Soda, energy drinks, candy, juice drinks, and any other foods with low-nutritional, low-satiety but high-caloric value.

TOP CHEFMD-APPROVED RECIPES FOR OBESITY
- Portuguese Caldo Verde (page 104)
- Red Pozole with Shredded Chicken and Avocado (page 124)
- Sardine and Arugula Salad with Ratatouille (page 129)

WATER-COOLER FACT: Fat around your waist acts like a hormone-producing organ. Fat on your hips, thighs, and arms is just storage. Fat around your waist triggers a chain of inflammatory activities, and men with waists of forty-three inches or more have more than twice the risk of colon cancer of men with normal waists. Cancers of the pancreas, esophagus, kidney, and post-menopausal breast are also linked to obesity. A pound is thirty-five hundred calories; cutting five hundred calories daily for a week will help you lose it.

OSTEOARTHRITIS

HOT DOGS MAKE MY KNEES HURT!

My patient Peggy had severe osteoarthritis. A retired schoolteacher and mother of five, she had knee pain that was so bad, she had a hard time walking, even with her cane. Except for the few blocks walk to the market, and the once-weekly shuttle to bridge or a matinee, she was virtually housebound.

"My doctor gives me pills," she told me. "But I forget to take them."

When I asked her about her diet, Peggy said she usually ate pastries for breakfast, tuna fish for lunch, a beef pot pie for dinner, and strawberry shortcake with whipped cream for dessert. She liked to cook, but didn't have the energy to do much more than poach an egg, or reheat leftovers.

Peggy's doctor had prescribed cyclooxygenase-2 (commonly known as COX-2) inhibitors, which I told her to put near her toothbrush so she would remember to take them. I explained that osteoarthritis was an inflammatory disease. Its pattern of pain and stiffness was predictable, so we could use food to treat and even prevent the pain. I prescribed an analgesic food for breakfast (berries), an antioxidant/anti-inflammatory food for lunch (fish, soy, ginger, or avocado), and an omega-3 rich food for dinner (fish, walnuts, or flax meal). And I told her not to eat foods with trans fats (they are inflammatory), starches and added sugars (they produce inflammatory cytokines), or red meat (the saturated fat adds to inflammation).

Three months after our first meeting she walked into my office without her cane, swearing that she had not felt so good in years. Then she said, "My daughter took me to a baseball game last week, and I had a hot dog. It was great! But I really paid for it. My knees were killing me for three days afterwards. But I went back on my program, and you know what? I feel so good I'm going to move north, where I can get some land." And she did: she now lives on twenty-four acres in Idaho, where she takes long walks with her two dogs.

WHAT IT IS: Osteoarthritis ("wear-and-tear arthritis"), the most common type in the United States, is a painful degenerative condition that occurs when cartilage (which cushions bone joints) becomes cracked and pitted.

YOU ARE AT INCREASED RISK IF YOU
- are obese
- have a family history of osteoarthritis
- have had an injury to a joint
- have had surgery on a joint
- have a hormonal disorder
- have osteoporosis

CULINARY MEDICINE
FOODS TO INCREASE
- Dairy foods. A Turkish study showed that people with osteoarthritis who drink the most milk have a decreased frequency of symptoms.
- Tea. It has also been shown to decrease the frequency of osteoarthritis, perhaps because of its anti-inflammatory compounds.

- Foods rich in vitamin C. People who eat the most foods rich in vitamin C (such as citrus fruits) have 70 percent less cartilage loss than those who eat the least and a threefold reduction in the progression of the disease.
- Avocado and soybeans. Their oils have both been found to be extremely effective in reducing the need for nonsteroidal anti-inflammatory drugs in people with osteoarthritis. The oils appear to stimulate collagen production and slow cartilage breakdown.
- Ginger. In a six-week study, its extract reduced the symptoms of osteoarthritis in the knee: ginger is a known anti-inflammatory.
- Fish oils. They may lubricate joints in people with osteoarthritis (or even prevent the condition) by keeping the joints lubricated.

FOODS TO AVOID

- Red meat, especially processed red meat such as sausage and hamburger. It has been shown to cause a higher risk of degenerative arthritis. In a study of people with moderate-to-severe knee osteoarthritis, those who eliminated red meat had the fewest painful attacks over a six- and twelve-week period, regardless of weight loss. Red meats are typically high in saturated fat and omega-6 fatty acids, which are inflammatory.
- Sugary and starchy foods. In the same study, people who limited their intake of processed baked goods had less pain after six and twelve weeks than those who did not.

TOP CHEFMD-APPROVED RECIPES FOR OSTEOARTHRITIS
- Cedar-Planked Roast Salmon with Candied Ginger and Berry Salsa (page 112)
- Grilled Citrus Trout over Crunchy Mediterranean Slaw (page 118)
- Honeyed Chinese Chicken Breasts (page 120)

WATER-COOLER FACT: It is estimated that 80 percent of the population will have osteoarthritis by the age of sixty-five, although almost half of those people will not have any symptoms.

PEPTIC ULCER DISEASE

WHAT IT IS: A peptic ulcer is a very painful sore in the stomach or small intestine's lining, usually caused by *H. pylori* bacteria.

YOU ARE AT INCREASED RISK IF YOU
- are under a lot of stress
- have a family history of peptic ulcer disease
- take steroidal anti-inflammatory drugs

CULINARY MEDICINE
FOODS TO INCREASE
Note: Make sure your food is from a clean source to try to minimize bacterial contamination.

- Fermented dairy products such as yogurt, cheese, and kefir. They have been shown to reduce the risk of ulcers by 18 percent, perhaps because of their probiotics. Probiotics reduce inflammation in the stomach.
- High-fiber fruits and vegetables. People who eat seven servings a day have a lower risk of duodenal (small intestine) ulcers than those who only eat three. An Italian study showed that people who ate the most vegetables had a 26 percent reduced risk of peptic ulcer.
- Foods rich in vitamin A. People who eat a diet rich in these foods have a 33 percent decreased risk of duodenal ulcer.
- Curcumin and ginger. They have been found to fight the growth of *H. pylori* in a laboratory setting.
- Chilies (including chili pepper, chili powder, or chili sauce). People who eat them frequently (twenty-four times a month) have 50 percent less risk than those who eat them less frequently (eight times a month).

FOODS TO AVOID
- Coffee. A German study showed that people who drink three or more cups a day are at almost 2.5 times the risk of *H. pylori* infection than people who drink less.
- Meats.

- Milk. A study of 1,135 people showed that a diet rich in regular (nonfermented) milk increases the risk of ulcer by 17 percent.

TOP CHEFMD-APPROVED RECIPES FOR PEPTIC ULCER DISEASE
- Butternut Barley Risotto with Goat Cheese and Toasted Almonds (page 111)
- Papaya Filled with Gingered Blueberries (page 142)
- Skillet Chilaquiles with Nopales, Eggs, and Kale (page 98)

WATER-COOLER FACT: Raise your glass in a toast to the fact that beer and wine help protect you against infection from *H. pylori* bacteria.

PROSTATE CANCER

WHAT IT IS: Prostate cancer is cancer of the prostate, a gland in men about the size and shape of a walnut that surrounds the urethra at the point where the urethra connects to the bladder.

YOU ARE AT INCREASED RISK IF YOU
- are a smoker
- are African American
- are over sixty-five
- are obese
- have elevated levels of testosterone in the blood
- have a family history of prostate cancer
- have an infection or inflammation of the prostate from a sexually transmitted disease

CULINARY MEDICINE
FOODS TO INCREASE
- Soy. Men who ate four slices of bread containing fifty grams of soy grits lowered their levels of prostate-specific antigens (PSAs), and the control group on ordinary bread raised theirs. Total PSA was down by 12.7 percent in the soy group versus up 40 percent in the control group. Soy contains isoflavones, natural substances that lower hormone production and inhibit the production of prostate cancer cells.

- Tomatoes. Eating them two or more times a week reduces the risk of prostate cancer by at least 23 percent, possibly because of the carotenoids.
- Fish oil. It increases the ratio of omega-3 to omega-6 fatty acid in the blood, reduces cyclooxygenase 2 (COX-2) inflammation and potentially slows the progression of prostate cancer.
- Pomegranate juice. Eight ounces daily slowed tumor doubling time by three in men without metastatic disease already treated with surgery or radiation. Pomegranate juice is rich in flavonoids.
- Flax meal. About three rounded tablespoons daily reduced tumor growth between 30 percent and 40 percent in men who took it for six months. PSA levels went down between an average of 5.72 nanograms per milliliter.
- Cruciferous vegetables, especially broccoli. A weekly serving of broccoli cut the risk of aggressive prostate cancer—stages III and IV—by 45 percent compared with just one serving per month. Broccoli's anticarcinogen, sulforaphane, turns on liver enzymes to detoxify carcinogens. Broccoli and cauliflower, another crucifer, alkalinize urine to accelerate carcinogen excretion.
- Foods rich in vitamin E. Eating foods such as nuts, seeds, spinach, peppers, and olive oil can reduce risk of advanced prostate cancer by 32 percent, as opposed to taking vitamin E supplements: in a study of over two hundred and ninety-five thousand men, the supplements had no effect.

FOODS TO AVOID

- Dairy foods. Men who eat five or more servings a week are at 65 percent increased risk of prostate cancer than those who eat few or none.
- Foods with a high glycemic index. These include doughnuts, pasta, crackers, white bread, potatoes, and jelly beans.
- Processed meat. Men who eat five or more servings a week of foods such as bacon, sausage, hot dogs, and salami are at more than twice the risk of prostate cancer than men who eat little or none.
- Red meat. The heme iron in meat is a catalyst of oxidative damage, and saturated fat is a risk factor, too. Well-done and

very well-done beef is especially risky, particularly for men with advanced prostate cancer, in part because carcinogenic heterocyclic amines are formed in well-done meat.

TOP CHEFMD-APPROVED RECIPES FOR PROSTATE CANCER
- Cioppino (page 114)
- Portuguese Caldo Verde (page 104)
- Spicy Gazpacho with Crab (page 137)

WATER-COOLER FACT: Prostate cancer is least common in Asia and most common in the United States. It is the most common cancer in American men and causes more deaths than lung cancer.

RHEUMATOID ARTHRITIS

WHAT IT IS: Rheumatoid arthritis is a chronic inflammatory autoimmune condition where the body attacks its own tissue, especially the joints, causing pain, tenderness, and swelling.

YOU ARE AT INCREASED RISK IF YOU
- have a family history of rheumatoid arthritis
- smoke

CULINARY MEDICINE
FOODS TO INCREASE

- The Mediterranean diet. Patients who adhered to it for twelve weeks had reduced inflammation, increased vitality, and better physical function of their affected joints. Those on the standard American diet showed no improvement.

- Cold-water fish. Patients with rheumatoid arthritis who reduced their ratio of omega-6 to omega-3 to two or three to one reduced their inflammation, and those who took at least 2.6 grams of fish oils had reduced dependence on anti-inflammatory medication.

- Extra-virgin olive oil. Eating it reduces your risk of rheumatoid arthritis by 61 percent, and two teaspoons, combined with three grams daily of fish oil, significantly improves morning stiffness, joint pain intensity, and onset of fatigue in rheumatoid arthritis patients after twelve weeks.

- Dairy products fortified with vitamin D. In a study of almost thirty thousand older women (ages fifty-five to sixty-nine), it was found that those who ate a diet rich in these foods had a 33 percent reduced risk of rheumatoid arthritis compared to those who ate few or none.

FOODS TO AVOID

- Any foods that cause personal allergic reactions, which may cause immune reactions in the joints.
- Peanut oil. It is high in arachidonic acid (an omega-6 fatty acid). An eight-month study of people with rheumatoid arthritis who ate a diet low in arachidonic acid (less than ninety milligrams a day) showed a reduction of swollen joints by 14 percent.
- Red meat (especially grain-fed steers), because of their omega-6 content, which is inflammatory. People who eat a diet rich in red meats are at almost twice the risk of developing rheumatoid arthritis compared with those who eat little or none.

TOP CHEFMD-APPROVED RECIPES FOR RHEUMATOID ARTHRITIS

- Cioppino (page 114)
- Cumin-Crusted Salmon over Silky Sweet Potatoes (page 115)
- Parmigiano Caesar Salad with Shrimp (page 121)

WATER-COOLER FACT: For reasons we do not understand, women under age sixty have three times the risk that men do, but after age sixty, both men and women are equally at risk.

ULCERATIVE COLITIS

WHAT IT IS: Ulcerative colitis is a chronic condition and type of inflammatory bowel disease. Tiny bleeding ulcers form on the surface of the lining of the colon and rectum.

YOU ARE AT INCREASED RISK IF YOU

- are related to someone with inflammatory bowel disease
- are white
- are Jewish, especially of European descent
- are a former smoker
- are a woman who has never breast-fed

- are under stress
- are sleep deprived
- take oral contraceptives

CULINARY MEDICINE
FOODS TO INCREASE

- Turmeric. Curcumin has improved symptoms in ulcerative proctitis, and four of five patients in a pilot study were able to reduce their medications. In a randomized double-blind placebo-controlled trial, two grams daily reduced clinical activity of the colitis and improved remission rates. Curcumin in turmeric inhibits the genes that control inflammation.

- Breakfast cereals. About seven ounces a week was found to reduce disease activity in people with ulcerative colitis.

- Foods that are low in fat.

- Fruits and vegetables. They may help reduce the risk of ulcerative colitis (although if you have cramping and diarrhea, this may be the result of the high-fiber content of the fruit, and you should reduce your intake).

- Oranges, kiwi, grapefruit, and other fruits rich in vitamin C. They reduce the risk for ulcerative colitis.

- Fish oil. Patients who took it for four months had improved symptoms, increased weight gain, and reduced levels of inflammation in the bowel and rectum.

- Fish. Ten ounces a week reduces disease activity.

- Low-fat active yogurt. It contains probiotics, including *Lactobacilli*, which have been found to prevent relapse, maintain remission, and reduce inflammation.

- Cheese. About 3.5 ounces a week has been found to reduce disease activity.

- Wheat grass juice. Taken daily, 3.3 ounces reduced severity of rectal bleeding and overall disease activity in a monthlong randomized placebo-controlled trial.

FOODS TO AVOID

- Alcohol. People with ulcerative colitis who drank the most alcohol had more than 2.5 times the rate of relapse compared with those who drank the least.

- Caffeinated drinks, such as coffee or tea. In a study women reported that these were common "trigger foods."
- Fast foods. People who ate fast foods at least twice weekly had nearly four times the risk of ulcerative colitis versus those who did not.
- Foods high in fat, specifically omega-6 fats such as corn, soy, sunflower, safflower, and red meat. A diet high in fat raises your risk of ulcerative colitis almost threefold.
- Red and processed meat. People with ulcerative colitis who ate the most red meat had more than three times the rate of relapse than those who ate the least.
- Foods high in sugar, especially sucrose or table sugar. A Japanese study found that people who eat the most sugary foods are at almost three times the risk of inflammatory bowel disease than those who eat few or none.

TOP CHEFMD-APPROVED RECIPES FOR ULCERATIVE COLITIS
- Grilled Citrus Trout over Crunchy Mediterranean Slaw (page 118)
- Pinto Bean and Cheese Enchiladas with Roasted Tomato Salsa (page 122)
- Sicilian Pasta with Swiss Chard, Goat Cheese, and Basil (page 130)

WATER-COOLER FACT: Stay at the water cooler. Drinking water can reduce the symptoms of ulcerative colitis.

Introduction

Stanton, R. A. 2006. Nutrition problems in an obesogenic environment. *Medical Journal of Australia* 184 (2): 76–79.

1. Enhancing Bioavailability: Absorb More of the Good Stuff

Brown, M. J., M. G. Ferruzzi, M. L. Nguyen, D. A. Cooper, A. L. Eldridge, S. J. Schwartz, and W. S. White. 2004. Carotenoid bioavailability is higher from salads ingested with full-fat than with fat-reduced salad dressings as measured with electrochemical detection. *American Journal of Clinical Nutrition* 80 (August): 396–403.

Fish, W. W., and R. D. Davis. 2003. The effects of frozen storage conditions on lycopene stability in watermelon tissue. *Journal of Agricultural and Food Chemistry* 51 (12): 3582–85.

Gibson, R. S., L. Perlas, and C. Hotz. 2006. Improving the bioavailability of nutrients in plant foods at the household level. *Proceedings of the Nutrition Society* 65 (2): 160–68.

Gil, M. I., F. Ferreses, and F.A. Tomás-Barberán. 1999. Effect of postharvest storage and processing on the antioxidant constituents (flavonoids and vitamin C) of fresh-cut spinach. *Journal of Agricultural and Food Chemistry* 47 (6): 2213–17.

Hunt, J. R. 2003. High-bioavailability but not low-bioavailability diets enable substantial control of women's iron absorption in relation to body iron stores, with minimal adaptation within several weeks. *American Journal of Clinical Nutrition* 78 (6): 1168–77.

Manach, C., G. Williamson, and C. Morand. 2005. Bioavailability and bioefficacy of polyphenols in humans. I. Review of 97 bioavailability studies. *American Journal of Clinical Nutrition* 81 (1 Suppl.): 230S–42S.

Ramesh, A., S. A. Walker, D. R. Hood, M. D. Gullien, K. Schneider, and E. H. Weyand. 2004. Bioavailability and risk assessment of orally ingested polycyclic aromatic hydrocarbons. *International Journal of Toxicology* 23 (5): 301–33.

Rosado, J. L., M. Díaz, A. Rosas, I. Griffit, and D. P. García. 2005. Calcium absorption from corn tortilla is relatively high and is dependent upon calcium content and liming in Mexican women. *Journal of Nutrition* 135 (November): 2578–81.

2. Avoiding Anti-Nutrients: Bad Guys in Your Food

Bateman, A. S., S. D. Kelly, and M. Woolfe. 2007. Nitrogen isotope composition of organically and conventionally grown crops. *Journal of Agriculture and Food Chemistry* 55 (7): 2664–70.

Brody, J. G., R. A. Rudel, K. B. Michels, K. B. Moysich, L. Berastein, K. R. Attfield, and S. Gray. 2007. Environmental pollutants, diet, physical activity, body size, and breast cancer: Where do we stand in research to identify opportunities for prevention? *Cancer* 109 (12 Suppl.): 2627–34.

Browning, L. M. 2006. Nutritional influences on inflammation and type 2 diabetes risk. *Diabetes Technology & Therapeutics* 8 (1): 45–54.

Felton, J. S., E. Fultz, F. A. Dolbeare, and M. G. Knize. 1994. Effect of microwave pretreatment on heterocyclic aromatic amine mutagens/carcinogens in fried beef patties. *Food Chemical Toxicology* 32 (10): 897–903.

Hughes-Fulford, M., L. Chai-Fei, J. Boonyaratanakornkit, and S. Sayyah. 2006. Arachidonic acid activates phosphatidylinositol 3-kinase signaling and induces gene expression in prostate cancer. *Cancer Research* 66 (February): 1427–33.

Mantovani, A., F. Maranghi, I. Furificato, and A. Marci. 2006. Assessment of feed additives and contaminants: An essential component of food safety. *Ann 1st Super Sanita* 42 (4): 427–32.

Willett, W. C. 2006. Trans fatty acids and cardiovascular disease-epidemiological data. *Atherosclerosis Supplement* 7 (2): 5–8.

3. The Science of Satiety: Feel Full Faster

Hetherington, M. M. 2007. Cues to overeat: Psychological factors influencing overconsumption. *Proceedings of the Nutrition Society* 66 (1): 113–23.

Kendall, C. W., et al. 2004. Resistant starches and health. *Journal of AOAC International* 87 (3): 769–74.

Leeman, M., E. Östman, and I. Björk. 2005. Vinegar dressing and cold storage of potatoes lowers postprandial glycemic and insulinemic responses in healthy subjects. Diabetes in control. *European Journal of Clinical Nutrition* 59:1266–71.

Mattes, R. D., and D. Rothacker. 2001. Beverage viscosity is inversely related to postprandial hunger in humans. *Physiology and Behavior* 74 (4): 551–57.

Rolls, B., L. Roe, and J. Mecays. 2004. Salad and satiety: Energy density and portion size of a first-course salad affect energy intake at lunch. *Journal of the American Dietetic Association* 104 (10): 1570–76.

Westerterp-Plantenga, M., K. Diepvers, A. Jooson, S. Bérubé-Parat, and A. Tremblay. 2006. Metabolic effects of spices, teas and caffeine. *Physiology & Behavior* 89 (1): 85–91.

4. The Kitchen Physician Prescription: Build Your Medicine Chest

Scarborough, P. 2007. Nutrition professionals' perception of the "healthiness" of individual foods. *Public Health Nutrition* 10 (4): 346–53.

BARLEY

Behall, K. M., D. J. Scholfield, and J. Hallfrisch. 2005. Comparison of hormone and glucose responses of overweight women to barley and oats. *Journal of the American College of Nutrition* 24 (3): 182–88.

McKee, L. H. 2000. Underutilized sources of dietary fiber: A review. *Plant Foods for Human Nutrition* 55 (4): 285–304.

OATS

Bazzano, L. A., J. He, L. G. Ogden, C. M. Loria, and P. K. Whelton. 2003. Dietary fiber intake and reduced risk of coronary heart disease in U.S. men and women: The National Health and Nutrition Examination Survey I Epidemiologic Follow-Up Study. *Archives of Internal Medicine* 163 (16): 1897–904.

Kelly, S. A., C. D. Summerbell, A. Brynes, V. Whittaker, and G. Frost. 2007. Wholegrain cereals for coronary heart disease. *Cochrane Database of Systematic Reviews* (2): CD005051.

BEANS

Agurs-Collins, T., D. Smoot, J. Afful, K. Makambi, and L. L. Adams-Campbell. 2006. Legume intake and reduced colorectal adenoma risk in African-Americans. *Journal of the National Black Nurses Association* 17 (2): 6–12.

Anderson, J. W., and A. W. Major. 2002. Pulses and lipaemia short- and long-term effect: Potential in the prevention of cardiovascular disease. *British Journal of Nutrition* 88 (Suppl 3): S263–71.

LENTILS

Kolonel, L. N., J. H. Hankin, A. S. Whittemore, A. H. Wu, R. P. Gallagher, L. R. Wilkens, E. M. John, et al. 2000. Vegetables fruits legumes and prostate cancer: A multiethnic case-control study. *Cancer Epidemiology Biomarkers & Prevention* 9 (8): 795–804.

Leterme, P. 2002. Recommendations by health organizations for pulse consumption. *British Journal of Nutrition* 88 (Suppl. 3): S239–42.

BROCCOLI

Canene-Adams, K., B. L. Lindshield, S. Wang, E. H. Jeffery, S. K. Clinton, and

J. W. Erdman, Jr. 2007. Combinations of tomato and broccoli enhance antitumor activity in dunning r3327-h prostate adenocarcinomas. *Cancer Research* 67 (2): 836–43.

Felton, J. S., M. G. Knize, L. M. Bennett, M. A. Malfatti, M. E. Colvin, and K. S. Kulp. 2004. Impact of environmental exposures on the mutagenicity/carcinogenicity of heterocyclic amines. *Toxicology* 198 (1–3): 135–45.

Rungapamestry, V., A. J. Duncan, Z. Fuller, and B. Ratcliffe. 2007. Effect of meal composition and cooking duration on the fate of sulforaphane following consumption of broccoli by healthy human subjects. *Proceedings of the Nutrition Society* 66 (1): 69–81.

BRUSSELS SPROUTS

Fowke, J. H., C. Longcope, and J. R. Hebert. 2000. Brassica vegetable consumption shifts estrogen metabolism in healthy postmenopausal women. *Cancer Epidemiology Biomarkers & Prevention* 9: 773–79.

McNaughton, S. A., and G. C. Marks. 2003. Development of a food composition database for the estimation of dietary intakes of glucosinolates, the biologically active constituents of cruciferous vegetables. *British Journal of Nutrition* 90 (3): 687–97.

Murray, S., B. G. Lake, S. Gray, A. J. Edwards, C. Springall, E. A. Bowey, G. Williamson, A. R. Boobis, and N. J. Gooderham. 2001. Effect of cruciferous vegetable consumption on heterocyclic aromatic amine metabolism in man. *Carcinogenesis* 22 (9): 1413–20.

CABBAGE

Fowke, J. H., F. L. Chung, F. Jin, D. Qi, Q. Cai, C. Conaway, J. R. Cheng, X. O. Shu, Y. T. Gao, and W. Zheng. 2003. Urinary isothiocyanate levels, brassica and human breast cancer. *Cancer Research* 63 (14): 3980–86.

Rungapamestry, V., A. J. Duncan, Z. Fuller, and B. Ratcliffe. 2006. Changes in glucosinolate concentrations, myrosinase activity, and production of metabolites of glucosinolates in cabbage (*Brassica oleracea* Var. *capitata*) cooked for different durations. *Journal of Agriculture and Food Chemistry* 54 (20): 7628–34.

KALE

De Azevedo, C. H., and D. B. Rodriguez-Amaya. 2005. Carotenoid composition of kale as influenced by maturity season and minimal processing. *Journal of the Science of Food and Agriculture* 85 (4): 591–97.

Higdon, J. V. 2007. Cruciferous vegetables and human cancer risk: Epidemiologic evidence and mechanistic basis. *Pharmacological Research* 55 (3): 224–36.

ONIONS

Galeone, C., C. Pelucchi, F. Levi, E. Negri, S. Franceschi, R. Talamini, A. Giacosa, and C. La Vecchia. 2006. Onion and garlic use and human cancer. *American Journal of Clinical Nutrition* 84 (5): 1027–32.

ROMAINE

Su, L. J., and L. Arab. 2006. Salad and raw vegetable consumption and nutritional status in the adult US population: Results from the Third National Health and Nutrition Examination Survey. *Journal of the American Dietetic Association* 106 (9): 1394–404.

SOYBEANS AND SOY FOOD

Blair, R. M., E. C. Henley, and A. Tabor. 2006. Soy foods have low glycemic and insulin response indices in normal weight subjects. *Nutrition Journal* 5:35.

V. Jayagopal, P. Albertazzi, E. S. Kilpatrick, E. M. Howarth, P. E. Jennings, D. A. Hepburn, and S. L. Atkin. 2002. Beneficial effects of soy phytoestrogen intake in postmenopausal women with type 2 diabetes. *Diabetes Care* 25: 1709–14.

SWEET POTATOES

Suda, I., F. Ishikawa, M. Hatakeyama, M. Miyawaki, T. Kudo, K. Hirano, A. Ito, O. Yamakawa, and S. Horiuchi. 2007. Intake of purple sweet potato beverage effects on serum hepatic biomarker levels of healthy adult men with borderline hepatitis. *European Journal of Clinical Nutrition* doi:10.1038/sj.ejcn.1602674.

SWISS CHARD

Bolkent, S., R. Yanardag, A. Tabakoglu-Oguz, and O. Ozsoy-Sacan. 2000. Effects of chard (Beta vulgaris L. var. Cicla) extract on pancreatic B cells in streptozotocin-diabetic rats: A morphological and biochemical study. *Journal of Ethnopharmacology* 73 (1–2): 251–59.

Gil, M. A., F. Ferreres, and F. A. Tomas-Barberan. 1998. Effect of modified atmosphere packaging on the flavonoids and vitamin C content of minimally processed swiss chard (*Beta vulgaris* subspecies *cycla*). *Journal of Agriculture and Food Chemistry* 46 (5): 2007–12.

TOMATOES

Ishida, B. K., and M. H. Chapman. 2004. A comparison of carotenoid content and total antioxidant activity in catsup from several commercial sources in the United States. *Journal of Agriculture and Food Chemistry* 52 (26): 8017–20.

Nkondjock, A. P. Ghadirian, K. C. Johnson, and D. Krewski. 2005. Dietary intake of lycopene is associated with reduced pancreatic cancer risk. *Journal of Nutrition* 135 (3): 592–97.

Reboul, E., P. Borel, C. Mikail, L. Abou, M. Charbonnier, C. Caris-Veyrat, P. Goupy, H. Portugal, D. Lairon, and M. J. Amiot. 2005. Enrichment of tomato paste with 6% tomato peel increases lycopene and {beta}-carotene bioavailability in men. *Journal of Nutrition* 135 (4): 790–94.

Sesso, H. D. S. Liu, J. M. Gaziano, and J. E. Buring. 2003. Dietary lycopene tomato-based food products and cardiovascular disease in women. *Journal of Nutrition* 133 (7): 2336–41.

WATERCRESS

Gill, C. I., S. Haldar, L. A. Boyd, R. Bennett, J. Whiteford, M. Butler, J. R. Pearson, I. Bradbury, and I. R. Rowland. 2007. Watercress supplementation in diet reduces lymphocyte DNA damage and alters blood antioxidant status in healthy adults. *American Journal of Clinical Nutrition* 85 (2): 504–10.

Hecht, S. S., F. I. Chung, J. P. Richie Jr., S. A. Akerkar, A. Borukhova, L. Showronski, and S. G. Carmella. 1995. Effects of watercress consumption on metabolism of a tobacco-specific lung carcinogen in smokers. *Cancer Epidemiology Biomarkers & Prevention* 4 (8): 877–84.

AÇAI BERRIES

Del Pozo-Insfran, D., S. S. Percival, and S. T. Talcott. 2006. Açai (Euterpe oleracea Mart.) polyphenolics in their glycoside and aglycone forms induce apoptosis of HL-60 leukemia cells. *Journal of Agriculture and Food Chemistry* 54 (4): 1222–29.

Schauss, A. G., X. Wu, R. L. Prior, R. Ou, D. Huang, J. Owens, A. Agarwal, G. S. Jensen, A. N. Hart, and E. Shanbrom. 2006. Antioxidant capacity and other bioactivities of the freeze-dried Amazonian palm berry Euterpe oleraceae mart. (acai). *Journal of Agriculture and Food Chemistry* 54 (22): 8604–10.

ARTICHOKES

Bundy, R, A. F. Walker, R. W. Middleton, G. Marakis, and J. C. Booth. 2004. Artichoke leaf extract reduces symptoms of irritable bowel syndrome and improves quality of life in otherwise healthy volunteers suffering from concomitant dyspepsia: A subset analysis. *Journal of Alternative and Complementary Medicine* 10 (4): 667–69.

Wang, M., J. E. Simon, I. F. Aviles, K. He, Q. Y. Zheng, and Y. Tadmor. 2003. Analysis of antioxidative phenolic compounds in artichoke (*Cynara scolymus L.*). *Journal of Agriculture and Food Chemistry* 51: 601–8.

AVOCADOS

Lopez Ledesma, R., A. C. Frati Munari, B. C. Hernandez Dominguez, S. Cervantes Montalvo, M. H. Hernandez Luna, C. Juarez, and S. Moran Lira. 1996. Monounsaturated fatty acid (avocado) rich diet for mild hypercholesterolemia. *Archives of Medical Research* 27 (4): 519–23.

Lu, Q. Y., J. R. Arteaga, Q. Zhang, S. Huerta, V. L. Go, and D. Heber. 2005. Inhibition of prostate cancer cell growth by an avocado extract: Role of lipid-soluble bioactive substances. *Journal of Nutritional Biochemistry* 16 (1): 23–30.

BLACKBERRIES

Seeram, N. P., L. S. Adams, Y. Zhang, R. Lee, D. Sand, H. S. Scheuller, and D. Heber. 2006. Blackberry, black raspberry, blueberry, cranberry, red raspberry, and strawberry extracts inhibit growth and stimulate apoptosis of human cancer cells in vitro. *Journal of Agriculture and Food Chemistry* 54 (25): 9329–39.

BLUEBERRIES

Rossi, M., E. Negri, R. Talamini, C. Bosetti, M. Parpinel, P. Gnagnarella, S. Franceschi, et al. 2006. Flavonoids and colorectal cancer in Italy. *Cancer Epidemiology Biomarkers & Prevention* 15 (8): 1555–58.

Seeram, N. P. L. S. Adams, Y. Zhang, R. Lee, D. Sand, H. S. Scheuller, and D. Heber. 2006. Blackberry, black raspberry, blueberry, cranberry, red raspberry, and strawberry extracts inhibit growth and stimulate apoptosis of human cancer cells in vitro. *Journal of Agriculture and Food Chemistry* 54 (25): 9329–39.

LIMES

Kawaii, S., Y. Tomono, E. Katase, K. Ogawa, and M. Yano. 1999. Antiproliferative effects of the readily extractable fractions prepared from various citrus juices on several cancer cell lines. *Journal of Agriculture and Food Chemistry* 47 (7): 2509–12.

Rodrigues, A., A. Sandström, T. Cá, H. Steinsland, H. Jensen, and P. Aaby. 2000. Protection from cholera by adding lime juice to food—results from community and laboratory studies in Guinea-Bissau West Africa. *Tropical Medicine & International Health* 5 (6): 418–22.

Tian, Q., E. G. Miller, H. Ahmad, L. Tang, and B. S. Patil. 2001. Differential inhibition of human cancer cell proliferation by citrus limonoids. *Nutrition and Cancer* 40 (2): 180–84.

OLIVES

Aguilera, C. M., M. C. Ramírez-Tortosa, M. D. Mesa, and A. Gil. 2001. Protective effect of monounsaturated and polyunsaturated fatty acids on the development of cardiovascular disease. *Nutrición hospitalaria* 2001 16 (3): 78–91.

Owen, R. W., R. Haubner, G. Wurtele, W. Hull, B. Spiegelhalder, and H. Bartsch. 2004. Olives and olive oil in cancer prevention. *European Journal of Cancer Prevention* 13 (4): 319–26.

OLIVE OIL

Beauchamp, G. K., R. S. J. Keast, D. Morel, J. Lin, J. Pika, Q. Han, C. H. Lee, A. B. Smith, and P. A. S. Breslin. 2005. Phytochemistry: Ibuprofen-like activity in extra-virgin olive oil. *Nature* 437:45–46.

Bondia-Pons, I., H. Schroder, M. I. Covas, A. I. Castellote, J. Kaikkonen, H. E. Poulsen, A. V. Gaddi, A. Machowetz, H. Kiesewetter, and M. C. Lopez-Sabater. 2007. Moderate consumption of olive oil by healthy European men reduces systolic blood pressure in non-Mediterranean participants. *Journal of Nutrition* 137 (1): 84–87.

POMEGRANATE

Aviram, M., M. Rosenblat, D. Gaitini, S. Nitecki, A. Hoffman, L. Dornfeld, and N. Volkova et al. 2004. Pomegranate juice consumption for 3 years by patients with carotid artery stenosis reduces common carotid intima-media thickness blood pressure and LDL oxidation. *Clinical Nutrition* 23 (3): 423–33.

Esmaillzadeh, A., F. Tahbaz, I. Gaieni, H. Alavi-Majd, and L. Azadbakht. 2004. Concentrated pomegranate juice improves lipid profiles in diabetic patients with hyperlipidemia. *Journal of Medicinal Food* 7 (3): 305–8.

CHEESE, LOWER FAT

Cornish, J. K., E. Callon, D. Naot, K. P. Palmano, T. Banovic, U. Bava, M. Watson, et al. 2004. Lactoferrin is a potent regulator of bone cell activity and increases bone formation in vivo. *Endocrinology* 145 (9): 4366–74.

Liu, S., Y. Song, E. S. Ford, J. E. Manson, J. E. Buring, and P. M. Ridker. 2005. Dietary calcium vitamin D and the prevalence of metabolic syndrome in middle-aged and older U.S. women. *Diabetes Care* 28:2926–32.

KEFIR

Lopitz-Otsoa, F., A. Rementeria, N. Elgnezabal, and J. Garaizar, 2006. Kefir: A symbiotic yeasts-bacteria community with alleged healthy capabilities. *Rievista Iberoamericana de Micología* 23 (2): 67–74.

Othman, M., J. P. Neilson, and Z. Alfirevic. 2007. Probiotics for preventing preterm labour. *Cochrane Database of Systematic Reviews* (1):CD005941.

PARMIGIANO-REGGIANO

Chavarro, J. E., Rich-Edwards, J. W. B. Rosner, and W. C. Willett. 2007. A prospective study of dairy foods intake and anovulatory infertility. *Human Reproduction* 22 (5): 1340–47.

Larsson, S., C. L. Bergkvist, and A. Wolk. 2005. High fat dairy food and conjugated linoleic acid intakes in relation to colorectal cancer incidence in the Swedish Mammography Cohort. *American Journal of Clinical Nutrition* 82 (4): 894–900.

YOGURT

Guarner, F., G. Perdigon, G. Corthier, S. Salminen, B. Koletzko, and L. Morelli. 2005. Should yoghurt cultures be considered probiotic? *British Journal of Nutrition* 93 (6): 783–86.

Manley, K. J., M. B. Fraenkel, B. C. Mayall, and D. A. Power. 2007. Probiotic treatment of vancomycin-resistant enterococci: a randomised controlled trial. *Medical Journal of Australia* 186 (9): 454–57.

Parvez, S., K. A. Malik, S. Ah Kang, and H. Kim. 2006. Probiotics and their fermented food products are beneficial for health. *Journal of Applied Microbiology* 100 (6): 1171–85.

ALMONDS

Hyson, D. A., B. O. Schneeman, and P. A. Davis. 2002. Almonds and almond oil have similar effects on plasma lipids and LDL oxidation in healthy men and women. *Journal of Nutrition* 132:703–7.

Tsai, C. J., M. F. Leitzmann, F. B. Hu, W. C. Willett, and E. L. Giovannucci. 2004.

A prospective cohort study of nut consumption and the risk of gallstone disease in men. *American Journal of Epidemiology* 160 (10): 961–68.

PECANS

Mukuddem-Petersen, J. 2005. A systematic review of the effects of nuts on blood lipid profiles in humans. *Journal of Nutrition* 135 (9): 2082–89.

Rajaram, S., K. Burke, B. Connell, T. Myint, and J. Sabate. 2001. A monounsaturated fatty acid–rich pecan-enriched diet favorably alters the serum lipid profile of healthy men and women. *Journal of Nutrition* 131 (9): 2275–79.

WALNUTS

Cortes, B., I. Nunez, M. Cofan, R. Gilabert, A. Perez-Heras, E. Casals, R. Deulofeu, and E. Ros. 2006. Acute effects of high-fat meals enriched with walnuts or olive oil on postprandial endothelial function. *Journal of American College of Cardiology* 48 (8): 1666–71.

Marangoni, F., C. Colombo, A. Martiello, A. Poli, R. Paoletti, and C. Galli. 2007. Levels of the n-3 fatty acid eicosapentaenoic acid in addition to those of alpha linolenic acid are significantly raised in blood lipids by the intake of four walnuts a day in humans. *Nutrition Metabolism and Cardiovascular Disease* 17 (6): 457–61.

CHILIES

Lejeune, M. P., E. M. Kovacs, and M. S. Westerterp-Plantenga. 2003. Effect of capsaicin on substrate oxidation and weight maintenance after modest body-weight loss in human subjects. *British Journal of Nutrition* 90 (3): 651–59.

Yoshioka, M., S. St.-Pierre, M. Suzuki, and A. Tremblay. 1998. Effects of red pepper added to high-fat and high-carbohydrate meals on energy metabolism and substrate utilization in Japanese women. *British Journal of Nutrition* 80 (6): 503–10.

CHOCOLATE

Engler, M. B. 2006. The emerging role of flavonoid-rich cocoa and chocolate in cardiovascular health and disease. *Nutrition Reviews* 64 (3): 109–18.

Taubert, D. 2007. Effect of cocoa and tea intake on blood pressure: A meta-analysis. *Archives of Internal Medicine* 167 (7): 626–34.

CINNAMON

Pham, A. Q. 2007. Cinnamon supplementation in patients with type 2 diabetes mellitus. *Pharmacotherapy* 27 (4): 595–99.

CLOVES

Khan, A., S. Qadir, K. Kattak, and R. A. Anderson. 2006. Cloves improve glucose cholesterol and triglycerides of people with type 2 diabetes mellitus [abstract]. *Journal of Federation of American Societies Experimental Biology* 20(5): A990#6405.

Shan, B., Y. Z. Cai, M. Sun, and H. Corke. 2005. Antioxidant capacity of 26 spice extracts and characterization of their phenolic constituents. *Journal of Agriculture and Food Chemistry* 53 (20): 7749–59.

CURRY POWDER AND TURMERIC

Ng, T. P., P. C. Chiam, T. Lee, H. C. Chua, L. Lim, and E. H. Kua. 2006. Curry consumption and cognitive function in the elderly. *American Journal of Epidemiology* 164 (9): 898–906.

Soni, K. B., and R. Kuttan. 1992. Effect of oral curcumin administration on serum peroxides and cholesterol levels in human volunteers. *Indian Journal of Physiology and Pharmacology* 36 (4): 273–75.

GARLIC

Lee, Y. L., T. Cesario, Y. Wang, E. Shanbrom, and L. Thrupp. 2003. Antibacterial activity of vegetables and juices. *Nutrition* 19 (11–12): 994–96.

Song, K., and J. A. Milner. 2001. The influence of heating on the anticancer properties of garlic. *Journal of Nutrition* 131:1054S–57S.

GINGER

Borrelli, F., R. Capasso, G. Aviello, M. H. Pittler, and A. A. Izzo. 2005. Effectiveness and safety of ginger in the treatment of pregnancy-induced nausea and vomiting. *Obstetrics & Gynecology* 105 (4): 849–56.

Wigler, I., I. Grotto, D. Caspi, and M. Yaron. 2003. The effects of Zintona EC (a ginger extract) on symptomatic gonarthritis. *Osteoarthritis Cartilage* 11 (11): 783–89.

HONEY

Molan, P. C. 2001. Potential of honey in the treatment of wounds and burns. *American Journal of Clinical Dermatology* 2 (1): 13–19.

Taormina, P. J., B. A. Niemira, and L. R. Beuchat. 2001. Inhibitory activity of honey against foodborne pathogens as influenced by the presence of hydrogen peroxide and level of antioxidant power. *International Journal of Food Microbiology* 69 (3): 217–25.

OREGANO

Lambert, R. J., P. N. Skandamis, P. J. Coote, and G. J. Nychas. 2001. A study of the minimum inhibitory concentration and mode of action of oregano essential oil thymol and carvacrol. *Journal of Applied Microbiology* 91 (3): 453–62.

Zheng, W., and S. Y. Wang. 2001. Antioxidant activity and phenolic compounds in selected herbs. *Journal of Agriculture and Food Chemistry* 49 (11): 5165–70.

ROSEMARY

Tapsell, L. C. I. Hemphill, L. Cobiac, D. R. Sullivan, M. Fenech, C. S. Patch, S. Rooderys, et al. 2006. Health benefits of herbs and spices: The past, the present, the future. *Medical Journal of Australia* 185 (Suppl. 4): S4–24.

Tsen, S. Y., F. Ameri, and J. S. Smith. 2006. Effects of rosemary extracts on the reduction of heterocyclic amines in beef patties. *Journal of Food Science* 71 (8): C469–73.

BEEF

Bray, G. A., M. Most, J. Rood, S. Redmann, and S. R. Smith. 2007. Hormonal responses to a fast-food meal compared with nutritionally comparable meals of different composition. *Annals of Nutrition and Metabolism* 51 (2): 163–71.

Wells, A. M., M. D. Haub, J. Fluckey, D. K. Williams, R. Chernoff, and W. W. Campbell. 2003. Comparisons of vegetarian and beef-containing diets on hematological indexes and iron stores during a period of resistive training in older men. *Journal of the American Diatetic Association* 103 (5): 594–601.

BISON OR BUFFALO

Marchello, M. J., W. D. Slanger, M. Hadley, D. B. Milne, J. A. Driskell. 1998. Nutrient composition of bison fed concentrate diets. *Journal of Food Composition and Analysis* 11 (3): 231–39.

SALMON

Morris, M. C., D. A. Evans, J. L. Bienias, C. C. Tangney, D. A. Bennett, R. S. Wilson, N. Aggarwal, J. Schneider. 2003. Consumption of fish and n-3 fatty acids and risk of incident Alzheimer disease. *Archives of Neurology* 60 (7): 940–46.

Mozaffarian, D., and E. B. Rimm. 2006. Fish intake, contaminants, and human health: Evaluating the risks and the benefits. *Journal of the American Medical Association* 296 (15): 1885–99.

SARDINES

Patin, R. V., M. R. Vítolo, M. A. Valverde, P. O. Carvalho, G. M. Pastore, and F. A. Lopez. 2006. The influence of sardine consumption on the omega-3 fatty acid content of mature human milk. *Journal of Pediatrics* 82 (1): 63–69.

Sanchez-Muniz, F. J., M. C. Garcia-Linares, M. T. Garcia-Arias, Bastida, S., and J. Viejo. 2003. Fat and protein from olive oil-fried sardines interact to normalize serum lipoproteins and reduce liver lipids in hypercholesterolemic rats. *Journal of Nutrition* 133:2302–8.

TURKEY

Baggio, S. R., E. Vicente, and N. Bragagnolo. 2002. Cholesterol oxides, cholesterol, total lipid and fatty acid composition in turkey meat. *Journal of Agriculture and Food Chemistry* 50 (21): 5981–86.

Yan, H. J., E. J. Lee, K. C. Nam, B. R. Min, and D. U. Ahn. 2006. Effects of dietary functional ingredients and packaging methods on sensory characteristics and consumer acceptance of irradiated turkey breast meat. *Poultry Science* 85 (8): 482–89.

COFFEE

Ascherio, A., S. M. Zhang, M. A. Hernán, I. Kawachi, G. A. Colditz, F. E. Speizer, and W. C. Willett. 2001. Prospective study of caffeine consumption and risk of Parkinson's disease in men and women. *Annals of Neurology* 50 (1): 56–63.

Higdon, J. V., and B. Frei. 2006. Coffee and health: A review of recent human research. *Critical Reviews in Food Science and Nutrition* 46 (2): 101–23.

TEA

Geleijnse, J. M., L. J. Launer, D. A. Van der Kuip, A. Hofman, and J. C. Witteman. 2002. Inverse association of tea and flavonoid intakes with incident myocardial infarction: The Rotterdam Study. *American Journal of Clinical Nutrition* 75 (5): 880–86.

Peters, U., C. Poole, and L. Arab. 2001. Does tea affect cardiovascular disease? A meta-analysis. *American Journal of Epidemiology* 154 (6): 495–503.

VEGETABLE JUICE

Dai, Q., A. R. Borenstein, Y. Wu, J. C. Jackson, and E. B. Larson. 2006. Fruit and vegetable juices and Alzheimer's disease: The Kame Project. *American Journal of Medicine* 119 (9): 751–59.

Watzl, B., A. Bub, K. Briviba, and G. Rechkemmer. 2003. Supplementation of a low-carotenoid diet with tomato or carrot juice modulates immune functions in healthy men. *Annals of Nutrition and Metabolism* 47 (6): 255–61.

WINE

Aggarwal, B. B., A. Bhardwaj, R. S. Aggarwal, N. P. Seeram, S. Shishodia, and Y. Takada. 2004. Role of resveratrol in prevention and therapy of cancer: Preclinical and clinical studies. *Anticancer Research* 24 (5A): 2783–840.

Carollo, C., R. Lo Presti, and G. Caimi. 2007. Wine, diet, and arterial hypertension. *Angiology* 58 (1): 92–96.

6. The Eight-Week Program for Optimal Health: Eat, Drink, and Be Healthier

Heber, D. 2004. Vegetables, fruits and phytoestrogens in the prevention of diseases. *Journal of Postgraduate Medicine* 50 (2): 145–49.

La Puma, J. 1996. Help your patients eat their way to health. *Managed Care*, S(6): 46–52.

Murphy, S. P., K. K. White, S. Park, and S. Sharma. 2007. Multivitamin-multimineral supplements' effect on total nutrient intake. *American Journal of Clinical Nutrition* 85 (1): 280S–84S.

Ogilvie, C. E. Foster, H. Rothnnie, N. Cavill, V. Hamilton, C. F. Fitzsimons, and N. Mutrie. 2007. Interventions to promote walking: systematic review. *British Medical Journal* 334 (7605): 1204.

Wansink, B. 2004. Environmental factors that increase the food intake and consumption volume of unknowing consumers. *Annual Review of Nutrition* 24:455–79.

Wansink, B., and M. Huckabee. 2005. De-marketing obesity. *California Management Review* 47 (4): 6–18.

7. What Do You Eat for That?

ACNE

Danby, F. W. 2005. Acne and milk, the diet myth, and beyond. *Journal of the American Academy of Dermatology* 52 (2): 360–62.

Liao, S. 2001. The medicinal action of androgens and green tea epigallocatechin gallate. *Hong Kong Medical Journal* 7 (4): 369–74.

ALLERGY

Enomoto, T., K. Xiao, and S. Shimazu. 2006. Suppression of allergy development by habitual intake of fermented milk foods, evidence from an epidemiological study. *Arerugi* 55 (11): 1394–99.

Nagel, G., A. Nieters, N. Becker, and J. Linseisen. 2003. The influence of the dietary intake of fatty acids and antioxidants on hay fever in adults. *Allergy* 58 (12): 1277–84.

ALZHEIMER'S

Durga, J., M. P. J. van Boxtel, and E. G. Shouten. 2007. Effect of 3-year folic acid supplementation on cognitive function in older adults in the FACIT trial: A randomized, double blind, controlled trial. *Lancet* 369 (9557): 208–16.

Morris, M. C., A. Evans, C. C. Tangney, J. L. Bienias, and R. S. Wilson. 2006. Associations of vegetable and fruit consumption with age-related cognitive change. *Neurology* 67 (8): 1370–76.

ANEMIA

Pynaert, I. 2007. Iron intake in relation to diet and iron status of young adult women. *Annals of Nutrition and Metabolism* 51 (2): 172–81.

Shi, Z., X. Hu, B. Yuan, X. Pan, et al. 2006. Association between dietary patterns and anaemia in adults from Jiangsu Province in Eastern China. *British Journal of Nutrition* 96 (5): 906–12.

ASTHMA

Chatzi, L., G. Apostolaki, I. Bibakis, I. Skypala, V. Bibaki-Liakou, N. Tzanakis, M. Kogevinas, and P. Cullinan. 2007. Protective effect of fruits, vegetables and the Mediterranean diet on asthma and allergies among children in Crete. *Thorax* 62:677–83.

Seif, O., J. Sterne, R. L. Thompson, C. E. Songhurst, B. M. Margetts, and P. Burney. 2001. Dietary antioxidants and asthma in adults. *American Journal of Respiratory and Critical Care Medicine* 164: 1823–28.

ATTENTION DEFICIT HYPERACTIVITY DISORDER

Itomura, M., K. Hamazaki, S. Sawazaki, M. Kobayashi, K. Terasawa, S. Watanabe, and T. Hanazaki. 2005. The effect of fish oil on physical aggression in schoolchildren—A randomized, double-blind, placebo-controlled trial. *Journal of Nutritional Biochemistry* 16 (3): 163–71.

Schab, D. W., and N. H. Trihn. 2004. Do artificial food colors promote hyperactivity in children with hyperactive syndromes? A meta-analysis of double-blind placebo-controlled trials. *Journal of Development and Behavioral Pediatrics* 25 (6): 423–34.

BENIGN BREAST DISEASE

Webb, P. M., C. Byrne, S. J. Schnitt, J. L. Connolly, T. W. Jacobs, H. J. Baer, W. C. Willett, and G. A. Colditz. 2004. A prospective study of diet and benign breast disease. *Cancer Epidemiology Biomarkers & Prevention* 13: 1106–13.

Galvan-Portillo, M. L. Torres-Sanchez, and L. Lopez-Carrillo. 2002. Dietary and reproductive factors associated with benign breast disease in Mexican women. *Nutrition and Cancer—An International Journal* 43 (2): 133–40.

BENIGN PROSTATIC HYPERPLASIA

Bravi, F., C. Bosetti, L. Dal Maso, R. Talamini, M. Montella, and E. Negri. 2006. Food groups and risk of benign prostatic hyperplasia. *Urology* 67 (1): 73–79.

Rorhmann, S E. Giovannucci, and W. Willett. 2007. Fruit and vegetable consumption, intake of micronutrients, and benign prostatic hyperplasia in US men. *American Journal of Clinical Nutrition* 85 (2): 523–29.

BREAST CANCER

Ambrosone, C. B., S. E. McCann, J. L. Freudenheim, J. R. Marshall, Y. Zhang, and P. G. Shields. 2004. Breast cancer risk in premenopausal women is inversely associated with consumption of broccoli, a source of isothiocyanates, but is not modified by GST genotype. *Journal of Nutrition* 134:1134–38.

Thiébaut, A. C., V. Kipnis, S. C. Chang, A. F. Subar, F. E. Thompson, P. S. Rosenberg, A. R. Hollaback, M. Leitzmann, and A. Schatzkin. 2007. Dietary fat and postmenopausal invasive breast cancer in the National Institutes of Health-AARP Diet and Health Study cohort. *Journal of the National Cancer Institute*, 99 (6): 451–62.

BRONCHITIS, CHRONIC

Celik, F., 2006. Nutritional risk factors for the development of chronic obstructive pulmonary disease (COPD) in male smokers. *Clinical Nutrition* 25 (6): 955–61.

Varraso, R., T. T. Fung, F. B. Hu, W. Willett, and C. A. Camargo. 2007. Prospective study of dietary patterns and chronic obstructive pulmonary disease among US men. *Thorax* 15.doi:10.1136/thx.2006.074534

CATARACTS

Brown, L. 1999. A prospective study of carotenoid intake and risk of cataract extraction in US men. *American Journal of Clinical Nutrition* 70 (4): 517–24.

Lu, M., E. Cho, A. Taylor, S. Harkinson, W. Willett, and P. F. Jacques. 2005. Prospective study of dietary fat and risk of cataract extraction among US women. *American Journal of Epidemiology* 161 (10): 948–59.

CELIAC DISEASE

Catassi, C., E. Fabiani, G. Iacono, C. D'Agate, R. Francavilla, F. Biaga, V. Volta, et al. 2007. A prospective, double-blind, placebo-controlled trial to establish a safe gluten threshold for patients with celiac disease. *American Journal of Clinical Nutrition* 85 (1): 160–66.

Dahele, A., and S. Ghosh. 2001. Vitamin B12 deficiency in untreated celiac disease. *American Journal of Gastroenterology* 96 (3): 745–50.

COMMON COLD

Rennard, B. O., R. F. Ertl, G. L. Gossman, R. A. Robbins, and S. I. Rennard. 2000. Chicken soup inhibits neutrophil chemotaxis in vitro. *Chest* 118 (4): 1150–57.

Takkouche, B., C. Reguira-Méndez, R. Garciá-Closas, A. Figneiras, J. J. Gestal-Otero, and M. A. Hernáq. 2002. Intake of wine, beer, and spirits and the risk of clinical common cold. *American Journal of Epidemiology* 155 (9): 853–88.

CONSTIPATION

Kim, T. I., S. J. Park, C. H. Choi, S. K. Lee, and W. H. Kim. 2004. Effect of ear mushroom (auricularia) on functional constipation. *Korean Journal of Gastroenterology* 44 (1): 34–41.

Koebnick, C., I. Wagner, P. Leitzmann, V. Stern, and H. J. Zunft. 2003. Probiotic beverage containing *Lactobacillus casei Shirota* improves gastrointestinal symptoms in patients with chronic constipation. *Canadian Journal of Gastroenterology* 17 (11): 655–59.

DEPRESSION

Lin, P. Y., and K Su. 2007. A meta-analytic review of double-blind, placebo-controlled trials of antidepressant efficacy of omega-3 fatty acids. *Journal of Clinical Psychiatry* 68 (7): 1056–61.

Strandberg, T. E., A. Y. Strandberg, K. Pitkälä, V. V. Salomaa, R. S. Tilvis, and T. A. Miettinen. 2007. Chocolate, well-being and health among elderly men. *European Journal of Clinical Nutrition* (February 28) doi:10.1038/sj.ejcn.1602707.

DIABETES

Frati, A. C. B. E. Gordillo, and P. Altamirano. 1991. Influence of nopal intake upon fasting glycemia in type II diabetics and healthy subjects. *Archivos de investigación médica* 22:51–56.

Montonen, J., R. Järvinen, P. Knekt, M. Heliövagra, and A. Reunanen. 2007.

Consumption of sweetened beverages and intakes of fructose and glucose predict type 2 diabetes occurrence. *Journal of Nutrition* 136 (6): 1447–54.

DIARRHEA

Pashapour, N., and S. Golmahammad. 2006. Evaluation of yogurt effect on acute diarrhea in 6–24-month-old hospitalized infants. *Turkish Journal of Pediatrics* 48 (2): 115–18.

Rabbani, G. H., T. Teka, B. Zaman, N. Majid, M. Khatun, and G. J. Fuchs. 2001. Clinical studies in persistent diarrhea: dietary management with green banana or pectin in Bangladeshi children. *Gastroenterology* 121 (3): 554–60.

DIVERTICULITIS

Alddori, W. 2002. Preventing diverticular disease. Review of recent evidence on high-fibre diets. *Canadian Family Physician* 48:1632–37.

White, J. A. 2006. Probiotics and their use in diverticulitis. *Journal of Clinical Gastroenterology* 40 (7 Suppl. 3): S160–62.

GALL BLADDER DISEASE

Tsai, C. J., M. F. Leitzmann, W. C. Willett, and E. L. Giovannucci. 2006. Fruit and vegetable consumption and risk of cholecystectomy in women. *American Journal of Medicine* 119:760–67.

Zhang, X. H., G. Andreotti, Y. T. Gao, J. Derg, E. Lin, A. Rashid, K. Wu, et al. 2006. Tea drinking and the risk of biliary tract cancers and biliary stones: a population-based case-control study in Shanghai, China. *International Journal of Cancer* 118 (12): 3089–94.

GOUT

Choi, H. K., K. Atkinson, E. Karlson, W. Willett, and G. Curham. 2004. Purine-rich foods, dairy and protein intake, and the risk of gout in men. *New England Journal of Medicine* 350 (110): 1093–1103.

Choi, H. K., and G. Curhan. 2004. Beer, liquor, and wine consumption and serum uric acid level: The Third National Health and Nutrition Examination Survey. *Arthritis Care & Research* 51 (6): 1023–29.

HAIR, SKIN, AND NAIL PROBLEMS

Black, H. S. and L. E. Rhodes. 2006. The potential of omega-3 fatty acids in the prevention of non-melanoma skin cancer. *Journal of Nutrition* 136 (6): 1565–69.

Heinrich, U., K. Nenkam, H. Tronnier, H. Sies, and W. Stahl. 2006. Long-term ingestion of high flavanol cocoa provides photoprotection against UV-induced erythema and improves skin condition in women. *Journal of Nutrition* 136 (6): 1565–69.

HEART DISEASE

Halton, T. L., W. Willett, S. Lin, J. Manson, C. Albert, K. Rexrode, and F. Hu.

2006. Low-carbohydrate-diet score and the risk of coronary heart disease in women. *New England Journal of Medicine* 355 (19): 1991–2002.

Kontogianni, M. D., D. B. Panagiotakos, C. Chrysohoon, C. Pitsavos, A. Zampelas, and C. Stefanadis. 2007. The impact of olive oil consumption pattern on the risk of acute coronary syndromes: The CARDIO2000 case-control study. *Clinical Cardiology* 30 (3): 125–29.

HEARTBURN

Austin, G. L., 2006. A very low-carbohydrate diet improves gastroesophageal reflux and its symptoms. *Digestive Diseases and Sciences* 51 (8): 1307–12.

Hamoui, N., R. V. Lord, J. A. Hagen, J. Theisen, T. R. de Meester, and P. F. Crookes. 2006. Response of the lower esophageal sphincter to gastric distention by carbonated beverages. *Journal of Gastrointestinal Surgery* 10 (6): 870–77.

HIGH CHOLESTEROL

Chisholm, A., K. Mc Anley, J. Mann, S. Williams, and M. Skeaff. 2005. Cholesterol lowering effects of nuts compared with a canola oil enriched cereal of similar fat composition. *Nutrition, Metabolism and Cardiovascular Disease* 15 (4): 284–92.

Ellegard, L. H., S. W. Andersson, A. J. Normen, and H. A. Andersson. 2007. Dietary plant sterols and cholesterol metabolism. *Nutrition Review* 65 (1): 39–45.

HIGH TRIGLYCERIDES

Deck, C., and K. Radack. 1989. Effects of modest doses of omega-3 fatty acids on lipids and lipoproteins in hypertriglyceridemic subjects. A randomized controlled trial. *Archives of Internal Medicine* 149 (8): 1857–62.

Gorinstein, S., A. Caspi, J. Libman, H. T. Lerner, D. Huang, H. Leontowicz, M. Leontowicz, et al. 2006. Red grapefruit positively influences serum triglyceride level in patients suffering from coronary atherosclerosis: Studies in vitro and in humans. *Journal of Agriculture and Food Medicine* 54 (5): 1887–92.

HYPERTENSION

Panagiotakos, D. B. 2007. Adherence to the Mediterranean food pattern predicts the prevalence of hypertension, hypercholesterolemia, diabetes and obesity, among healthy adults; the accuracy of the MedDietScore. *Preventative Medicine* 44 (4): 335–40.

Takahashi, Y. 2006. Blood pressure change in a free-living population-based dietary modification study in Japan. *Journal of Hypertension* 24 (3): 451–58.

INSOMNIA

Afaghi, A., H. O'Connor, and C. M. Chow. 2007. High-glycemic-index carbohydrate meals shorten sleep onset. *American Journal of Clinical Nutrition* 85:426–30.

Harada, T., M. Hirotani, M. Maeda, H. Nomura, and H. Takeuchi. 2007. Correlation between breakfast tryptophan content and morning-evening in Japanese infants and students aged 0–15 yrs. *Journal of Physiological Anthropology* 26 (2): 201–7.

IRRITABLE BOWEL SYNDROME

Parisi, G. C., M. Zilli, M. P. Miani, M. Carrara, E. Bottona, G. Verdianelli, G. Battaglia, et al. 2002. High-fiber diet supplementation in patients with irritable bowel syndrome (IBS): A multicenter, randomized, open trial comparison between wheat bran diet and partially hydrolyzed guar gum (PHGG). *Digestive Diseases and Sciences* 47 (8): 1697–1704.

Uz, E., C. Turkay, S. Avtac, and N. Bavbek. 2007. Risk factors for irritable bowel syndrome in Turkish population: Role of food allergy. *Journal of Clinical Gastroenterology* 41 (4): 380–83.

KIDNEY STONES

Curhan, G. C., W. C. Willett, F. E. Speizer, and M. J. Stampfer et al. 1998. Beverage use and risk for kidney stones in women. *Annals of Internal Medicine* 128 (7): 534–40.

McHarg, T., A. Rodgers, and K. Charlton. 2003. Influence of cranberry juice on the urinary risk factors for calcium oxalate kidney stone formation. *BJU International* 92 (7): 765–68.

MACULAR DEGENERATION

Seddon, J. M., J. Cote, and B. Rosner. 2003. Progression of age-related macular degeneration: Association with dietary fat, transunsaturated fat, nuts, and fish intake. *Archives of Ophthalmology* 121 (12): 1728–37.

Van Leeuwen, R., S. Boekhoorn, J. R. Vingerling, J. C. Witteman, C. C. W. Klaver, A. Hofman, and P. T. V. M. de Jong. 2005. Dietary intake of antioxidants and risk of age-related macular degeneration. *Journal of the American Medical Association* 294 (24): 3101–7.

MALE INFERTILITY

Dickman, M. D., C. K. M. Leung, and M. K. H. Leung. 1998. Hong Kong male subfertility links to mercury in human hair and fish. *Science of the Total Environment* 214 (1–3): 165–74.

Eskenazi, B., S. A. Kidd, A. R. Marks, E. Sloter, G. Block, and A. J. Wyrobek. 2005. Antioxidant intake is associated with semen quality in healthy men. *Human Reproduction* 20 (4): 1006–12.

METABOLIC SYNDROME

Elwood, P. C., J. E. Pickering, and A. M. Fehily. 2007. Milk and dairy consumption, diabetes and the metabolic syndrome: The Caerphilly prospective study. *Journal of Epidemiology and Community Health* 61:695–98.

Panagiotakos, D. B., C. Pitsavos, Y. Skoumas, and C. Stefanadis. 2007. The association between food patterns and the metabolic syndrome using principal components analysis: The ATTICA Study. *Journal of the American Dietetic Association* 107 (6): 979–87.

MIGRAINE

Kelman, L. 2007. The triggers or precipitants of the acute migraine attack. *Cephalagia* 27 (5): 394–402.

Kohlenberg, R. J. 1982. Tyramine sensitivity in dietary migraine: A critical review. *Headache* 22 (1): 30–34.

MULTIPLE SCLEROSIS

Munger, K. L., L. I. Levin, B. W. Hollis, N. S. Howard, and A. Ascherio. 2006. Serum 25-hydroxyvitamin D levels and risk of multiple sclerosis. *Journal of the American Medical Association* 296:2832–38.

Weinstock-Guttman, B., M. Baier, Y. Park, J. Feichter, P. Lee-Kwen, E. Gallagher, J. Venkatraman, et al. 2005. Low fat dietary intervention with omega-3 fatty acid supplementation in multiple sclerosis patients. *Prostaglandins, Leukotrienes and Essential Fatty Acids* 73 (5): 397–404.

OBESITY

Gardner, C. D., A. Kiazand, S. Alhassan, S. Kim, R. S. Stafford, R. R. Balise, H. C. Kraemer, and A. C. King. 2007. Comparison of the Atkins, Zone, Ornish, and LEARN diets for change in weight and related risk factors among overweight premenopausal women: The A to Z Weight Loss Study: A randomized trial. *Journal of the American Medical Association* 297:969–77.

Kinsell, L. W., B. Cunnino, C. O. Michaels, S. E. Cox, and C. Lemon. 1964. Calories do count. *Metabolism* 13:195.

OSTEOARTHRITIS

Hailu, A., S. F. Knutsen, and G. E. Fraser. 2006. Associations between meat consumption and the prevalence of degenerative arthritis and soft tissue disorders in the Adventist Health Study. *Journal of Nutrition, Health & Aging* 10 (1): 7–14.

Kagar, C., et al. 2004. The association of milk consumption with the occurrence of symptomatic knee osteoarthritis. *Clinical and Experimental Rheumatology* 22 (4): 473–76.

PEPTIC ULCER DISEASE

Kang, J. Y., K. G. Yeoh, H. P. Chia, H. P. Lee, Y. W. Chia, R. Guan, and I. Yap. 1995. Chili—Protective factor against peptic ulcer? *Digestive Diseases and Sciences* 40 (3): 576–79.

Misciagna, A. M. Cisternino, and J. Freudenheim. 2000. Diet and duodenal ulcer. *Digestive and Liver Disease* 32 (6): 468–72.

PROSTATE CANCER

Giovannucci, E., E. B. Rimm, Y. Lin, M. J. Stampfer, W. C. Willett. 2002. A prospective study of tomato products, lycopene, and prostate cancer risk. *Journal of the National Cancer Institute* 94 (5): 391–98.

Kurahashi, N., M. Iwasaki, S. Sasazuki, T. Otani, and M. Inoune. 2007. Soy product and isoflavone consumption in relation to prostate cancer in Japanese men. *Cancer Epidemiology Biomarkers & Prevention* 16:538–45.

RHEUMATOID ARTHRITIS

Adam, O., C. Beringer, T. Kless, C. Lenmen, A. Adam, M. Wisenan, P. Adam, R. Klimmek, and W. Forth. 2003. Anti-inflammatory effects of a low arachidonic acid diet and fish oil in patients with rheumatoid arthritis. *Rheumatology International* 23 (1): 27–36.

Linos, A., V. G. Kaklamani, E. Kaklamani, Y. Koumantaki, E. Giziaki, S. Papazoglou, and C. S. Mantzoros. 1999. Dietary factors in relation to rheumatoid arthritis: A role for olive oil and cooked vegetables? *American Journal of Clinical Nutrition* 70 (6): 1077–82.

ULCERATIVE COLITIS

Holt, P. R., S. Katz, and R. Kirshoff. 2005. Curcumin therapy in inflammatory bowel disease: A pilot study. *Digestive Diseases and Sciences* 50 (11): 2191–93.

Shah, S. 2007. Dietary factors in the modulation of inflammatory bowel disease activity. *MedGenMed* 9 (1): 60.

avocados (*cont.*)
  Warm Beef Tenderloin Salad with
    Mango and Avocado, 133

B
bacteria, in food, 22–23
bananas
  Açai Berry and Banana Dessert
    Soup, 139
  resistant starch in, 42
  Walnut-Scented Dessert Pancakes
    with Bananas and Agave
    Nectar, 145
barbecue sauce, buying, 89–90
barley
  about, 53
  Butternut Barley Risotto with
    Goat Cheese and Toasted
    Almonds, 111–12
  buying, 89
  health benefits, 53–54
beans
  about, 55
  canned, buying, 90
  health benefits, 55
  Pasta e Fagioli (Pasta and Bean)
    Soup, 102–3
  Pinto Bean and Cheese
    Enchiladas with Roasted
    Tomato Salsa, 122–23
  resistant starch in, 42
  in Rosemary Grilled Chicken and
    Summer Vegetables, 127–28
  Saffron Scallop, Shrimp, and
    Chickpea Paella, 128–29
  Shrimp and Egg Burritos with
    White Beans and Corn, 106
  soaking, 55
  soybeans, 59–60
  Spicy and Rich Sausage and
    Kidney Bean Chili, 107
  storing, 84
  in Teriyaki Tofu, Vegetables, and
    Buckwheat Noodles, 108
  Toasted Walnut and Creamy
    White Bean Pitas, 109
beef
  buying, 22
  corn-fed, 22

dietary fats in, 22
  grass-fed, 22, 78–79
  health benefits, 78–79
  Healthy Real Hamburgers, 119–20
  storing, 85
  Warm Beef Tenderloin Salad with
    Mango and Avocado, 133
bell peppers
  carotenoids in, 10
  organic, buying, 11
  Roasted Red Pepper, Wine, and
    Red Lentil Soup, 105
  in Spicy Gazpacho with Crab,
    137
  in Teriyaki Tofu, Vegetables, and
    Buckwheat Noodles, 108
benign breast disease (BBD), 197–98
benign prostatic hyperplasia,
    198–200
berries. *See also specific berries*
  Cedar-Planked Roasted Salmon
    with Candied Ginger and Berry
    Salsa, 112–13
  frozen, buying, 91
  Maple Syrup Triple Berry Parfait,
    141–42
beta-carotene
  in carrots, 16
  defined, 52
  in multivitamins, 182
  in sweet potatoes, 60
  in tomatoes, 61
  in watermelon, 5–6
betacyanin, defined, 52
beta-sitosterol, defined, 52
betaxanthin, defined, 52
beverages. *See also* coffee; tea;
    vegetable juice; water; wine
  Chocolate Blackberry Breakfast
    Smoothie, 95–96
  Cinnamon Orange Dreamsicle,
    141
  drinking, from tall glass, 45–46
  Strawberry Pomegranate Blender
    Blaster, 144
  Tangy and Cool Buttermilk and
    Avocado Breakfast Smoothie,
    99–100
  thick, effect on satiety, 41

bioavailability
  barricades to, 7–8
  definition of, 5
  effect of cooking methods on,
    15–17
  effect of food combinations on,
    12–15
  effect of food quality on, 9–12
  maximizing, importance of, 5–6
  quiz on, 3–4
bison
  about, 79
  Bison Steak and Broccoli Salad,
    110–11
  buying, 22
  health benefits, 79
  storing, 85
blackberries
  about, 64
  Blackberry, Kiwi, and Mango
    Fruit Salad, 140
  Chocolate Blackberry Breakfast
    Smoothie, 95–96
  health benefits, 64–65
  in Warm and Nutty Cinnamon
    Quinoa Cereal, 100
blueberries
  about, 65
  health benefits, 65
  Papaya Filled with Gingered
    Blueberries, 142–43
bottled water, 32–33
bread, whole-grain, buying, 43
bread dough, potassium bromate
    in, 28
breast cancer
  culinary medicine, 200–203
  fermented cabbage and, 38
  flavonoids and, 17
  inflammation and, 21
  rBST and, 24
  risk factors, 200
  breast disease, benign (BBD),
    197–98
broccoli
  about, 56
  best cooking methods, 56
  Bison Steak and Broccoli Salad,
    110–11

fibrocystic breast disease. *See* benign
    breast disease (BBD)
filtered tap water, 32
fish. *See also* salmon; sardines
    Cioppino, 114–15
    Grilled Citrus Trout over Crunchy
        Mediterranean Slaw, 118–19
    storing, 85
    flavonoids
    defined, 52
    in lettuce, 6
    in olives, 66
    in red onions, 58
    in romaine, 59
    in tea, 17
flax, omega-3s in, 17
folate. *See also* folic acid
    in cauliflower, 13
    foods rich in, 183
    in green beans, 13
    in leeks, 13
    maximal intake, 181
folic acid
    deficiency, culinary medicine for,
        192
    in yogurt, 70
food
    aroma of, 37–38
    combining, to increase
        bioavailability, 12–15
    food poisoning, 22–23
    mouthfeel of, 38
    processing methods, 15
    sight of, 38–39
    sound of, 39
    unhealthy, hiding, 45
free radicals, defined, 52
fruit. *See also specific fruits*
    buying whole, 6
    conventionally grown, 11
    high in pesticide contaminants, 11
    increasing intake of, 44
    locally grown, 12
    nutritional loss in, 6
    organically grown, 11–12
    phytonutrients in, 12–15
    preparing sauce for, 27
    presliced, vitamin loss in, 6
    shopping for, 10–12

storing, 45, 85
vitamin C in, 6
water content of, 44
fungicides, 31

G

gallbladder disease, 221–23
garlic
    about, 75–76
    Garlicky Potato Salad with
        Spinach and Lemon, 135
    health benefits, 8, 23, 76
gastroesophageal reflux disease
    (GERD), 231–32
genetically modified foods, xiv
genetic influences, 7
genistein, in soy foods, 60
ghrelin, 28, 36, 41
ginger
    about, 76
    Cedar-Planked Roasted Salmon
        with Candied Ginger and Berry
        Salsa, 112–13
    Ginger Peanut Grilled Chicken
        with Sweet Potatoes and Sugar
        Snap Peas, 117–18
    health benefits, 76
    Papaya Filled with Gingered
        Blueberries, 142–43
    products, buying, 91–92
    Quick Steel-Cut Oats with Apples,
        Ginger, and Walnuts, 97–98
gingivitis, 46
glasses, drinking, 45–46
glossary, kitchen prescription, 52–53
GLP-1 (glucagon-like peptide 1), 41
glucosinolates
    in broccoli, 13, 56
    in brussels sprouts, 56, 57
    in cabbage, 38, 57
    defined, 52
    in kale, 58
glutamate, in ketchup, 61
glycemic index, of rice, 13–14
gout, 223–25
grains, whole. *See also* barley; oats;
        quinoa; rice
    in breads, 43
    buying, 95

in cereals, 43
fiber in, 43
pan-toasting, xv
resistant starch in, 42
storing, 84
grapes, organic, buying, 11
Greek-style yogurt, buying, 92
green beans, folate in, 13
greens. *See also specific greens*
    absorbing carotenoids from, 7–8
    Bison Steak and Broccoli Salad,
        110–11
    grilling, ways to make safe, 22
growth hormones, 22–23
Guacamole, Fresh Tomatillo, 138

H

H. pylori bacteria, 43
hair, skin, and nail problems,
        225–27
Hamburgers, Healthy Real, 119–20
heartburn, 231–32
heart disease
    culinary medicine, 229–31
    inflammation as cause of, 21
    lean protein consumption and, 41
    patient story, 227–28
    risk factors, 228–29
herbicides, 31
heterocyclic amines (HCAs), 22
high blood pressure, 238–40
high-fructose corn syrup, 27–29
high triglycerides
    (hypertriglyceridemia), 236–38
honey
    about, 76–77
    health benefits, 77
    Honeyed Chinese Chicken
        Breasts, 120–21
hormones, growth, 22–23
hypercholesterolemia, 232–36
hypertension (high blood pressure),
        238–40
hypertriglyceridemia, 236–38

I

indole-3 carbinol, 53, 56
infertility, male, 246–48
insoluble fiber, 43

sauerkraut
    health benefits, 38, 57
    Sauerkraut with Onion, Apple,
        and Toasted Caraway, 136
sausages, chicken
    buying, 90–91
    Spicy and Rich Sausage and
        Kidney Bean Chili, 107
sausages, meatless
    buying, 94
    in Portuguese Caldo Verde, 104
scallops
    Cioppino, 114–15
    Saffron Scallop, Shrimp, and
        Chickpea Paella, 128–29
selenium, 181, 183
sex, health benefits from, 47
shellfish. See crabmeat; scallops;
    shrimp
shrimp
    Parmigiano Caesar Salad with
        Shrimp, 121
    Saffron Scallop, Shrimp, and
        Chickpea Paella, 128–29
    Shrimp and Egg Burritos with
        White Beans and Corn, 106
    Stir-Fried Giant Shrimp, Baby
        Bok Choy, and Portobellos,
        131–32
silymarin, defined, 53
skin, hair, and nail problems,
    225–27
skin cancer, 11, 82
smoothies
    Chocolate Blackberry Breakfast
        Smoothie, 95–96
    Tangy and Cool Buttermilk and
        Avocado Breakfast Smoothie,
        99–100
sodium nitrates, 26
soluble fiber, 43, 53, 54
soups
    Açai Berry and Banana Dessert
        Soup, 139
    boxed, buying, 94
    Cioppino, 114–15
    effect on weight loss, 44
    Pasta e Fagioli (Pasta and Bean)
        Soup, 102–3

Portuguese Caldo Verde, 104
Red Pozole with Shredded
    Chicken and Avocado, 124
Roasted Red Pepper, Wine, and
    Red Lentil Soup, 105
Spicy Gazpacho with Crab, 137
soybeans
    about, 59
    health benefits, 59–60
soy foods. See also tofu
    about, 59
    health benefits, 59–60
    meatless sausages, buying, 94
    in Portuguese Caldo Verde, 104
    soy-based mayonnaise, buying, 94
    Soyrizo, buying, 94
speed scratch cooking, 15–16
spices. See also specific spices
    storing, 85
spinach
    Garlicky Potato Salad with
        Spinach and Lemon, 135
    organic, buying, 11
    vitamin K in, 16
squash
    Butternut Barley Risotto with
        Goat Cheese and Toasted
        Almonds, 111–12
    in Rosemary Grilled Chicken and
        Summer Vegetables, 127–28
stair-climbing, 173
stanol esters, defined, 53
staph infections, 26
starch. See resistant starch
stearic acid, 21
strawberries
    organic, buying, 11
    Strawberry Pomegranate Blender
        Blaster, 144
strength training, 175
stretching, 169–70, 171
stroke, 41
sugar, 27–29
sulforaphane
    in broccoli, 10, 56
    defined, 53
super-bugs, 25–26
supplements, vitamin and mineral,
    179–80

sweeteners, artificial, 28–29
sweet potatoes
    about, 60
    Cumin-Crusted Salmon over
        Silky Sweet Potatoes,
        115–16
    Ginger Peanut Grilled Chicken
        with Sweet Potatoes and Sugar
        Snap Peas, 117–18
    health benefits, 60
    in Portuguese Caldo Verde, 104
swiss chard
    about, 61
    health benefits, 61
    in Portuguese Caldo Verde, 104
    Sicilian Pasta with Swiss Chard,
        Goat Cheese, and Basil, 130–31
synthetic chemicals, 24–25

T
tea
    about, 82
    buying, 94
    health benefits, 11, 17
    heath benefits, 82–83
teeth, brushing, 46
teriyaki sauce, buying, 94
Teriyaki Tofu, Vegetables, and
    Buckwheat Noodles, 108
testosterone, 31
texture, of food, 38
tofu
    about, 59–60
    buying, 94
    Cheese Ravioli with Tofu and
        Baby Peas, 113–14
    in Chocolate Blackberry Breakfast
        Smoothie, 95–96
    in Roasted Winter Vegetables with
        Cranberry-Studded Quinoa,
        126–27
    Teriyaki Tofu, Vegetables, and
        Buckwheat Noodles, 108
Tomatillo Guacamole, Fresh, 138
tomatoes
    about, 61
    canned, buying, 90
    Cherry Tomato and Mozzarella
        Morsel Salad, 134

DR. JOHN LA PUMA is the "food as medicine doc." A board-certified specialist in internal medicine, a professionally trained chef, and a best-selling author, Dr. La Puma hosts "What's Cookin' with ChefMD?" every Sunday morning on the national TV series *Health Corner*, airing on the cable TV network Lifetime. Thousands of viewers have joined ChefMD.com, receive the free ChefMD Recipe of the Week, and view the award-winning TV clips online.

A Phi Beta Kappa graduate of the University of California in creative studies and a graduate of the Baylor College of Medicine, he performed his residency in internal medicine at the West L.A. Veterans Administration Medical Center and UCLA and completed the first postgraduate fellowship in internal medicine and clinical medical ethics in the United States, at the University of Chicago. He was appointed to the associate faculty for six years and has authored or co-authored more than fifty peer-reviewed scientific papers and two hundred articles and book chapters.

Dr. La Puma is also a graduate of the Cooking and Hospitality Institute of Chicago, a Le Cordon Bleu School, and taught the first Nutrition and Cooking Course for medical students in the United States. The founder of CHEF Clinic®, he served as a Professor of Nutrition at Kendall School of Culinary Arts and cooked for nearly four years once weekly at Chef Rick Bayless's Topolobampo in Chicago. Dr. La Puma contributed recipes to the number-one bestseller *You: The Owner's Manual* and has consulted with companies such as CIGNA, Caremark, and Kraft.

Dr. La Puma's first popular book, *The RealAge Diet: Make Yourself*

Younger with What You Eat, became a *New York Times* bestseller; his first cookbook, *Cooking the RealAge Way,* became an Amazon #1 Cookbook. Both were coauthored with Michael Roizen, M.D. RealAge has been featured on *Oprah, Good Morning America, Today, Montel,* and dozens of other national shows. The *New England Journal of Medicine,* the *Journal of the American Medical Association,* the *Encyclopaedia Britannica,* the *Wall Street Journal,* and the *New York Times* have published Dr. La Puma's work. *Eating Well, Health, Martha Stewart Living, Men's Journal, More, Newsweek, Parade, Prevention, Reader's Digest, Self, Shape,* and *Vogue* have also featured his work.

Named "One of America's Top Physicians" by the Consumers' Research Council and a "Secret Weapon" by the *Wall Street Journal,* Dr. La Puma received the National Association of Medical Communicators' Award of Excellence in 2007. He has delivered more than 300 keynotes and designed conference menus of meeting planners. He practices medicine with the Santa Barbara Institute for Medical Nutrition & Healthy Weight and is based in Santa Barbara, California, and at www.DrJohnLaPuma.com.

REBECCA POWELL MARX is a ChefMD co-founder and partner, a writer, a marketing executive, and a medical television producer. In 2007, she won a prestigious FREDDIE Award for ChefMD.com as the International Health and Medical Media's best website. Since 1990 she has overseen the production of one hundred-plus hours of health and medical television. As a journalist, Rebecca has researched and written on many topics, but her first love has always been food.

Rebecca graduated from the University of Wisconsin in 1979 with a degree in home economics and a minor in journalism. Her first job after college was as "Alice in Dairyland"—the Wisconsin Department of Agriculture's goodwill ambassador and spokesperson. She traveled throughout the country and internationally, speaking about the healthy benefits of quality, natural foods. This work became the foundation for her realization that food can be delicious medicine.

Rebecca is married with three children and lives in beautiful, rural Wisconsin. Her family is her passion.